Methodological Advances in Health Services Research

Gordon H. DeFriese,
Thomas C. Ricketts, III,
Jane S. Stein,
Editors

Methodological Advances in Health Services Research

health administration press · PERSPECTIVES ·

Health Administration Press Ann Arbor, Michigan 1989

Library of Congress Cataloging-in-Publication Data

Methodological advances in health services research.

Articles reprinted from various issues of the journal, Health services research, with new introductions.
Bibliography: p.
1. Public health—Research—Methodology. I. DeFriese, Gordon H. II. Ricketts, Thomas C. III. Stein, Jane S. IV. Health services research. [DNLM: 1. Health Services Research—trends—United States—collected works. W 84.3 M5912]
RA440.85.M47 1988 362.1'072073 88-32819
ISBN 0-910701-42-3 (soft)

Health Administration Press
A Division of the Foundation of the
American College of Healthcare Executives
1021 East Huron Street
Ann Arbor, Michigan 48104-9990
(313)764-1380

TABLE OF CONTENTS

Section Two: Modeling Health Care Use and System Performance

Section Three: Modeling Clinical Decision Making

Reprint Information

All articles in this book are reprinted from *Health Services Research*, copyright by the Hospital Research and Educational Trust. *HSR* is the official journal of the Association for Health Services Research.

Chapter One: Norma I. Gavin. An Application of Statistical Matching with the Survey of Income and Education and the 1976 Health Interview Survey. *HSR* 20(2):183–98, June 1985.

Chapter Two: Joel L. Weissfeld, Bruce M. Brock, John P. Kirscht, and Victor M. Hawthorne. Reliability of Health Belief Indexes: Confirmatory Factor Analysis in Sex, Race, and Age Subgroups. *HSR* 21(6): 777–93, February 1987.

Chapter Three: John R. Griffith, Peter A. Wilson, Robert A. Wolfe, and Diane P. Bischak. Clinical Profiles of Hospital Discharge Rates in Local Communities. *HSR* 20(2):131–51, June 1985.

Chapter Four: Wilbert M. Gesler and Melinda S. Meade. Locational and Population Factors in Health Care-Seeking Behavior in Savannah, Georgia. *HSR* 23(3):443–62, August 1988.

Chapter Five: Steven L. Gortmaker, Colleen J. G. Clark, Stanley N. Graven, Arthur M. Sobol, and Arline Geronimus. Reducing Infant Mortality in Rural America: Evaluation of the Rural Infant Care Program. *HSR* 22(1):91–116, April 1987.

Chapter Six: Pamela A. Gray-Toft and James G. Anderson. Organizational Stress in the Hospital: Development of a Model for Diagnosis and Prediction. *HSR* 19(6):753–74, February 1985, Part I.

Chapter Seven: Kyle L. Grazier, William C. Richardson, Diane P. Martin, and Paula Diehr. Factors Affecting Choice of Health Care Plans. *HSR* 20(6):659–82, February 1986, Part I.

Chapter Eight: Richard A. Elnicki and John P. Schmitt. Contribution of Patient and Hospital Characteristics to Adverse Patient Incidents. *HSR* 15(4):397–414, Winter 1980.

Chapter Nine: John M. Kuder and Gary S. Levitz. Visits to the Physician: An Evaluation of the Usual-Source Effect. *HSR* 20(5):579–96, December 1985.

Chapter Ten: Jerry Cromwell and Janet B. Mitchell. An Economic Model of Large Medicaid Practices. *HSR* 19(2):197–218, June 1984.

Chapter Eleven: Mark J. Young, John M. Eisenberg, Sankey V. Williams, and John C. Hershey. Comparing Aggregate Estimates of Derived Thresholds for Clinical Decisions. *HSR* 20(6):763–80, February 1986, Part I.

Mark J. Young, Lisbeth S. Fried, John Eisenberg, John Hershey, and Sankey Williams. Do Cardiologists Have Higher Thresholds for Recommending Coronary Arteriography than Family Physicians? *HSR* 22(5):623–35, December 1987.

Chapter Twelve: William A. Sollecito and Dennis B. Gillings. The Assessment of Health Policy Changes Using the Time-Reversed Crossover Design. *HSR* 20(6):705–36, February 1986, Part I.

Chapter Thirteen: Randall S. Brown. The Evaluation of the National Long Term Care Demonstration: 2. Estimation Methodology. *HSR* 23(1):23–49, April 1988.

Chapter Fourteen: Harold S. Luft. Health Services Research as a Scientific Process: The Metamorphosis of an Empirical Research Project from Grant Proposal to Final Report. *HSR* 21(4):563–84, October 1986.

Health Services Research is published six times a year by Health Administration Press for the Hospital Research and Educational Trust in cooperation with the Association for Health Services Research.

Acknowledgments

A number of people have helped to make this volume possible. First of all, there are the authors of the papers assembled here. Without the diligent efforts they made in the first place to put these papers into the formal literature of the field, there would not have been such an accumulation of methodological work upon which we could draw for a volume such as this. Then there are the anonymous peer reviewers of each of these manuscripts whose careful attention to the details of method, presentation, and execution has substantially contributed to each of these papers in the process of their development. As editors of *Health Services Research*, we are constantly aware of the enormous sacrifice our reviewers make on a daily basis, and we are very proud of the quality of the reviews that prospective authors have generally received when their manuscripts have been reviewed by *HSR*.

The idea for this book came from Health Administration Press, which publishes *Health Services Research* for the Hospital Research and Educational Trust. The book was shaped and more clearly articulated by the professional staff of the Press, most particularly by Nancy J. Moncrieff, in conversations with the editors of *HSR*. At Health Administration Press, Kathleen A. Malone, the Managing Editor of *HSR*, has been a constant influence on the quality and readability of all of the manuscripts that eventually are published in the pages of this journal. In this volume one can see the results of her craft on every page. We are forever grateful to her for what she has done for *HSR* and for the field.

Also of importance to the production of this volume was Amy L. Kragnes, managing editor for books of Health Administration Press.

Finally, we wish to acknowledge the efforts of Pheobe Lindley, Assistant to the Editor of *HSR*, and Cheryl McDade, also an Assistant to the Editor, who have worked with us on a daily basis to service the administrative and clerical needs of the journal.

Preface

The field of health services research has experienced in recent years an extraordinarily rapid growth and development worldwide, attracting large numbers of scholars, policy analysts, and health services providers. The term "health services research," relatively new and not widely used in the early 1960s, has become widely accepted in these past twenty-five years as the interdisciplinary study of structures and processes through which personal health care services are organized, financed, delivered, and used. The essence of this interdisciplinary field has developed into finding ways to provide *as much* quality health care for *as many* people as possible. It has found its place as a vital adjunct to the functions of health sector management and policy development.

Health services research draws upon the theory and methods of a wide variety of disciplines, ranging from the clinical health sciences to the social and behavioral sciences, law, administrative science, and management. Although persons who work in this field may be trained in a single discipline, they may find that a range of methodological techniques and approaches derived from a variety of other fields is relevant to their work. The interdisciplinary nature of much of this work makes it necessary that ways be found for integrating these different theoretical perspectives, methodological skills, and interests in a single project.

This volume is intended as an overview of examples illustrating the wide variety of methodological approaches currently being taken within the field of health services research to the study and understanding of fundamental health care issues and problems. All of the chapters in this volume were originally published as articles in *Health Services Research*, the official peer-reviewed journal of the Association for Health Services Research in the United States. These articles therefore represent the work of health services research in a single, developed nation. They represent some of the best examples of ways in which teams of well-respected scholars have struggled with the methods they have chosen in attempting to derive valid and useful answers to concrete questions of concern to this field.

The methods illustrated in this volume cover a wide range of techniques currently in use in the broad field of health services research. No attempt has been made to assemble a comprehensive overview of the methods of the field. Nor should one assume that the methods illustrated here are those most preferred by the people editing or reviewing papers submitted to *Health Services Research*. What we have tried to do in this volume is to provide a concise, easily accessible compendium of methodologically interesting papers which, taken together, illustrate some of the more innovative approaches to common research problems in this field.

As diverse as the methods themselves are the substantive problems or research questions addressed by the papers. These include the effects of population sociodemographic composition on health services utilization; the relationship between the population-based clinical distribution of disease conditions and patterns of hospital service use; the reliability of standard measures of health beliefs; consumer choices among health care plans; the contribution of patient and hospital characteristics to the frequency of adverse patient incidents; tests of alternative theoretical relationships between having a usual source of care and patterns of personal health services use; a study of the effect of organizational climate, supervisory practices, and work-group relations on the amount of role conflict and ambiguity experienced among hospital nurses; the behavior and performance of large Medicaid practices; the problems of reducing infant mortality in rural areas; the effect of a consumer cost-sharing provision on health services utilization among members of a prepaid insurance plan; the evaluation of the impact of a demonstration program designed to provide home health care services in lieu of nursing home care for an elderly population; the effects of selection factors and competition on HMO performance in selected markets; the geographical characteristics of users of health care services; and the thresholds of clinical decision making among physicians with respect to coronary arteriography.

The articles we have selected for this volume are arranged to represent a sequence of considerations in the research process. The volume begins with a series of articles that describe methods for ensuring that the most appropriate data are usable for addressing a research question of interest; for developing scales and other measurement strategies for the variables of importance to research; and for using descriptive data in interpreting the patterns of utilization for hospital service areas, including the use of modern techniques from the field of medical geography.

Section Two includes six articles that illustrate various quantitative approaches to the development of models for health services use and system performance. Among these articles are descriptions of the use of techniques such as time-series regression, structural equation and path analysis approaches to model building, stepwise regression and discriminant function analysis, ordinary least-squares regression, recursive and non-recursive models, and probit economic models.

Section Three consists of two articles by the same group of researchers who use weighted least-squares regression analysis in the study of clinical decision making as applied to complex diagnostic testing. This pair of articles illustrates the development of a specific methodology and its subsequent application.

The fourth section, another set of two studies, focuses on the special problems of large-scale health program evaluation and illustrates the use of statistical techniques appropriate for quasi-experimental evaluations and randomized trials of health program experiments.

The final section in this volume is represented by one article, a paper rare in the annals of health services research. It presents the chronological case study of a single research project from beginning (the grant proposal) to end (publication of the study results). This paper, we feel, provides a fitting last chapter for a volume of this kind.

Two of us are editors of *Health Services Research*. In preparing for the publication of this volume, we examined nearly 100 papers published in the journal over the past several years, and we became more convinced than ever that our field has achieved high scientific standards. Standards of research in health services are deserving of healthy respect from all who care about the issues addressed by the authors represented here and by other workers in this field. As editors of one of the major journals in this field, we take pride in these papers, in our journal, and in our field.

The articles in this volume speak for themselves, but we have added a brief editorial introduction to each to make the reason for its selection clear to the reader. It is our hope that this collection of some of the most interesting and important work to appear in *Health Services Research* in recent years will serve as a useful text for students preparing for careers in this field and as a convenient review for those who are experienced in this line of research. In addition, we are hopeful that some of those we have hoped to influence, who occupy important positions in public and private health sector agencies, will find these articles useful in their attempts at better understanding and subsequent use of the products and information generated through health services research.

Gordon H. DeFriese
Thomas C. Ricketts, III
Jane S. Stein

Chapel Hill, July 1988

SECTION ONE

Descriptive Data Analysis

CHAPTER ONE

Database Development

One of the first decisions that researchers need to make, given a well-defined problem or hypothesis, is whether to use primary or secondary data. Several factors are brought to bear on the increasing use of secondary data in health services research. The cost of primary data collection is high, and the search for support for such research is very time and resource consuming. It is particularly difficult to obtain support for longitudinal research, since funders are wary of committing resources for more than a few years. As the field of health services research has come of age, the availability of good sources of secondary data has increased. In particular, many national, population-based data collection efforts have been mounted by the National Center for Health Statistics and the National Center for Health Services Research and Health Care Technology Assessment. These national databases have sophisticated designs, are often linkable from year to year (if not longitudinally), and are both readily available and extremely well documented.

Norma Gavin's article presents a technique that allows data from different sources to be combined into one research database. Her intent was to combine health care utilization data, available in the Health Interview Survey, with information on income and employment from the Survey of Income and Education, in order to estimate eligibility for medical assistance programs. She also set out to make state-specific estimates, which are not possible using data from the Health Interview Survey alone due to its size.

The technique she describes, statistical matching, has been refined by statisticians and economists; however, it is complex and requires a great deal of insight and methodological sophistication. Although the decisions she describes are based on the questions raised by the research at hand, the technique can be used to create generally useful databases from existent data. National agencies can multiply the usefulness of their data collection efforts by creating merged research databases. Longitudinal databases can be generated from cross-sectional ones. If these are well documented and available, they will increase the amount of secondary data analysis and, thereby, the "cost effectiveness" of large, national data collection efforts.

An Application of Statistical Matching with the Survey of Income and Education and the 1976 Health Interview Survey

Norma I. Gavin

This article outlines an alternative procedure to household surveys for obtaining individual observation-level data. The procedure, called statistical matching, integrates data on an individual observation from one source with data on a different observation identified as the "best matching" or "most similar" record from a second source. The best match is determined by objective statistical criteria. Also reported is a significant application of the procedure between the Survey of Income and Education and the 1976 National Health Interview Survey. The success of merging these two large, nationally representative data files shows statistical matching as a viable method of creating databases for health services research.

Studies have shown that not only the size but also the demographic composition, socioeconomic status, and geographic distribution of the population have a significant effect on the use of health services and the related expenditures. Therefore, the current and future characteristics of the consumer-patient population are of great concern to health planners, policy analysts, and health care providers. Population-based files of health care utilization and expenditure data on individual observations can help answer many of their questions.

The project reported in this article was conducted while the author was at Mathematica Policy Research, Inc., under contract with the Health Care Financing Administration and the Office of the Assistant Secretary for Planning and Evaluation, U.S. Department of Health and Human Services pursuant to contract numbers HCFA-500-74-60 and HEW-100-79-0161.

Address correspondence and requests for reprints to Norma I. Gavin, M.A., Research Assistant, Economics Department, Duke University, Durham, NC 27706. Ms. Gavin is also a Health Data Analyst at Blue Cross and Blue Shield of North Carolina, Durham, NC 27702.

Household survey files are the usual source of such data. However, surveys are time-consuming and costly and often cannot be made for every research need. Regular and periodic surveys, such as the National Health Interview Survey and those conducted by the Center for Health Administration Studies and the National Opinion Research Center at The University of Chicago, while rich with information, often lack a critical variable for a particular study.

This paper outlines an alternative procedure for obtaining the required database. The procedure, called statistical matching, is a method of integrating data on individual observations from one source with data on similar but different observations from a second source. It is used to add variables to records in a data file in which they did not exist before and to correct or adjust the distributions of variable values on a data file where there is reason to believe that the distribution on one file is superior to that on the other.

The procedure has been used by analysts to construct more comprehensive and accurate databases from existing ones for estimates of the distributions of income, taxes, wealth, energy consumption, and the costs and effects of changes in government programs [1–12]. However, its potential use in developing databases for health services research has not been fully evaluated. A pioneering statistical match between the Survey of Income and Education (SIE) and the 1976 Health Interview Survey (HIS) is described.[1] It is hoped that the presentation will provide a base for discussion on the appropriateness of statistical matching in creating databases to study certain health care issues.

A Description of the Procedure

In a statistical match, composite data records are created by selecting a record from one file that best matches a given record on a second file and appending information on that record to the record in the second file. The best match is determined by an objective statistical criterion, such as the minimization of a distance function of the differences between values of variables common to the two files or the maximization of a score where points are given for matches on the values of the common variables.

Alternative statistical techniques, such as regression analysis, can also be used to impute variables contained in one file to another file or to adjust the values of certain variables on a file. However, where a substantial number of imputations or adjustments are required and where the joint distributions among the imputed variables are important, a statistical match may be more appropriate.

A precondition for a statistical match, then, is the existence of two or more data files, which together contain the data needed for the analysis and which have variables in common on which to base the match, and sample populations which are consistent or can be aligned.

BRINGING ABOUT THE SIE/HIS MATCH

Several years ago, the expected congressional interest in Medicaid reform and other national health insurance programs revealed the need for a database that could provide comparable estimates of eligibles, participants, and costs of the various proposed plans. A population-based data file of records on individuals representative of the U.S. population to which the various program rules could be applied in a microsimulation model was needed.

Household surveys existing at the time lacked either the required income data to determine program eligibility among the sample population or the required health care utilization and/or expenditure data to determine program costs. Furthermore, sample sizes were too small to support state-specific analyses. State estimates are important for determining the geographic distribution of gainers and losers in a new program and are particularly relevant in comparing the current Medicaid program—in which the eligibility and benefit rules vary by state—to a federalized Medicaid program with a single set of rules.

No existing database had all of these features. However, some of the variables needed for the analysis were on the SIE file, while others were on the HIS file.

The SIE, conducted by the Census Bureau in the spring of 1976, is a national survey of approximately 151,000 households designed to give reliable state estimates of the number of children 5–17 years of age living in poverty. The file contains detailed information on income and employment necessary for the determination of eligibility for medical assistance programs, as well as certain sociodemographic data, such as age, sex, education, family income, and health insurance coverage, that are comparable to information gathered in the HIS.

The HIS is conducted annually by the National Center for Health Statistics and is composed of information on a national sample of about 42,000 households. It is designed to provide national estimates of acute illnesses and injuries, disability days, and measures of health care utilization. The utilization data are needed to determine the benefit or transfer amounts in studies of the comparative costs of medical assistance programs.

Because the two files contained several variables in common and their sample universes were the same, a statistical match was possible.

Before the statistical properties of the variables common to the two files could be examined to determine their use in a match, their definitions had to be reconciled. The alignment of the common variables on the SIE and HIS files was fairly easy. In all cases, an attempt was made to preserve the maximum possible amount of significant detail. The distributions over the variable values were nearly identical on the two files for all of the variables, except census division and state. The different geographic distributions were expected and are due to the different sampling designs of the surveys.

Reporting errors on the surveys were discovered from comparisons with administrative program data. The underreporting of income, private health insurance, and the receipt of cash welfare payments was slightly more pronounced in the HIS, while the underreporting of the receipt of Medicaid benefits was more pronounced on the SIE. These differences can also be explained from the different survey designs. The SIE is designed to obtain income and employment data; therefore, the questionnaire contains probes to elicit more accurate information relating to these items. On the other hand, the HIS is designed to elicit accurate health care utilization data, which include Medicaid benefits. The differences did not affect the match itself because they were small and because an exact match on all of the variable values was not required.

The matching of these two files allows analysts access to the best information from both surveys. The most reliable survey data on income, employment, and health care utilization are available on a single file without unduly burdening survey respondents.

The Design of a Match

Among the major elements of a match are the direction, the matching unit, the variables to be used to stratify the files and those to be used in the matching algorithm (e.g., the distance function), the weights of these latter variables, and constraints imposed on the number of times a record can be used.

THE DIRECTION

The direction of the match is determined by which data file serves as the base file and which one serves as the non-base file. The unique information from the non-base file records is transferred to the base file records; the population distributions on the final merged file will be those of the base file. Therefore, the decision on the direction of the match depends on the intended use of the output file.

The SIE and HIS data files are both representative samples of the U.S. population, but only the SIE is large enough to give reliable state estimates. Because we wanted a file that gave estimates of health care utilization and program eligibility by state, the SIE was chosen as the base file and the HIS as the non-base file in our match.

THE MATCHING UNIT

Matching is performed on a single common unit or level of observation. The data files may have different units of observation, or they may have more than one common unit. When the files have no common unit, a corresponding unit must be made by combining or dividing records on one or both of the files.

Both the SIE and HIS files have multiple observation levels, with household and/or family records for each household interviewed and person records for each household member.[2] The SIE/HIS match was made at the person level; that is, person records from the HIS were chosen to match the person records in the SIE. The choice of persons for the matching unit, rather than the family, substantially increased the cost of the match. But the choice was made because, although family characteristics have a significant influence in determining the utilization of health care services by family members, the influence of personal characteristics, such as age and sex, is much greater. Furthermore, a person match allows the analyst greater flexibility in redefining filing units for modeling alternative medical assistance programs.

THE MATCH VARIABLES

Match variables are the variables common to both files on which the matching criteria are based. They are typically grouped into stratification and weighted match variables. The stratification variables define matching cells. Only non-base file records in the cell corresponding to the base file record's cell are searched to determine the best match for a record on the base file. The use of cells greatly reduces the cost of the match; in many applications, it would be exorbitantly expensive to search every non-base file record for every base file record. The weighted match variables then are chosen from the remaining variables common to the two files and are assigned either a weight for use in a distance function or points which are awarded for matches between the two files.

Stratifying the files into cells is equivalent to giving the stratification variables extremely high weights so that the best matching records would always match on them. Ideally, the most important determinants of the variables to be appended to or adjusted on the base file serve as stratification variables.

The desired stratification variables for the SIE/HIS match were those that are the most important determinants of health care utilization and participation in medical assistance programs. However, other factors, such as the cell sizes on the HIS and the similarity of the variable distributions on the two files, important to retain the aggregate values and distributions of the utilization variables on the merged file, were also considered. Regression analysis on the major health care utilization variables in the HIS file was used to ascertain the relative importance of the potential matching variables.

The variables chosen to stratify the files were census division, age, sex, and family size. The family size categories varied across the cells. In addition, a high-low family income flag and a disability flag were used to break down further the remaining large cells of persons under 65 years of age, and all cells of persons over age 65 were stratified by the disability flag.

THE WEIGHTS

Once the stratification variables are identified, a matching algorithm or rule can be specified, and the weights or scores for the remaining common variables can be determined. In the SIE/HIS match a scoring system was used. Each match variable was assigned a certain number of points, which were accumulated in a total score for each of the HIS records in a cell if that record and the SIE record had the same variable value. The HIS record with the highest total score greater than a minimum allowable value was determined to be the best match.

The points assigned to each of the match variables was based on their relative importance in determining the information to be appended to or adjusted on the base file. To compute the points assigned to the variables in the SIE/HIS match, we ran least-squares regression equations on the HIS doctor visit variable. This variable was chosen over other utilization data on the file because it had fewer zero responses; therefore, the bias resulting from the use of the least-squares method is smaller than it would be with the other variables. Furthermore, because much of the utilization of health care services is either induced by the physician or naturally follows visits to physicians, the use of the number of doctor visits to represent overall health care utilization is not without a theoretical base [13,14].

The independent variables of the equation included the stratification variables and a potential scored variable. A regression equation was run for each potential scored-match variable. In addition, because of widely different health care needs and motivational factors in seeking care, separate sets of equations were run for children (0–16 years old), non-aged adults (17–64 years old), and the aged (65 or more years old).

The individual variable scores then were derived from the square of the partial correlation coefficient between the potential scored variables and the doctor-visit variable in these equations, r^2. These values represent the proportional reduction of the variation in physician visits not explained by the stratification variables.

Note that this is not the only way to determine the variable weights or scores. In most previous matches, these values were determined subjectively, based on the analysts' knowledge of the relative importance of the variables [3–5,7,8,10–12]. However, other statistical criteria have also been used [1].

The resulting r^2 values for the potential match variable are shown in Table 1. They varied considerably among the three age groups. However, the most significant variable by far for all three groups was the disability flag. State of residence and the different insurance coverage variables were also among the more significant explanatory variables for the three groups.

For the most part, the r^2 values were directly translated into the individual variable scores. However, the scores for several variables that were considered more highly correlated with participation in a medical assistance or national health insurance program or dimensions of health care utilization not reflected in the doctor visit variable were adjusted to account for these relationships. Furthermore, for continuous variables, partial points were awarded if the variable values were within a tolerance range but did not match exactly.

CONSTRAINTS

Statistical matches are usually one of two types—totally constrained or totally unconstrained. In an unconstrained match, often called matching with replacement, emphasis is made on picking the best matching

Table 1: Proportional Reduction of the Variation in the Number of Doctor Visits with the Different Potential Scored-Match Variables

	Children	*Non-aged Adults*	*Aged Adults*
State	.00363	.00171	.00689
Health insurance			
No insurance flag	.00237	.00080	.00004
Type of insurance coverage	.00389	.01813	.00487
Private insurance flag	.00003	.00266	.00004
Medicaid coverage flag	.00246	.01689	.00490
Medicare coverage flag	.00002	.00088	.00004
Military insurance flag	.00004	.00034	.00000
Type of private insurance with private insurance flag	—	.00000	.00003
Medicaid beneficiary flag with Medicaid coverage flag	.00057	.00136	.00141
Disability			
Disability flag	.04066	.06564	—
Duration of disability with disability flag	—	.00579	.00042
Family characteristics			
Family income	.00107	.00228	.00000
Education of head	.00242	.00266	.00062
Family size	.00166	.00000	.00015
Number of children under six	.00011	.00267	.00000
Children under six flag	.00029	.00239	.00000
Family structure	.00068	—	—
Personal characteristics			
Age	.00451	.00012	.00015
Infant flag (age under 2)	.01209	—	—
Race	.00049	.00138	.00054
Marital status	—	.00347	.00071
Family relationship	—	.00221	.00025
Welfare recipient flag with Medicaid coverage flag	.00002	.00004	.00368

record from the non-base file for each record in the base file. Therefore, after a non-base file record is chosen to match a base file record, it is replaced in the non-base file and may be selected as the best match for any number of base file records. There is no constraint on the number of times a given non-base file record can be chosen. What may occur in these instances is that certain records are chosen many times and others are not chosen at all. Consequently, the aggregate values and distributions of the non-base file variables on the matched file may not be the same as the values and distributions on the original non-base file.

When it is important that the aggregate totals and distributions of these variables be maintained, a constrained match, or match without replacement, is used. In this procedure, all of the records on the non-base file must be matched to base file records, and their sample weight in the merged file must equal their original sample weight. To do this requires record splitting or other, similar techniques, and some nonoptimum matches for individual records will occur to keep the whole picture unbiased.[3]

Thus, the trade-off lies between obtaining an unbiased overall match and obtaining unbiased matches for individual records and subgroups of the population. Little is known about the relative magnitudes of these biases. They are functions of the statistical properties of the two samples, the sample sizes, and the matching method [15,16].

In the SIE/HIS match, unbiased individual records were needed, because the rules of the various Medicaid reforms and national health insurance plans were to be applied at the individual record level. At the same time, it was considered important to maintain the aggregate values of the health care utilization variables found on the HIS file. Although these variables are known to contain considerable underreporting, there is no evidence to suggest that one subgroup of the population is a better or worse reporter than another [17].

The method chosen to match the SIE and HIS files was a compromise in which the records in the non-base file were partially constrained so that they would not be chosen more than a given number of times unless they were much better matches than any of the other records: penalty points were added to a record's score if it was chosen as the best match for a given number of base file records. The penalty increased the more times a record was chosen beyond the acceptable number.

Results of the SIE/HIS Match

The SIE/HIS match was accomplished in two passes of the SIE file. In the first pass, almost all of the SIE records were successfully matched—we were able to find an HIS record with a score greater than the minimum allowable score for more than 99.7 percent of the SIE records. Nearly all of the unmatched records were for disabled persons, and most were for children 11–16 years of age. Geographically, almost

40 percent of the unmatched records were for persons residing in the Mountain-states region.

In a comparison of mean health care utilization figures from the matched file with those from the HIS file, we found a considerable undercount among the adult population, particularly among the aged. The reason was found to be differing distributions of disability over the three age groups in the two files. Although the files have approximately the same number of disabled persons, the SIE has more disabled children records (5.2 percent compared to 3.8 percent on the HIS), slightly fewer disabled non-aged adult records (13.4 percent compared to 14.2 percent), and considerably fewer disabled aged adult records (36.9 percent compared to 45.2 percent). The use of health care services increases significantly with age, and in each age group, the disabled utilize considerably more health care services than do the nondisabled. Therefore, in the merged file from the first-pass match, where all successful matches were forced to have identical disability codes, health care utilization was underestimated.

To correct the undercount, SIE records of nondisabled adults with low match scores were selected to be rematched with the unmatched records from the first pass. In the second-pass match, all rematched and unmatched SIE records for adults were forced to match HIS records of disabled persons. At the same time, some of the unmatched records of disabled children were forced to match HIS records of nondisabled children.

The second-pass match was successful. The frequency of matches of the scored-match variables in the final output file are shown in Table 2 by age group. Each of the variables matched on a vast majority of the records. Variables with higher numbers of points had higher percentages of matches.

But the real success of the match is judged by how well the distributions of the health care utilization measures on the HIS are reproduced on the matched file with the SIE population weights. The totals, means, standard deviations, and the incidence of non-zero values for the major utilization variables on the HIS file compared to those on the matched file are shown in Table 3.

None of the totals on the matched file differ more than 1–2 percent from the total on the HIS file. In addition, the distributions of the health care measures are almost identical on the two files as judged by their means and standard deviations, as well as by the percentages of persons with positive values.

Also compiled were detailed tables of the percentage of disabled persons, the mean number of doctor visits, and the number of hospital-

Table 2: Frequency of Matches on the Scored-Match Variables in the Final Matched File by Age Group

	Children	*Non-aged Adults*	*Aged Adults*
State	77.2	62.1	87.4
Health insurance			
No insurance flag	96.3	96.3	97.0
Type of insurance coverage	88.8	92.3	68.0
Private insurance flag	—	95.6	—
Medicaid coverage flag	97.0	99.1	92.1
Disability flag	99.5	99.0	91.6
Family characteristics			
Family income category			
Exact match	70.3	73.2	69.6
Tolerance match	12.3	11.0	14.6
Education of head	74.5	80.3	60.8
Family size			
Exact match	76.5	81.1	76.4
Tolerance match	15.4	11.6	14.8
Number of children under 6	—	90.8	—
Children under 6 flag	78.7	95.1	—
Family structure	86.7	—	—
Personal characteristics			
Age			
Exact match	39.6	25.9	12.1
Tolerance match	33.4	26.1	39.5
Infant flag (age under 2)	99.8	—	—
Race	84.5	86.8	90.8
Marital status	—	90.6	78.6
Family relationship	—	92.1	81.3
Welfare recipient flag	95.5	—	97.1

days per 100 persons on the matched file compared to the HIS file broken down by sex, more detailed age categories, health insurance coverage, census division, and state [18]. In general, these tables show that the match was successful in reproducing the distributions of the HIS health care measures on the new file. Not surprisingly, distributions broken down by stratification variables are more closely reproduced than those broken down by scored-match variables.

To the extent that the SIE gives a better distribution of sample persons over the different age groups, and given that the distributions of the health care utilization measures for these age groups are closely

Table 3: Comparison of the Major Health Care Utilization Estimates from the 1976 HIS and the Matched SIE/HIS Files by Age Group

	Children		*Non-aged Adults*		*Aged Adults*	
	HIS	*SIE/HIS*	*HIS*	*SIE/HIS*	*HIS*	*SIE/HIS*
Outpatient doctor visits						
Total number (in 000's)	179,480	181,994	505,245	504,742	122,094	120,857
Mean number	2.95	2.99	3.94	3.94	5.63	5.57
Standard deviation	7.17	6.59	9.68	9.49	13.38	13.06
Percentage of population with one or more visits	74.8	75.8	76.2	76.6	80.3	80.1
Short-term hospital stays						
Total number (in 000's)	3,824	3,833	18,318	18,570	5,290	5,171
Mean number per 100 persons	6.29	6.30	14.30	14.50	24.39	23.84
Percentage of population with one or more stays	5.4	5.5	11.7	11.7	17.8	17.6
Short-term hospital days						
Total number (in 000's)	20,025	19,850	130,967	130,454	57,710	57,104
Mean number per 100 persons	32.9	32.7	102.2	101.8	266.1	263.3
Standard deviation	285.9	305.7	546.1	532.7	292.3	295.7
Dental visits						
Percentage of population with one or more visits	50.5	51.4	51.5	52.7	29.9	30.7

reproduced on the merged file, estimates of total utilization from the matched file may be an improvement over the HIS estimates.

However, the matching procedure may have introduced other biases in the estimates and, thus, they may be less reliable. The relative sizes of these biases are unknown, but there is no evidence that the matching procedure introduced any sizable bias.

CONCLUSION

A synthetic file for health services research was created by statistically matching the 1976 HIS file with records in the SIE file. The new file consists of records for the households and persons in the SIE sample containing all of the information collected on them in that survey. In addition, each person record is linked with the health information for an individual in the HIS sample with characteristics most nearly identical to the SIE individual.[4] No significant biases in the distributions of the health care data using the SIE population weights were found. Thus, the merged file successfully combines the most reliable, nationally representative survey data on income and employment with the most reliable, nationally representative survey data on health care utilization.

This population-based file can be used to help answer many questions facing health planners, policy analysts, and health care providers. For example, the file can be used in a microsimulation model in which the rules of various alternative medical assistance or national health insurance programs are sequentially applied to the information on each person to determine his or her eligibility, participation, and program utilization and expenditures. Aggregating these data over the sample individuals would give total program eligibility, participation, utilization, and costs for comparative analyses. Many equity and target efficiency questions can be addressed in this fashion.

The file can also be used in a broader context to estimate total national health care utilization and expenditures among the civilian, noninstitutionalized population and to give a breakdown of these estimates by state. The file could be aged by adjusting the population weights to equal the projected population in some future year and then used to project future health care utilization and expenditures. If the aging adjustments are made by state, age, and sex or by some other geographic and demographic breakdown, the effects of population shifts on health care utilization can be estimated.

For example, such an analysis could show the extent to which health care demand might grow as the baby boom-era cohorts swell the ranks of the older population groups. An aged SIE/HIS file could also be used to estimate the growth in the share of health expenditures paid by the government as more and more people become eligible for Medicare benefits.

Thus, the success of the match shows that statistical matching of health care data to a large census file on an individual-record level is a viable method of creating a flexible database for health services research. The matching procedures are expensive and time-consuming. But when judged against the alternative of conducting a full-scale household survey, statistical matching may prove to be more efficient and more economical.

Furthermore, the procedure need not be restricted to building population-based files. It is easy to imagine a scenario where a file with records for different health facilities or health care services could be created from a statistical match.

ACKNOWLEDGMENTS

The author wishes to thank Dr. Harold Beebout and Dr. Constance Citro of Mathematica Policy Research, Inc., and Dr. Rodney Erickson and Dr. Edward Budd of The Pennsylvania State University, for comments on earlier drafts.

NOTES

1. The statistical match between the SIE and the 1976 HIS was performed by Mathematica Policy Research, Inc. and Social and Scientific Systems, Inc., under contract with the Health Care Financing Administration and the Office of the Assistant Secretary for Planning and Evaluation of the U.S. Department of Health and Human Services. For further information on the procedures used to create the merged database or on its availability, contact Mathematica Policy Research, Inc., 600 Maryland Avenue S.W., Suite 550, Washington, DC 20024.
2. The HIS actually consists of five record types—household records for each household interviewed, person records for each household member, and condition, hospital episode, and doctor visit records for each incidence of these among the household members. The SIE contains three record types—household records for each household interviewed, family records for each family in the household, and person records for each family member. Extracts of these files with only one record type per person were made for the match.
3. In record splitting, when the sample weights of matching records from the

two files are not equal, the record with the larger weight is split into two records, identical except for their sample weights. One of the new records is given the weight of the matching record in the other file and is matched with it. The other is given a weight equal to the difference in the original record weight and the matching record from the other file, and is replaced in the file of unmatched records for subsequent matching.

4. The actual output of the match is a series of files. One file contains the identification numbers of the SIE records and the matching HIS records. Another contains the original HIS records sorted by the identification number of the SIE records to which they were matched. From these files variables can be extracted and appended to the original SIE file.

REFERENCES

1. Alter, H. Creation of a synthetic data set by linking records of the Canadian Survey of Consumer Finances with the Family Expenditure Survey. *Annals of Economic and Social Measurement* 373–94, April 1974.
2. Barr, R. S., and J. S. Turner. A New Linear Programming Approach to Microdata File Merging. *1978 Compendium of Tax Research*. Office of Tax Analysis, U.S. Department of Treasury. Washington, DC: U.S. Government Printing Office, 1978, pp. 131–49; Reply, pp. 152–55.
3. Boulding, W. Creation of a New Data Base Using the Survey of Income and Education and the Annual Housing Survey. Draft final report to Division of Housing and Demographic Analysis, U.S. Department of Housing and Urban Development. Washington, DC: Mathematica Policy Research, June 29, 1979.
4. King, J. A. The Distributional Impact of Energy Policies: Development and Application of the Phase I Comprehensive Human Resources Data System. Final report to Federal Energy Administration. Washington, DC: Mathematica Policy Research, June 1977.
5. Okner, B. Constructing a new data base from existing microdata sets: The 1966 merge file. *Annals of Economic and Social Measurement* 325–42, July 1972.
6. Radner, D. B. The Development of Statistical Matching in Economics. Paper presented at the 1978 meetings of the American Statistical Association, Social Statistics Section. San Diego, CA: August 16, 1978.
7. Radner, D. B. An example of the use of statistical matching in the estimation and analysis of the size distribution of income. *Review of Income and Wealth* 211–42, September 1981.
8. Radner, D. B. The Statistical Matching of Microdata Sets: The BEA 1964 CPS-TM Match. Unpublished Ph.D. dissertation, Yale University, May 1974.
9. Radner, D. B., and H. J. Muller. Alternative Types of Record Matching: Costs and Benefits. *Proceedings of the 1977 Meetings of the American Statistical Association, Social Statistics Section*, 1977, pp. 756–61.
10. Ruggles, N., and R. Ruggles. A strategy for merging and matching microdata sets. *Annals of Economic and Social Measurement* 353–72, 1974.
11. Ruggles, N., R. Ruggles, and E. Wolff. Merging microdata: Rationale,

practice, and testing. *Annals of Economic and Social Measurement* 407–28, 1977.

12. Springs, R., and H. Beebout. The 1973 Merged SPACE/AFDC File: A Statistical Match of Data from the 1970 Decennial Census and 1973 AFDC Survey. Final report to Social and Rehabilitation Service, U.S. Department of Health, Education, and Welfare. Washington, DC: Mathematica Policy Research, March 1976.
13. Fuchs, V. R. *Who Shall Live? Health, Economics, and Social Choice.* New York: Basic Books, 1974.
14. Feldstein, M. S. Econometric studies of health economics. In M. D. Intriligator and D. A. Kendrick (eds.). *Frontiers of Quantitative Economics*, Vol. II. Amsterdam: North Holland Publishing Co., 1974, pp. 377–434.
15. Kadane, J. B. Some Statistical Problems in Merging Data Files. *1978 Compendium of Tax Research.* Office of Tax Analysis, U.S. Department of Treasury. Washington, DC: U.S. Government Printing Office, 1978, pp. 159–71; Reply, pp. 177–79.
16. Hollenbeck, K. M., and P. Doyle. Distributional Characteristics of a Merged Microdata File. Paper presented at the annual meetings of the American Statistical Association. Washington, DC, August 13–16, 1979.
17. National Center for Health Statistics. *A Summary of Studies of Interviewing Methodology.* Vital and Health Statistics, Series 2, No. 69. U.S. Department of Health, Education, and Welfare, Public Health Service. Washington, DC: U.S. Government Printing Office, 1979, pp. 4–17.
18. Pappas, N. G. The Statistical Match Between the 1976 Health Interview Survey and the Survey of Income and Education. Final report to Health Care Financing Administration. Washington, DC: Mathematica Policy Research, November 1979.

CHAPTER TWO

Confirmatory Factor Analysis in Scale Construction

In the course of putting together questionnaires for use in measuring complex dimensions and concomitants of health behavior, researchers look for items and scales that have been shown to be reliable, valid, stable across subpopulations, and used in other research. However, much of the theory in this area is evolving, and it is sometimes difficult to identify extant items and reliable and valid scales that pertain to the specific problem at hand.

Clearly, the issues involved in item selection extend beyond the realm of health behavior. There is a movement toward, if not the standardization of measures, at least an agreement on the domains of major measures. This trend is reflected in the excellent book, *Measuring Health: A Guide to Rating Scales and Questionnaires*, by Ian McDowell and Claire Newell (1987). The health services research community is well served by such efforts, since the ability to compare a study population with groups from other studies on similar measures can enhance the generalizability of findings.

This next article uses secondary data, collected for another purpose, to derive scales designed to reflect the Health Belief Model and to establish the reliability and stability of these scales across populations. It provides a creative use of secondary data and a thorough discussion of the techniques used in each phase. The authors take a structured approach to the development of their final instrument. The first step is exploratory factor analysis on a random half sample. They validate the derived factors using confirmatory factor analysis, and apply a measurement of stability across the other half of the sample and in other population subgroups. The tests for goodness of fit and estimates of scale reliability using the Omega coefficient are indicative of the organized approach the authors have chosen. Their confidence in the scales is supported by appropriate inclusion of the tables summarizing the factor development process, and the indexes and tests of reliability.

REFERENCE

McDowell, Ian, and Claire Newell. *Measuring Health: A Guide to Rating Scales and Questionnaires*. Oxford University Press, 1987.

Reliability of Health Belief Indexes: Confirmatory Factor Analysis in Sex, Race, and Age Subgroups

Joel L. Weissfeld, Bruce M. Brock, John P. Kirscht, and Victor M. Hawthorne

Despite frequent reference to the Health Belief Model (HBM), few studies address the internal consistency (within questionnaires) or the stability across populations of scales used to measure HBM variables. As part of a 1983 Michigan statewide blood pressure survey, trained interviewers administered 32 health belief questionnaire items to 2,802 randomly selected adult Michigan residents. Exploratory common factor analysis was used to examine the structure of these questionnaire items. Six correlated factors, which corresponded closely with theoretical constructs, appeared. Guided by these results, we developed a confirmatory common factor model. The model's fit was examined in random population halves and in univariate sex, race, and age subgroups. Except perhaps in the oldest age group, the model's fit appeared constant. Reliabilities estimated for HBM factor scales formed with these questionnaire items appeared independent of age, race, or sex.

The Health Belief Model (HBM) is one of several psychosocial models developed to explain preventive health behavior, compliance with medical regimens, and health care utilization [1]. Although varied by dif-

---

This work was supported, under contract with the Michigan Department of Public Health, by the National Heart, Lung, and Blood Institute (Grant No. N01-HV-92914).

Address correspondence and requests for reprints to Joel L. Weissfeld, M.D., M.P.H., Instructor of Internal Medicine (Ambulatory Care), Ann Arbor Veterans Administration Hospital, 2215 Fuller Road, Ann Arbor, MI 48105. Bruce M. Brock, Ph.D., M.P.H. is President of Information Transfer Systems, Inc. and Executive Director of DataStat, Inc., both in Ann Arbor; John P. Kirscht, Ph.D., M.A. is Professor of Health Behavior and Health Education, University of Michigan; and Victor M. Hawthorne, M.D. is Professor of Epidemiology, University of Michigan.

ferent writers, a widely used version of the HBM associates an individual's health behavior with five psychological variables: general health motivation, susceptibility, severity, benefits, and barriers. General health motivation is defined as the nonspecific tendency for an individual to engage, across situations, in healthful behavior. Susceptibility refers to an individual's estimate of his chance of acquiring a disease or of suffering the ill-effects of disease. Severity refers to an individual's perception of the seriousness of a given disease or of disease in general. Benefits and barriers refer to an individual's assessment of the value and cost, respectively, of alternative behaviors. Under the model, other variables (e.g., environmental cues, and sociodemographic and social support variables) are thought to affect behavior through health beliefs.

Although many published studies provide empirical support for the HBM [2], only a few have examined the formal psychometric properties of health belief indexes [3–7]. Most such methodologic studies employ specialized and nonrepresentative populations [5,6]. While some investigators compare the distribution of health beliefs among population subgroups [6,7], none confirm that the structure and reliability of health belief indexes remain invariant with respect to the variables used to characterize the subgroups.

The 1983, population-based Michigan Blood Pressure Survey included many health belief questionnaire items. In a representative and generally healthy population, this present study aimed at assessing the structure and internal consistency (i.e., reliability) of health belief measures. Further, structure and internal consistency were compared across major population subgroups. Equivalent structure and reliability are important psychometric properties if scales formed from these measures are to be used to compare mean health beliefs across population subgroups.

METHODS

The 1983 Michigan Blood Pressure Survey was designed to measure the prevalence of undiagnosed, diagnosed, treated, and controlled hypertension in the Michigan adult population and in its major sociodemographic subgroups. Other health-related information, including health beliefs, was also collected. A probability sample of Michigan households was selected by means of a stratified multistage cluster sample design. In each sampled household, one adult, 18 years or older, was randomly selected by means of the Kish selection tables [8]. Between July 1983 and March 1984, face-to-face interviews were successfully completed in 74.4 percent of eligible households. A total of 2,802 adults were interviewed (1,184 men, 1,618 women; 73.6 percent white, 24.4 percent black, 1.9 percent other; 49.8, 27.2, and 23.0 percent aged 18–39 years, 40–59 years, and greater than 59 years, respectively).

All interviewers received standard training, which included written procedure manuals, lectures, group practice sessions, role playing, and mock interviews. Procedures were established to minimize nonresponse, missing data, coding errors, data entry errors, and falsification of interview data.

Thirty-two questionnaire items measured hypothesized HBM constructs. The questionnaire employed a closed, Likert-type format (some items without a middle category), with four to six ordinally scaled options per item. With the exception of the barriers construct, the HBM dimensions were represented by several items. In order to assess the reliability of scales formed from these questionnaire items, exploratory and confirmatory factor analytic techniques were employed. Data exploration and model building were initially performed on a random half of the study population. Exploratory common factor analysis employed the OSIRIS IV computer program package [9]. The Pearson product-moment correlation matrix was formed for the 32 HBM questionnaire items. With communalities placed in the diagonal of the correlation matrix, factors were extracted by means of the principle-axis method of Hotelling [10]. The number of factors to retain in the factor solution was determined by application of the Scree test [11]. The factor solution was examined after Varimax and Oblimin rotations.

Confirmatory factor analyses employed the LISREL VI computer program package [12]. The polychoric correlation matrix was formed for the 32 HBM questionnaire items. Polychoric correlations were felt to be more appropriate in light of the noninterval nature of the health belief measures [12]. Confirmatory common factor models, with each questionnaire item loaded singly, were specified. Since the distribution of responses to the HBM questionnaire items departed from multinormality, unweighted least-square parameter estimation (instead of maximum likelihood estimation) was employed [12].

Using the factor loading and factor correlation patterns developed for the first random population half, parameters for the same common factor model were estimated for the second random half and for univariate sex, race, and age subgroups. The adequacy and comparability of these models were assessed by examination of: (1) the parameter estimates; (2) the amount of variance, in the pool of questionnaire items, explained by the entire model and by each common factor; (3) the reliability of factor scales formed under the model; and (4) the LISREL VI Goodness of Fit Index (GFI) [12]. The GFI, a global measure of how well the model reproduces the sample correlation matrix, approaches unity for models with good fit. Coefficient omega was employed to estimate the reliability of scales formed by simple addition of normalized questionnaire item responses [13].

RESULTS

We used exploratory factor analysis to guide development of a confirmatory common factor model, in which each hypothesized HBM questionnaire item loaded on only one factor. Then, factor loading and factor correlation estimates, percentage of variance explained by each factor and by all factors, and global measures of the model's goodness of fit were directly compared across mutually exclusive population subgroups. If such a parsimonious model fits the data adequately, then scales can be constructed with each questionnaire item contributing to only one scale [14]. Further, if the model's fit is stable across population subgroups, one can then compare each scale's reliability estimate across these subgroups.

The 32 HBM questionnaire items and the theoretical HBM dimension each represents are listed in Appendix A. Items were assigned to theoretical HBM dimensions by consensus between two authors (J. L. W. and B. M. B.) and prior to any statistical analysis. Appendix B shows the Oblimin-rotated, exploratory factor analysis solution for one random population half. Interpretation based on the Varimax rotation gave similar results. The solution contained six significant factors (Scree test). For interpretation, all factor loadings, except for each item's largest loading, were ignored. (Item 25 had large loadings on two factors. The second-highest loading, felt to have greater face validity, was retained.) These six factors were entitled, General Health Motivation/Concern, General Health Threat, Susceptibility, Severity, Benefit of Medical Care, and Self-help Benefit (benefit of self-help behaviors) (Appendix A, under Empirical Constructs). After Oblimin rotation, three factor pairs—Benefit of Medical Care and Self-help Benefit, General Health Motivation/Concern and Benefit of Medical Care, and General Health Motivation/Concern and Self-help Benefit—were modestly correlated (Appendix B).

These exploratory factor analysis results guided development of a six-factor confirmatory factor analysis model. In all models examined, each HBM questionnaire item was forced to load only on the factor with which it associated in the exploratory factor analysis. When all 15 factor intercorrelations were allowed to vary, only four intercorrelations were large (> 0.25). Three of these four intercorrelations (Benefit of Medical Care and Self-help Benefit, General Health Motivation/Concern and Benefit of Medical Care, and General Health Motivation/Concern and Self-help Benefit) were observed in the Oblimin rotated exploratory factor analysis. In confirmatory factor analysis, General Health Motivation/Concern and Susceptibility represented a fourth large factor intercorrelation. All subsequent confirmatory factor analysis models allowed correlation between each of these four factor pairs. Correlation between any other factor pair was not allowed.

In each random population half and in univariate sex, race, and age subgroups, Table 1 shows the factor-loading estimates for the final confirmatory common factor model. Except for item 23, the only theoretical barrier item available for study, loadings for all items in all models exceeded 0.3, a level conventionally considered "important" [14].

Because a statistical test has not been developed [12], apparent differences in the magnitude of parameter estimates were interpreted cautiously. In general, factor loadings (Table 1) and factor intercorrelations (not shown for the confirmatory factor analysis models) were similar. However, in blacks compared to whites, a question measuring "blood pressure concern" (item 4) loaded on the latent Health Motivation/Concern construct more heavily than a question measuring the belief "in the importance that people take special care of their health" (item 3, Table 1). Similarly, in older age groups, questions measuring "thinking about health" (item 1) and "concern about health" (item 2) loaded on the Health Motivation/Concern construct less heavily than a question measuring the belief "in the importance that people take special care of their health" (item 3, Table 1).

In subgroup comparisons, the percent of variance explained by each factor and the percent of variance explained by all factors were construed as summary measures of the comparability of factor loadings within factors and over all factors, respectively. Generally, these measures were comparable (Table 2). In black-white comparisons, however, these measures tended to be slightly larger in blacks.

In a common-factor analysis, the Goodness of Fit Index (GFI) was construed as a global measure of how well the factors and their correlations reproduced all off-diagonal elements in the sample correlation matrix. The model appeared to deteriorate in older age groups

Table 1: Factor Loadings (Confirmatory Factor Analysis Model) for Two Random Population Halves and Sex, Race, and Age Subgroups

	1st Random Half	*2nd Random Half*	*Men*	*Women*	*Whites*	*Blacks*	*Age 18–39*	*Age 40–59*	*Age > 59*
Sample Size	1429	1373	1184	1618	2057	683	1393	761	643
General Health Motivation/Concern									
1.	0.57	0.54	0.58	0.55	0.53	0.50	0.66	0.56	0.39
2.	0.65	0.72	0.72	0.67	0.66	0.64	0.75	0.67	0.59
3.	0.67	0.78	0.75	0.65	0.80	0.34	0.67	0.72	0.82
4.	0.67	0.61	0.63	0.68	0.56	0.78	0.61	0.67	0.60
General Health Threat									
5.	0.76	0.72	0.76	0.72	0.70	0.90	0.68	0.81	0.81
6.	0.63	0.59	0.53	0.66	0.60	0.61	0.63	0.62	0.56
Susceptibility									
7.	0.38	0.36	0.36	0.37	0.33	0.48	0.39	0.38	0.35
8.	0.77	0.76	0.80	0.76	0.75	0.80	0.81	0.71	0.74
9.	0.82	0.84	0.83	0.82	0.84	0.82	0.85	0.81	0.82
10.	0.60	0.62	0.63	0.60	0.61	0.68	0.57	0.64	0.68
11.	0.56	0.54	0.59	0.53	0.54	0.66	0.55	0.53	0.63
Severity									
12.	0.85	0.85	0.85	0.85	0.85	0.84	0.89	0.83	0.79
13.	0.93	0.93	0.93	0.93	0.93	0.93	0.93	0.90	0.94
14.	0.84	0.84	0.83	0.85	0.84	0.84	0.85	0.81	0.85
15.	0.82	0.85	0.82	0.85	0.84	0.84	0.82	0.89	0.80
16.	0.41	0.36	0.38	0.38	0.39	0.36	0.42	0.34	0.37

Benefit of Medical Care									
17.	0.41	0.37	0.43	0.33	0.40	0.30	0.34	0.44	0.42
18.	0.58	0.52	0.59	0.53	0.54	0.62	0.49	0.53	0.66
19.	0.52	0.48	0.49	0.51	0.47	0.61	0.44	0.51	0.57
20.	0.63	0.70	0.64	0.70	0.65	0.68	0.65	0.63	0.72
21.	0.53	0.46	0.46	0.55	0.50	0.56	0.55	0.50	0.46
22.	0.70	0.73	0.72	0.65	0.69	0.71	0.71	0.69	0.78
23.	0.24	0.19	0.18	0.25	0.22	0.30	0.22	0.18	0.24
Self-help Benefit									
24.	0.58	0.59	0.54	0.61	0.61	0.61	0.60	0.58	0.60
25.	0.54	0.53	0.52	0.58	0.53	0.61	0.61	0.54	0.54
26.	0.58	0.63	0.57	0.62	0.62	0.58	0.56	0.63	0.66
27.	0.59	0.58	0.55	0.59	0.59	0.57	0.53	0.63	0.64
28.	0.70	0.68	0.67	0.66	0.64	0.77	0.64	0.77	0.68
29.	0.68	0.61	0.60	0.67	0.63	0.64	0.64	0.66	0.61
30.	0.65	0.62	0.61	0.65	0.67	0.65	0.65	0.64	0.61
31.	0.61	0.64	0.60	0.61	0.59	0.69	0.61	0.69	0.57
32.	0.56	0.55	0.53	0.54	0.54	0.55	0.52	0.62	0.55

Table 2: Percent of Variance (in the Pool of Questionnaire Items) Explained by Each Factor, Percent of Variance Explained by All Factors, and Goodness of Fit Index for Confirmatory Factor Analysis Models Fitted to Each of Two Random Population Halves and Sex, Race and Age Subgroups

	1st Random Half	*2nd Random Half*	*Men*	*Women*	*Whites*	*Blacks*	*Age 18–39*	*Age 40–59*	*Age > 59*
Percent of variance explained by factor									
General Health Motivation/Concern	5.16	5.96	5.71	5.07	5.25	4.30	5.68	5.42	4.80
General Health Threat	3.06	2.70	2.66	2.96	2.67	3.68	2.70	3.23	3.02
Susceptibility	6.56	6.55	7.00	6.30	6.32	7.62	6.70	6.23	6.83
Severity	9.78	9.82	9.69	9.93	9.86	9.78	10.14	9.53	9.43
Benefit of Medical Care	6.24	5.95	6.09	6.01	5.89	6.99	5.72	5.91	7.32
Self-help Benefit	10.58	10.35	9.42	10.63	10.26	11.23	10.09	11.63	10.37
Percent of variance explained by all factors	41.38	40.97	40.57	40.90	40.26	43.60	41.04	41.95	41.78
Goodness of Fit Index	0.917	0.897	0.898	0.910	0.908	0.906	0.920	0.895	0.864

(Table 2). This finding suggested that a six-common-factor model, with four correlated factor pairs and with each questionnaire item loaded singly, provided a relatively poor fit in the oldest age group.

Finally, once the model was accepted, Table 3 shows reliability estimates (coefficient omega), a measure of internal consistency, for factor scales (Appendix C) formed with questionnaire items loading on a given factor. The reliabilities were acceptable in magnitude and generally stable when examined across subgroups (Table 3). An alternative reliability coefficient based on the Spearman-Brown formula [13] gave nearly identical results.

DISCUSSION

An exploratory factor analysis of 32 health belief questionnaire items yielded a factor structure that corresponded fairly closely with the conceptual form of the Health Belief Model. That is, the health belief questionnaire items consistently loaded, in that pattern suggested by theory, on common factors with HBM interpretations. Subsequently, we formed the confirmatory common factor model suggested by the results of the exploratory factor analysis. The model's fit and the scales' estimated reliabilities appeared to be relatively independent of sex, race, and age. These findings suggested that the questionnaire items and the resulting scales represented not only internally consistent measures with respect to Health Belief Model theory, but also psychological measures of similar constructs in different sex, race, and age subgroups.

The primary purpose of this article was to examine, in different demographic subgroups, psychometric properties of health belief questionnaire items. In addition, the exploratory factor analysis solution shown in Appendix B permitted comment on the possible nature of the six factors identified. Two questionnaire items, one measuring general susceptibility, the second general severity, formed the General Health Threat dimension. In contrast, disease-specific items formed distinct susceptibility and severity dimensions. Past work has been largely ambiguous regarding the relationship between susceptibility and severity. One previous study, a factor analysis of a telephone survey of Michigan adults, produced a similar factor which combined general disease susceptibility and severity items [3]. In the study presented here, the General Health Threat factor had substantial loadings from several items having a self-help benefit interpretation. The pattern of loading suggested that individuals perceiving a greater threat from

Table 3: Reliability (Coefficient Omega) Estimated for Factor Scales (Appendix C)

	1st Random Half	*2nd Random Half*	*Men*	*Women*	*Whites*	*Blacks*	*Age 18–39*	*Age 40–59*	*Age > 59*
General Health Motivation/Concern	0.74	0.76	0.77	0.73	0.74	0.66	0.77	0.75	0.72
General Health Threat	0.65	0.60	0.59	0.64	0.60	0.73	0.60	0.68	0.64
Susceptibility	0.77	0.77	0.79	0.76	0.76	0.82	0.78	0.76	0.78
Severity	0.89	0.89	0.88	0.89	0.89	0.89	0.90	0.88	0.88
Benefit of Medical Care	0.72	0.72	0.72	0.72	0.71	0.75	0.70	0.71	0.66
Self-help Benefit	0.84	0.84	0.82	0.84	0.84	0.86	0.83	0.86	0.79

disease were less likely to perceive health value in a balanced diet or regular exercise. This observation suggested that the general disease susceptibility and severity items and several self-benefit items formed polar extremes of a dimension which represented an individual's sense of control over subsequent health.

The benefit questionnaire items formed two correlated dimensions. One dimension appeared to measure the perceived value of medical care and the medical care system. The second appeared to measure the perceived value of more personal health behaviors. Further, the General Health Motivation/Concern dimension correlated with each of the benefit dimensions. This confirmed Maiman's [4] observation, in mothers of obese children, of a similar correlation between health concern and belief in a physician's ability to cure illness.

The paucity of theoretical barrier questionnaire items in the 1983 Michigan Blood Pressure Survey severely limited our ability to determine whether benefits and barriers form separate psychological dimensions. The only barrier item (item 23, Appendix A) loaded weakly with benefit items. This observation is too weak to clarify a previous suggestion that benefits and barriers form polar extremes of a single dimension [5].

Factor analytically derived reliability estimates must be interpreted cautiously [13]. In our study, response-set bias may explain part of the observed inter-item correlations. Although the 32 HBM questionnaire items were dispersed in a 424-item questionnaire, items measuring the same theoretical HBM construct tended to use similar question formats and to appear together in the questionnaire.

Development of a standard, flexible, widely useful instrument to measure HBM variables has not been fruitful. In part, this is because of the need to target the content of questionnaires to specific health behaviors, disease states, and populations. Most studies, in fact, do not examine the degree to which the theoretical components are represented in the actual measures. We were able to identify only eight published studies which addressed the psychometrics of health beliefs [3-7, 15-17]. Several, however, incorporated constructs (e.g., locus of control, social support) not conventionally considered health beliefs [6,15]. Populations studied included random samples of healthy adults [3,15] or children [7], mothers of obese children [4], diabetics [17], and availability samples (e.g., hospital employees [6] and graduate students [5]). Most employed factor-analytic methods to develop internally consistent scales with acceptable reliabilities. Only two studies validated results in a second sample [3,17]. On very small nonrandom subsamples, only two studies examined the instrument's test-retest reliability [6,16]. Without examining the scales' appropriateness in different population subgroups, two studies examined the manner in which values for factor scales were distributed according to age, sex, marital status, or education [6,7]. Thus, only limited information has been available concerning measurement issues in research on health beliefs. This article represents an initial step toward the development of standard health belief scales which generalize for men and women, blacks and whites, and perhaps different age groups.

APPENDIX A

HBM QUESTIONNAIRE ITEMS

	Theoretical Construct	*Empirical Construct*
1. How often do you think about your health?	Motivation	Motivation/ Concern
2. How concerned are you about your health?	Motivation	Motivation/ Concern
3. How important do you think it is that people take special care of their health?	Motivation	Motivation/ Concern
4. How concerned are you about the possible future effects of high blood pressure on your health? How concerned are you about health problems that high blood pressure could cause for you?*	Motivation	Motivation/ Concern
5. Compared to other people your age, would you say that you get sick much more often, more often, as often, less often, or much less often?	Susceptibility	General Health Threat
6. Compared to other people your age, when you do get sick, would you say you get much more sick, more sick, as sick, less sick, or much less sick?	Severity	General Health Threat
7. How likely do you think it is that you will get high blood pressure sometime in your life? One year from now, how likely do you think it is that you will have elevated blood pressure levels where your pressure is not in good control?*	Susceptibility	Susceptibility
8. How likely is it that you will have a heart attack in the future?	Susceptibility	Susceptibility
9. How likely is it that you will have a stroke in the future?	Susceptibility	Susceptibility

Continued

Appendix A: Continued

	Theoretical Construct	*Empirical Construct*
10. How likely is it that you will have kidney disease in the future?	Susceptibility	Susceptibility
11. How likely is it that you will have cancer in the future?	Susceptibility	Susceptibility
12. How serious a health problem would high blood pressure be for you? How serious a health problem do you think high blood pressure will be for you in the future?*	Severity	Severity
13. How serious a health problem would having a heart attack be for you?	Severity	Severity
14. How serious a health problem would having a stroke be for you?	Severity	Severity
15. How serious a health problem would having kidney disease be for you?	Severity	Severity
16. How serious a health problem would having cancer be for you?	Severity	Severity
17. Overall, how helpful are doctors when you are ill?	Benefit	Benefit of Medical Care
18. Overall, how effective do you think medical treatment is in preventing illness from the effects of high blood pressure?	Benefit	Benefit of Medical Care
19. More specifically, how effective do you think blood pressure medicines are in preventing illness from the effects of high blood pressure?	Benefit	Benefit of Medical Care
20. What about special diets?	Benefit	Benefit of Medical Care
21. What about exercise programs for high blood pressure?	Benefit	Benefit of Medical Care
22. How important do you think controlling high blood pressure is?	Benefit	Benefit of Medical Care
23. Overall, how easy or difficult is it to get medical care when you want it?	Barrier	Benefit of Medical Care
"Now I'll read you a list of things some people think help their health. Tell me if you think each one I read helps a person's health a great deal, a large amount, a fair amount, a little, or if it doesn't help at all."		
24. . . . eating a balanced diet?	Benefit	Self-help Benefit
25. . . . getting regular physical activity?	Benefit	Self-help Benefit
26. . . . being at the ideal weight for a person's height?	Benefit	Self-help Benefit
27. . . . avoiding getting tense and anxious?	Benefit	Self-help Benefit

Continued

Appendix A: Continued

	Theoretical Construct	*Empirical Construct*
28. . . . getting regular medical checkups?	Benefit	Self-help Benefit
29. . . . getting the right amount of sleep?	Benefit	Self-help Benefit
30. . . . avoiding cigarettes?	Benefit	Self-help Benefit
31. . . . avoiding alcohol?	Benefit	Self-help Benefit
32. . . . leading a spiritually good life?	Benefit	Self-help Benefit

*Alternative questionnaire item for respondents reporting a history of high blood pressure.

APPENDIX B

EXPLORATORY FACTOR ANALYSIS SOLUTION, SIX FACTORS, OBLIMIN ROTATION, FIRST RANDOM POPULATION HALF

The factor pattern and the factor intercorrelation matrixes follow. Only factor loadings with values greater than 0.175, in absolute value, are shown.

	Factor					
Questionnaire Items	*Motivation Concern*	*Threat*	*Susceptibility*	*Severity*	*Medical Benefit*	*Self-help*
1. Health think	0.58					
2. Health concern	0.74					
3. Special care	0.28					
4. BP concern*	0.50					
5. Sick often		-0.34	0.25			
6. Sick severe		-0.23	0.23			
7. HTN likely			0.38			
8. MI likely			0.72			
9. Stroke likely			0.75			
10. Kid dis likely			0.52			
11. Cancer likely			0.50			
12. HTN serious				0.73		
13. MI serious				0.83		
14. Stroke serious				0.74		
15. Kid dis serious				0.66		
16. Cancer serious	0.24			0.29		
17. Doctors helpful		-0.18			0.25	
18. Medical treatment					0.71	
19. BP medicines					0.70	
20. Prescr diet					0.42	
21. Prescr exercise		0.30			0.38	

Continued

Appendix B: Continued

Questionnaire Items	*Factor*					
	Motivation Concern	*Threat*	*Susceptibility*	*Severity*	*Medical Benefit*	*Self-help*
22. BP control					0.18	
23. Care barrier					0.18	
24. Diet		0.35				0.39
25. Exercise		0.45				0.39
26. Ideal weight		0.19				0.47
27. Anxiety		0.19				0.48
28. Checkups	0.18				0.19	0.46
29. Sleep						0.57
30. Cigarettes						0.53
31. Alcohol						0.59
32. Good life						0.49
	Motivation Concern	*Threat*	*Susceptibility*	*Severity*	*Medical Benefit*	*Self-help*
Motivation/Concern	1.00	0.02	0.09	0.08	0.11	0.20
Threat		1.00	-0.01	0.02	0.03	0.01
Susceptibility			1.00	0.06	-0.01	0.03
Severity				1.00	0.05	0.10
Medical Benefit					1.00	0.26
Self-help Benefit						1.00

*BP = blood pressure; HTN = hypertension; MI – myocardial infarction; kid dis = kidney disease; prescr = prescribed.

APPENDIX C

HEALTH BELIEF SCALES

Each scale is scored by summing the items indicated. Before summation, each item is standardized against its mean and standard deviation. Means and standard deviations provided were not weighted to reflect the study's sample design. Sample sizes used to estimate means and standard deviations vary because of missing responses.

Questionnaire Item	*Sample Size*	*Range*	*Mean*	*Standard Deviation*
Motivation/Concern				
1. Health think	2794	1-6	2.91	1.26
2. Health concern	2791	1-4	1.65	0.82
3. Special care	2792	1-4	1.14	0.41
4. BP concern	2773	1-4	1.87	1.03

Continued

Appendix C: Continued

Questionnaire Item	*Sample Size*	*Range*	*Mean*	*Standard Deviation*
Threat				
5. Sick often	2724	1-5	3.92	0.92
6. Sick severe	2681	1-5	3.45	1.00
Susceptibility				
7. HTN likely	2617	1-4	2.62	0.91
8. MI likely	2590	1-4	2.85	0.87
9. Stroke likely	2579	1-4	2.91	0.82
10. Kid dis likely	2603	1-4	3.04	0.80
11. Cancer likely	2535	1-4	2.76	0.89
Severity				
12. HTN serious	2687	1-4	2.01	0.97
13. MI serious	2690	1-4	1.33	0.70
14. Stroke serious	2702	1-4	1.25	0.62
15. Kid dis serious	2694	1-4	1.40	0.75
16. Cancer serious	2708	1-4	1.23	0.61
Benefits of Medical Care				
17. Doctors helpful	2761	1-4	1.56	0.74
18. Medical treatments	2639	1-4	1.63	0.67
19. BP medicines	2571	1-4	1.57	0.65
20. Prescribed diet	2670	1-4	1.50	0.64
21. Prescribed exercise	2559	1-4	1.68	0.76
22. BP control	2782	1-4	1.08	0.31
23. Care barrier	2772	1-4	1.70	0.74
Self-help Benefit				
24. Diet	2789	1-5	1.45	0.76
25. Exercise	2783	1-5	1.53	0.80
26. Ideal weight	2768	1-5	1.74	0.91
27. Anxiety	2768	1-5	1.70	0.95
28. Checkups	2780	1-5	1.82	1.03
29. Sleep	2783	1-5	1.75	0.89
30. Cigarettes	2753	1-5	1.41	0.80
31. Alcohol	2752	1-5	1.85	1.03
32. Good life	2748	1-5	2.07	1.24

REFERENCES

1. Becker, M. H. (ed.). The Health Belief Model and Personal Health Behavior. *Health Education Monographs* 2(4):324–508, Winter 1974.
2. Janz, N. K., and M. H. Becker. The health belief model: A decade later. *Health Education Quarterly* 11:1–47, 1984.

3. Jette, A. M., et al. The structure and reliability of health belief indices. *Health Services Research* 16(1):81-98, 1981.
4. Maiman, L. A., et al. Scales for measuring health belief model dimensions: A test of predictive values, internal consistency, and relationships among beliefs. *Health Education Monographs* 5(3):215-30, Fall 1977.
5. Cummings, K. M., A. M. Jette, and I. M. Rosenstock. Construct validation of the health belief model. *Health Education Monographs* 6(4):394-405, Winter 1978.
6. Elder, J. P., et al. Multivariate evaluation of health attitudes and behaviors: Development and validation of a method for health promotion research. *Preventive Medicine* 14(1):34-54, 1985.
7. Dielman, T. E., et al. Dimensions of children's health beliefs. *Health Education Quarterly* 7(3):219-38, 1980.
8. Kish, L. *Survey Sampling*. New York: John Wiley and Sons, 1965.
9. Survey Research Center. *OSIRIS IV User's Manual*. Ann Arbor: University of Michigan, Institute for Social Research, 1981.
10. Hotelling, H. Analysis of a complex of statistical variables into principle components. *Journal of Educational Psychology* 24(6):417-441, 498-520, 1933.
11. Cattel, R. B. The Scree test for the number of factors. *Multivariate Behavioral Research* 1(2):245, 1966.
12. Joreskog, K. G., and D. Sorbom. *LISREL VI: Analysis of Linear Structural Relationships by Maximum Likelihoods, Instrumental Variables, and Least Square Methods*. Mooresville, IN: Scientific Software, Inc., 1984.
13. Carmines, E. G., and R. A. Zeller. *Reliability and Validity Assessment*. Beverly Hills, CA: Sage Publications, Inc., 1979.
14. Kim, J., and C. W. Mueller. *Factor Analysis: Structural Methods and Practical Issues*. Beverly Hills, CA: Sage Publications, Inc., 1978.
15. Berkanovic, E., C. Telesky, and S. Reeder. Structural and social psychological factors in the decision to seek medical care for symptoms. *Medical Care* 19(7):693-709, 1981.
16. Champion, V. L. Instrument development for health belief model constructs. *Advances in Nursing Science* 6(1):73-85, 1984.
17. Given, C. W., et al. Development of scales to measure beliefs of diabetic patients. *Research in Nursing and Health* 6(1):127-41, 1983.

Chapter Three

Descriptive Statistical Profiles of Hospital Service Areas

Hospital discharge abstract data files have become a major source of secondary data for researchers concerned with practice variations. Questions about quality of care and cost of care are being investigated in the context of wide variations among geographic areas in rates of procedures and hospitalizations. The article by Griffith, Wilson, Wolfe, and Bischak presents a step in the incremental use of discharge files to explain these prevalent variations.

It had been established by previous research that significant differences were occurring, by community, in admission rates for medical patients in Michigan. The authors wished to explore whether certain clinical categories or activities might explain these differences, or whether these variations were nonspecific in these regards. By establishing that clinical differences did not, in general, explain the variation, they took one more step in this line of research.

Much secondary data analysis—both epidemiological analysis and research on services utilization—involves rates and proportions (or percentages). The article by Griffith et al. provides examples of some nonparametric techniques used in such analyses. It includes a justification for the selection of the secondary database, an explanation of a procedure for geographic clustering, a careful statement of hypotheses, the use of multiple clinical dimensions in an attempt to be comprehensive, the use of multiple techniques to strengthen their findings, and varied tabular and graphical representation of their findings. The analysis is essentially descriptive, but it points out the care with which descriptive data must be organized and presented to draw conclusions and suggest further research.

Clinical Profiles of Hospital Discharge Rates in Local Communities

John R. Griffith, Peter A. Wilson, Robert A. Wolfe, and Diane P. Bischak

Using comprehensive 1980 data for hospitalization of the 9 million citizens of Michigan's lower peninsula, the authors have previously demonstrated that the discharge rates of local communities differ by a range of 2 to 1. This article seeks to identify differences in the clinical profile of high-use compared to low-use communities. Population-based rates and percentages of total discharges were studied for major clinical activity groups, such as cardiovascular disease, frequent diagnoses, rarely occurring diagnoses, short- and long-stay diagnoses, certain surgical procedures, and major organ groups of the diagnostic classification system. Although high-use communities tend to admit proportionately fewer surgical cases and proportionately more nonsurgical cases, few other such patterns could be demonstrated.

BACKGROUND

Various investigators have developed measures of hospital use for geographically identified communities defined by the population's tendency to use a set of community general hospitals located in the trade center of the community. The usual finding from such research is a

---

This article is supported in part by the Health Care Financing Administration, DHHS Grant No. 05-P-97227/5.

Address all correspondence and requests for reprints to John R. Griffith, Andrew Pattullo Collegiate Professor and Chair, Department of Health Services Management and Policy, School of Public Health II, 1420 Washington Heights, The University of Michigan, Ann Arbor, MI 48109. Peter A. Wilson, Ph.D. is Senior Vice President, Michigan Hospital Association; Robert A. Wolfe, Ph.D., is Associate Professor of Biostatistics at The University of Michigan School of Public Health; and Diane P. Bischak is Assistant Professor at North Carolina State University, Industrial Engineering Department.

wide variation among ostensibly similar communities. When measured in nonobstetric discharges per thousand population, communities within a single state vary from 100 discharges per 1,000 population to over 200. These variations persist after age adjustment and careful efforts to adjust for patient traffic into and out of the areas in question [1-4].

Papers seeking explanations for this widespread variation in various measures of hospital use have been published for several decades. A large number of contributing factors have been hypothesized and tested.

One obvious explanation of the finding of variation would be that citizens of high-use communities have a demonstrably higher need for hospitalization and treatment. Several authors have investigated this hypothesis, although more of the work has focused on surgical use. Only one could find support for need as an explanation of rate variation; three studies disagreed. Mitchell and Cromwell, reporting on 350 primary sampling units of the Health Interview Survey, had concluded:

> What [explains] these small area variations are large differences in demand and supply factors. However, the reduced form surgery equations show that variables such as medical need, ability to pay, and substitute sources of care were all important determinants of surgical utilization. Health status as measured by both age and disability data has made a significant contribution to small areas of surgical variation. Sicker persons demand more operations, particularly non-elective ones [5].

A study by Wennberg, also using health interview survey data, concluded the opposite for the total discharge rate [6]. An international study of rates for several surgical procedures also contradicted the Mitchell and Cromwell conclusion [7]. Roos and Roos, working with surgery rates of elderly patients in rural communities in Manitoba and using more detailed individual health characteristics, such as activities of daily living, life satisfaction, and socioeconomic status, concluded that "the data do not support a needs model . . . high rate areas were not characterized by an elderly population that was disabled and in ill health" [8].

In fact, much prior work assumes that variation in use is a function of health care system variables. Lembcke noted that surgical volumes and surgical deaths were associated [9], and went on to devise ways to amend surgeons' behavior [10]. Roemer concluded that use was related to the supply of beds [11]. Many studies have associated surgical use with the supply of surgeons. This work was summarized and documented in Roos and Roos [8].

The difficulty with the "Roemer's Law" approach—basically that supply generates demand—is that it begs the question of why supply should be higher in one community than in another one which is ostensibly similar. The problem is particularly obvious with hospital beds—a community with twice the patient-day rate of another must have nearly twice as many beds. (In Michigan, no community routinely fills all of the beds accessible to it. On the average in 1980, 1.5 empty beds were available, and 3.3 were filled for every 1,000 persons. Higher levels of empty beds were associated with increased use, especially in small communities.) But why did one community build substantially more beds than another? Some reason should emerge for such large variations. Income and related economic factors are often cited, but these are by no means uniform in their action. The reason may lie in attitudes toward hospitalization. For reasons good or bad, one community may want twice as much hospital use as another.

Recently, attention has turned to attitudinal factors: perceptions of the desirability of hospitalization as opposed to need or supply. Wennberg concludes that surgeons develop "profiles" of procedures [3]. Roos believes that "hysterectomy-prone" surgical practice style is a valid concept in explaining small area variations in Manitoba [12]. Rosenblatt and Moscovice report that nonmedical factors affecting hospitalization patterns of general and family practitioners include practice characteristics, such as the scope of outpatient services used and how busy the doctor is, as well as patient characteristics, such as age and average income of the county of the doctor's office [13]. While little is reported on patient attitudes, one suspects that they also enter into the decision.

In prior work on the Michigan database, Wilson and Tedeschi demonstrated that discharge rates vary far more than the length of stay, and that within the total discharge rate, variation in nonsurgical use is more important than variation in surgical use. Although the two discharge rates are almost equal for Michigan as a whole, near 75 per 1,000 population per year, the standard deviation and range of the nonsurgical discharge rates across communities are approximately twice those of surgical rates [14].

This leads to the question explored here. This article examines variations in discharge rates among categories defined by morbidity type or by organ system in the ICD-9-CM classification; among common or rare first-listed diagnoses in hospital admissions; among exceptionally long-stay or exceptionally short-stay patients; among identifiable subcategories of disease, such as cardiovascular disease, carcinoma, trauma, and diabetes; and among certain common surgical procedures. The theory to be tested is that the tendency to high use is pervasive across most such groups rather than reflecting a diverse pattern of high and low use for differing categories. One might infer that if the theory is rejected, diverse patterns of use reflect different kinds of patients with different needs. If the theory is supported, consistently high or low use reflects some characteristic of practice which is community related, such as a general economic or health status condition, a common set of attitudes among patients or physicians toward hospitalization, or an insurance or supply system encouraging use.

METHODS AND DATA

THE DATABASE

We used 1980 data from all short-term general hospitals in Michigan's lower peninsula, grouped into 60 market-defined communities or "clusters" serving 9 million people who used 1.35 million discharges within that year. The "cluster" is arguably a hospital service community; we use the terms interchangeably. (Uncomplicated obstetrics, totaling 180,000 admissions, have been removed from the data studied here.) A *Note* at the end of this article amplifies the description of the database.

So far as we can determine, 1980 was a reasonably typical year for hospital use. Total state statistics had shown only modest changes for some years. Costs were increasing at a rate below the national averages. Length of stay had been falling and discharges had been increasing. Unemployment was rising, but most industrial workers retained their health care benefits. No major epidemics of hospitalized diseases were reported, and overall rates of medical and surgical discharges were within a few percentage points of 1978 statewide values. When classified by discharge rate, most of the communities in the high and low quartiles were in the same quartiles in 1978. We believe the relative ranking had obtained for some years.

Nineteen eighty was also an exceptional year for data quality. A major effort to gain completeness captured about 98 percent of the known discharges, and missing data could be closely approximated. The census count yielded the most accurate possible denominators for rate calculations.

SERVICE AREAS

The theory implies that a "cluster" is an identifiable hospital care community. Clusters consist of all zip code populations where a plurality of hospital discharges are from the local hospitals. Obviously, clusters are not totally self-contained. Only four to six of the clusters are capable of full tertiary service. The others must refer for complex care, and people self-select their source of care to a surprising extent. The average cluster had 66 percent of its discharges from its associated hospitals, with a range from 45 percent to 91 percent. It is possible to study only core areas having majority percentages to the local hospitals. Core areas tend to contain the bulk of the population and to have discharge rates which are highly correlated with the larger "plurality" areas studied here. We have chosen to study the larger plurality areas because they include the entire Michigan population. Presumably, comparative relationships we see in the plurality clusters would be strengthened by limiting the analysis to core areas.

These patterns of hospital selection appear to be stable over time. For the 43 communities with complete data in both 1978 and 1980, the maximum shift in local hospital market share was only 6 percent. To the degree practically possible, we believe we have identified medical care "systems" in the sense that the population and the medical care resources are substantially committed to each other.

DIAGNOSTIC CLASSIFICATION

Diagnostic classification was obtained using the Commission on Professional and Hospital Activities (CPHA) "List A," a set of 391 clinically related groups of ICD-9-CM codes using the primary listed diagnosis [15]. These codes were placed into 16 morbidity groupings (omitting complications originating in the perinatal period), as shown in Table 1, using the classification found in ICD-9-CM. The diagnostic frequency groups—common, middle, and rare—were established by dividing the rank-ordered List A categories into thirds. Thus, the "common" group was the 27 most frequent List A diagnoses, comprising 450,000 admissions. The "rare" was the 307 least frequent diagnoses also comprising 450,000 admissions, and the "middle" group is the 57 other diagnoses. Short- and long-stay cases were developed by rank-ordering List A groups according to their statewide average length of stay and selecting those List A groups with an average length of stay less than 3 days and those List A groups with an average length of stay equal to or greater than 11 days. Six common surgical procedures have been identified, based on the literature, particularly Wennberg's surgical profile [16]. The six were appendectomy, cholecystectomy, hemorrhoidectomy, hysterectomy, prostatectomy, and tonsillectomy and adenoidectomy. Each of the procedures was identified by its CPHA List B

Table 1: Classification of Diseases and Injuries

Morbidity Group Number	*Description*	*ICD-9-CM Coding*	*Number of Discharges*	*Percent of Total Discharges (%)*
1.	Infectious and parasitic diseases	001–139	11,930	1.7
2.	Neoplasms	140–239	86,872	7.5
3.	Endocrine, nutritional, and metabolic diseases and immunity disorders	240–279	34,074	2.9
4.	Diseases of the blood and blood-forming organs	280–289	9,701	0.8
5.	Mental disorders	290–319	49,254	4.2
6.	Diseases of the nervous system and sense organs	320–389	58,147	5.0
7.	Diseases of the circulatory system	390–459	137,759	11.8
8.	Diseases of the respiratory system	460–519	115,981	9.9
9.	Diseases of the digestive system	520–579	153,922	13.2
10.	Diseases of the genitourinary system	580–629	130,638	11.2
11.	Complications of pregnancy, childbirth, and the puerperium	630–676	25,628	2.2
12.	Diseases of the skin and subcutaneous tissue	680–709	19,766	1.7
13.	Diseases of the musculoskeletal system and connective tissue	710–739	86,084	7.4
14.	Congenital anomalies	740–759	11,655	1.0
15.	Certain conditions originating in the perinatal period	760–779	2,489	0.2
16.	Symptoms, signs, and ill-defined conditions	780–799	51,176	4.4
17.	Injury and poisoning	800–999	115,409	9.9
	Noncoded or unreadable		57,410	4.9
	Total		1,165,895	99.9

Procedure Code. (Appendectomies incidental to another procedure were excluded.)

RATE AND PERCENTAGE CALCULATION

Two measures were constructed to evaluate the profiles of use in the communities. Discharge rates were constructed on an age-specific basis and standardized to the Michigan statewide age distribution. Percentages of discharges took the category in question as numerator and all nonobstetric discharges for the community as denominators. In both cases numerators and denominators were complete counts for the cluster communities, independent of the site of hospitalization.

HYPOTHESES AND MODEL

Our general hypothesis is that high use is pervasive across discharges grouped by different clinical descriptors. It can be evaluated by testing two null hypotheses:

H^1_0: There is no association between a community's total nonobstetric age-adjusted *discharge rates* and its use in each of the following discharge categories:

a. Sixteen different morbidity groups
b. Short- and long-stay lengths of stay
c. Common, medium, and rare diagnoses
d. A number of specific diagnoses and surgical procedures.

H^2_0: There is no association between a community's total nonobstetrical discharges and the *percentage* of those discharges occurring in each of the following communities with respect to each of the following discharge categories:

a. Sixteen different morbidity groups
b. Short- and long-stay lengths of stay
c. Common, medium, and rare diagnoses
d. A number of specific diagnoses and surgical procedures.

Rejection of the first null hypothesis, H^1_0, indicates that high- and low-use communities, defined in terms of overall nonobstetrical hospital use, are also different with respect to hospital use for the specific discharge type or clinical category. Rejection of the second null hypothesis, H^2_0, indicates that the difference in use in the specific category is not commensurate with the difference in overall hospital use, i.e., the proportionality is not maintained. In combination, the two hypotheses allow an exploration of the detailed comparative anatomy of high and low hospital-use communities.

We tested the first hypothesis by examining the statistical correlation for the 60 communities between each of the categorical rates and the total rate. This was pursued by correlating the age-adjusted categorical rates against the rank order of the age-adjusted nonobstetric discharge rate, using the Friedman two-way analysis of variance for the categorical rates [16]. To test the second hypothesis, a correlation analysis was performed to relate the percentages of the nonobstetric rate falling in each category to the total rate and the rank order of the total rate. One should note that these percentages are not inherently related to the total rate as the component rates themselves are.

In addition, the quartiles of the age-adjusted nonobstetrical discharge rate were identified, and the Student's t-test for the equality of means was performed on the high and low quartiles ($n = 30$) for both age-adjusted and age-specific rates within the different discharge groupings. To reduce inequalities of variances, the variables were transformed to logarithms and the test repeated. The Mann-Whitney U-test was also performed on the rates and percentages.

Table 2 describes the high- and low-quartile communities in terms of a number of key demographic and medical care supply characteristics. In Michigan in 1980, there is a clear relationship between community size and discharge rate. High-use communities tend to be smaller, although there are a number of exceptions to this generalization. High-

Table 2: Characteristics of High- and Low-Use Communities, 1980

Characteristic	*High Quartile* (n = 15)	*Low Quartile* (n = 15)
Population		
<50,000	4 communities	11 communities
≥50,000	11 communities	4 communities
Mean	121,570*	257,080
Median	28,834	99,519
Age distribution		
0–44 years	68.5%	70.6%
45 + years	31.5%	29.4%
Median per capita income		
Mean	$8,168†	$9,449
Unemployment		
Mean	14.3%†	10.7%
Discharges by payment source		
Medicare	26.7%†	29.5%
Medicaid	12.6%†	7.7%
Blue Cross	28.9%†	24.8%
Total	68.2%†	62.0%
Physicians per 10,000 population (mean)		
Nonsurgeons	6.87	6.25
Surgical specialties	3.40	3.30
Acute beds per 1,000 population		
Mean	5.65†	3.63
Range	4.45–8.45	2.86–4.55
Hospital use (age-adjusted nonobstetrical means)		
Patient-days per 1,000 population	1,235†	897
Discharges per 1,000 population	175†	117
Average length of stay	7.2	7.7

*High and low quartiles significantly different at .05 using Mann-Whitney nonparametric test.

†High and low quartiles significantly different at .05 using Student's *t*-test.

use communities have a significantly lower median income and a higher unemployment rate. However, in Michigan, as elsewhere in the United States, the financial barrier to hospital care has been substantially mitigated by government insurance programs. In Michigan, three major reimbursers, Medicare, Medicaid, and Blue Cross, paid on a cost basis in 1980. High-use communities have a significantly higher percentage of patients with Medicaid, a significantly lower Medicare percentage, and significantly higher cost-based reimbursement overall. Other government programs are relatively insignificant in Michigan and could not be identified reliably from this data set. Given the mixed pattern of response, it is difficult to draw conclusions about the impact of insurance coverage. Finally, high-use communities have a somewhat older age distribution. However, since our use rates are age adjusted, this difference in distribution does not explain the observed differences in hospital use.

Turning to the medical care system characteristics of the communities, the high- and low-use quartiles have roughly the same physician supply in both surgical and nonsurgical specialties. There is, however, a striking difference between their supplies of acute care beds and the Michigan hospital license counts. The high-use quartile has a mean in excess of 50 percent greater than the low-use quartile, and the ranges have virtually no overlap. This bed supply difference is implied by the differences in hospital use. Occupancy rate tends to be similar in both high- and low-use communities.

With very few exceptions, the same findings occur in comparing high- and low-use quartiles as with the correlation and Friedman analysis. The quartile comparisons are presented as a useful comparison.

FINDINGS: ORGAN GROUPS

FRIEDMAN ANALYSIS

The 16 age-adjusted discharge rates were positively associated with each other (Friedman's Chi-square = 524, df = 72, $p < .001$). This indicates that communities that have a high rate of discharge in one organ group also tend to have high rates of discharge in other organ groups. Kendall's coefficient of concordance was equal to 0.455 for these data. The average Spearman rank correlation between pairs of the 16 measures was equal to 0.419. This indicates a high degree of positive interdependence among the 16 discharge rates.

Correlation analysis between two measures of overall discharge rates and 33 percentage measures of patterns of discharge yielded the results in Table 3. The percentage of discharges in organ groups were, with the exceptions noted below, only weakly correlated with the ranking by overall discharge rate. For 11 of the 16 organ groups, the correlation between percent of discharges and average discharge rate was less than 0.25 in magnitude. The strongest correlations were for organ system 2 (neoplasms), 8 (respiratory), 14 (congenital anomalies), and 6 (nervous system), with correlations of -0.79, +.46, -.46, and -.38, respectively. This indicates that high discharge-rate communities tend to have a relatively larger fraction involving respiratory disease than do low discharge-rate communities. When other approaches to categorization of disease (cardiovascular, trauma, adverse effects, carcinoma, and diabetes) are examined, similar findings emerge. Only carcinoma, a subset of organ group 2, is significantly different in percent of discharges.

HIGH AND LOW QUARTILES

Tables 4 and 5 indicate the findings for the high and low quartiles. The first null hypothesis, H^1_0, that there is no difference in discharge rates by clinical subsets, is almost universally rejected, as was the case with the correlation analysis. Communities which have high rates of hospitalization overall have high rates in almost every group.

The high quartile of communities has an overall mean discharge rate of 50 percent higher than the low quartile, which is statistically significant, and this significant difference persists through 15 of the 16 morbidity groups tested. The single exception, group 11—Complications of Pregnancy, Childbirth, and the Puerperium—is sex specific and found principally in the age group 15–29. The Student's *t*-test applied to that age specific group shows a significant difference ($p < .05$).

The five other disease categories show findings similar to the Friedman analysis, except that a significant but small shift appears in cardiovascular disease as well as in carcinoma.

FINDINGS: OTHER CHARACTERISTICS

As Table 3 shows, the six surgical procedures selected for study are negatively associated with total use, but only one is significant. The interquartile comparisons (Table 5) show increased rates for three of six procedures but equal or (for hysterectomies) reduced percentages. This

Table 3: Correlation Matrix of Patient Category Percentage

Patient Category	*Correlation with Rank Order*	*Correlation with Adjusted Rate*
1. Org. grp. 1	.1323	.1165
2. Org. grp. 2*	-.7930	-.7930
3. Org. grp. 3	.0206	.0135
4. Org. grp. 4	.0767	.0995
5. Org. grp. 5	-.1149	-.1177
6. Org. grp. 6*	-.3710	-.3818
7. Org. grp. 7	-.2088	-.2199
8. Org. grp. 8*	.4647	.4589
9. Org. grp. 9	.1352	.1481
10. Org. grp. 10	.0031	.0116
11. Org. grp. 11	-.0774	-.0595
12. Org. grp. 12	-.0196	-.0393
13. Org. grp. 13	-.1870	-.2112
14. Org. grp. 14*	-.4652	-.4608
15. Org. grp. 16	.1827	.2077
16. Org. grp. 17	.1318	.1029
17. Short stay	-.2129	-.2120
18. Long stay*	-.6539	-.6713
19. Medium stay*	.6608	.6755
20. Cardiovascular	-.1627	-.1704
21. Trauma	.1007	.0758
22. Adverse effects	-.1854	-.1896
23. Carcinoma*	-.7482	-.7591
24. Diabetes	.1271	.1133
25. Tonsillectomy; adenoidectomy	-.1433	-.1441
26. Hysterectomy*	-.6307	-.6125
27. Appendectomy	-.2083	-.2017
28. Prostatectomy	-.3015	-.3069
29. Hemorrhoidectomy	-.0469	-.0135
30. Cholecystectomy*	-.5226	-.5199
31. Common diagnoses*	.4121	.4254
32. Medium diagnoses	-.1921	-.1861
33. Rare diagnoses*	-.4531	-.4792

*Significant at $p < .01$ (both columns).
$N = 60$ $DF = 58$ $R.0500 = .2542$ $R.0100 = .3301$.

is one of the few places where the findings are inconsistent between the quartile and Friedman analysis.

Between common, medium, and rare diagnoses, it is clear that higher-use communities admit proportionately fewer rare and proportionately more common cases. This is significant in both analyses. Between short-, medium-, and long-stay diagnoses, higher-use communities admit a significantly higher percentage of medium-stay cases,

Table 4: Morbidity Groupings—Means for High- and Low-Quartile Communities

Morbidity Group	Age-Adjusted Discharge Rate		Percent of Total Discharges*	
	High Quartile (Standard Deviation)	*Low Quartile (Standard Deviation)*	*High Quartile (Standard Deviation)*	*Low Quartile (Standard Deviation)*
1	3.2§ (0.73)	1.9 (0.61)	1.8 (0.44)	1.6 (0.47)
2	9.9§ (1.14)	9.0 (0.91)	5.7§ (0.76)	7.8 (0.97)
3	5.4§ (1.17)	3.6 (0.48)	3.1 (0.72)	3.1 (0.37)
4	1.3§ (0.56)	0.8 (0.18)	0.8 (0.29)	0.7 (1.30)
5	5.3§ (2.24)	3.8 (1.58)	3.1 (1.34)	3.2 (1.22)
6	7.3§ (0.72)	5.6 (0.66)	4.2§ (0.52)	4.8 (0.65)
7	24.0§ (3.70)	16.8 (1.95)	13.8 (2.16)	14.4 (1.31)
8	23.2§ (5.45)	11.6 (1.47)	13.3§ (2.81)	9.9 (1.13)
9	24.6§ (3.91)	15.7 (1.80)	14.0 (1.64)	13.4 (1.11)
10	18.3§ (3.17)	12.3 (1.77)	10.4 (1.38)	10.5 (1.17)
11	2.8 (1.46)	2.0 (0.84)	1.6 (0.81)	1.7 (0.67)
12	2.6§ (0.58)	1.7 (0.25)	1.5 (0.33)	1.4 (0.19)
13	11.7§ (1.99)	8.4 (1.37)	6.7§ (0.96)	7.2 (1.47)
14	1.4§ (0.26)	1.2 (0.19)	0.8§ (0.13)	1.0 (0.16)
15†	—	—	—	—
16	7.8§ (11.7)	5.4 (1.31)	6.1 (6.3)	4.6 (0.98)
17	17.8§ (3.08)	11.2 (1.67)	10.2 (1.51)	9.6 (1.09)
Total	166.6§	111.0	95.5*	94.9*
Cardiovascular disease‡	41.3§ (6.51)	29.3 (4.26)	23.7§ (4.08)	25.0 (2.68)
Trauma	17.1§ (2.78)	10.9 (2.07)	9.8 (1.39)	9.3 (1.49)
Adverse effects	7.8§ (1.79)	5.5 (1.55)	4.5 (1.05)	4.7 (1.20)
Carcinoma	7.2§ (0.93)	6.8 (0.82)	4.2§ (0.68)	5.9 (0.85)
Diabetes	3.4§ (1.00)	2.2 (0.36)	1.9 (0.52)	1.9 (0.28)

*Discharge percentages do not add to 100 percent because of noncoded or nonsense-coded discharges.
†Analysis omitted because of the small number of discharges in this category.
‡Age adjusted for the population aged 45 or older.
§Significantly different at .05 using Student's t-test, and Student's t-test on log transform $N(1) = N(2) = 15$.

Table 5: Duration of Hospital Stay, Commonality of Diagnosis, and Surgical Use for High- and Low-Quartile Communities

	Age-Adjusted Discharge Rate		*Percent of Total Discharges*	
Characteristics	*High Quartile (Standard Deviation)*	*Low Quartile (Standard Deviation)*	*High Quartile (Standard Deviation)*	*Low Quartile (Standard Deviation)*
Length of Stay				
Long (≥ 11 days)	28.8† (3.26)	23.2 (2.27)	16.6† (2.37)	19.9 (1.60)
Medium	176.23† (12.7)	117.0 (8.12)	77.8† (2.81)	73.8 (1.23)
Short (< 3 days)	10.5† (1.96)	7.3 (1.31)	6.0† (1.12)	6.3 (1.18)
Diagnosis Frequency				
Common third	64.4† (11.36)	41.5 (316)	37.0† (4.8)	33.7 (1.2)
Medium third	58.9† (6.48)	40.6 (3.88)	32.0 (2.5)	33.0 (1.6)
Rare third	56.5† (5.26)	40.9 (3.12)	30.8† (2.5)	33.2 (1.6)
Procedures				
Hysterectomy*	4.6 (1.09)	4.3 (0.58)	2.6† (0.54)	3.6 (0.50)
Appendectomy	1.7† (0.63)	1.2 (0.16)	0.9 (0.31)	1.0 (0.16)
Prostatectomy*	2.4 (0.84)	2.0 (0.44)	1.3 (0.43)	1.7 (0.43)
Hemorrhoidectomy	0.8 (0.47)	0.6 (0.24)	0.5 (0.25)	0.5 (0.20)
Cholecystectomy	2.4† (0.47)	1.9 (0.27)	1.4 (0.28)	1.6 (0.26)
Tonsillectomy and adenoidectomy	3.4† (1.79)	2.4 (1.10)	2.0 (0.98)	2.1 (1.11)
Surgical discharge	85†	64	48†	55
Medical discharge	90†	53	52†	45

*Hysterectomy and prostatectomy rates are sex specific.

†Significantly different at .05 using Student's *t*-test, and using Student's *t*-test on log transform.

avoiding both extremes, but a significantly lower percentage of long-stay diagnoses (Tables 3 and 5).

In summary, the clinical characteristics of communities with higher discharge rates can be described as follows:

- The general pattern is to admit proportionately more of all categories of patients studied.
- The characteristics where high-use communities tend to focus their increased admission activity (i.e., admit proportionately more patients) are respiratory diseases, common diagnoses, and medium length-of-stay diagnoses.
- The characteristics where high-use communities tend to avoid increasing admissions (i.e., admit proportionately fewer patients) are carcinoma, diseases of the nervous system, rare diagnoses, and those with long stay.

DISCUSSION

Beyond the fact that hospital use varies tremendously from community to community, little is understood about the details of that difference, much less the explanation of it. In large part this reflects the difficulty of constructing appropriate databases, an activity that is taxing in both the political and technical dimensions.

Earlier explorations of the Michigan inpatient database established a number of interesting findings: that communities differed more substantially in admission rates than in average length of stay; that communities differed more in their use of hospitals for medical patients than for surgical patients; that high use was ubiquitous in the sense that a community with a high medical or surgical discharge rate or length of stay tends to be high on the rest of those dimensions; and, finally, that there is a significant correlation of levels of hospital use across a community by age groups and payment sources [16].

In this article, we extended the articulation of high hospital-use communities into a number of clinically descriptive dimensions: diagnostically defined categories, selected surgical procedures, and characteristics of length of stay and frequency of diagnosis. Our expectation, based upon the earlier work, was that high use would be a generic, nonspecific phenomenon extending across clinical dimensions as it had earlier extended across age groups, insurance sources, and discharge rates and length of stay, both medical and surgical.

Our expectation was fulfilled, with findings that both confirmed and extended the previous work. High-use communities have a 50 percent greater propensity to hospitalize overall, and this percentage recurs in many of the dimensions explored. There are two principal exceptions to the latter finding. First, for a number of morbidity groupings where surgery is the predominant intervention, the difference in hospital use is closer to 30 percent. Second, high-use communities have a tendency to focus upon common diagnoses (up 60 percent), respiratory discharges (up 100 percent), and medium-stay discharges (up 44 percent). The groups which differ are sufficiently small in total not to lend much support to the hypothesis that high-use communities are such simply because of an emphasis upon "bread and butter" hospitalizations. The results fail to support explanations based upon "excess surgery."

Figures 1 through 4 show graphically how high- and low-use communities differ. Although the rates of individual case groups are not exactly parallel between the high quartile and the low quartile, they are clearly similar, with the two middle quartiles between. A test for parallelism fails, apparently because of slight differences as well as the impact of the groups which are obviously approached quite differently [17]. On the graphs showing percentages of cases (Figure 2), no orderly pattern emerges. In many cases the percentages of two or more quartiles were too close to graph separately.

The findings are consistent with any community-wide or disease-independent phenomenon. They appear to be inconsistent with specific disease-dependent phenomena, because it is hard to conceive why all disease incidences—from pregnancy-related complications to heart disease—would be correlated. Community-wide differences include income, education, poverty, and insurance. They may include smoking and drinking behavior, health care beliefs, and care-seeking practices. They may also include factors related to the care "systems," such as availability and access of hospitals, availability and access of doctors and care substitutes, and, as Wennberg suggests, the attitudes of physician gatekeepers [18].

NOTE

CALCULATIONS OF COMMUNITY POPULATION-BASED MEASURES OF HOSPITAL USE

The quantity of hospital care used by groups of individuals is calculated as a use rate—either discharges or patient-days in the numerator,

Figure 1: Profile of Discharge Rates by Organ Group

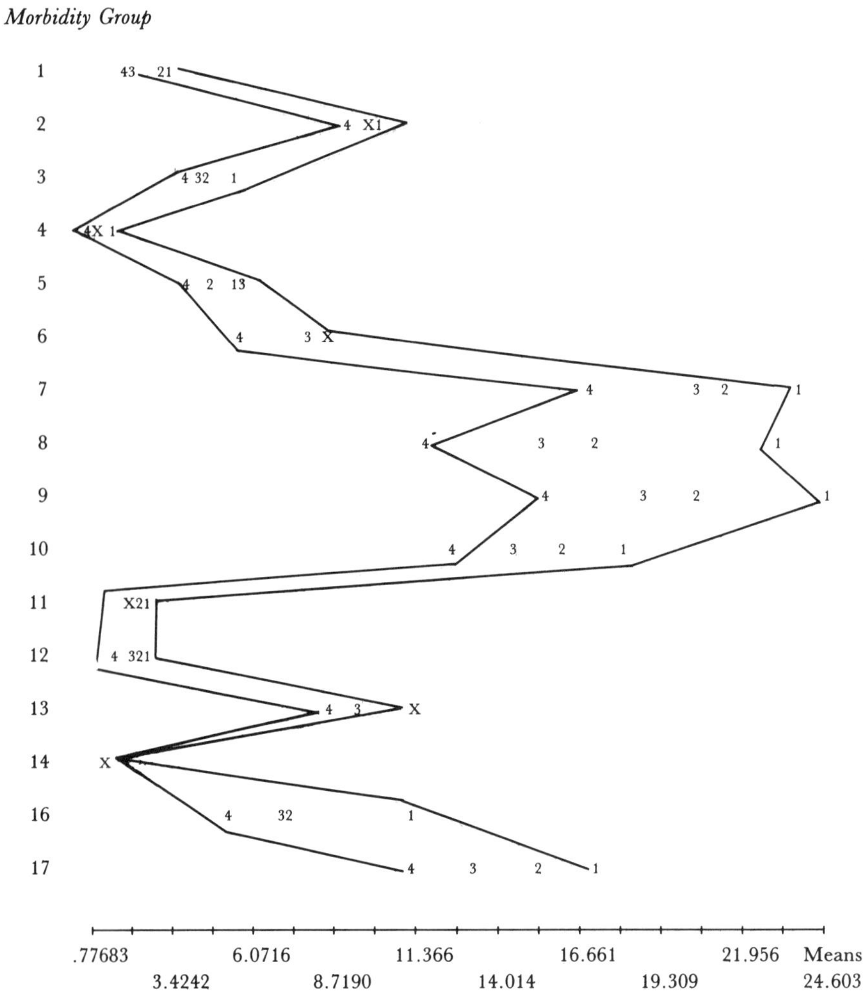

and the population in the denominator. Calculations of community use rates involve the assignment of all short-term general hospital discharges for a year to the residence of the patient, in a convenient geographic subunit such as postal code area or minor civil division. For each of these "micro" areas, the population and the discharges must be known for at least four age categories.

Figure 2: Profile of Percent of Discharges by Organ Group

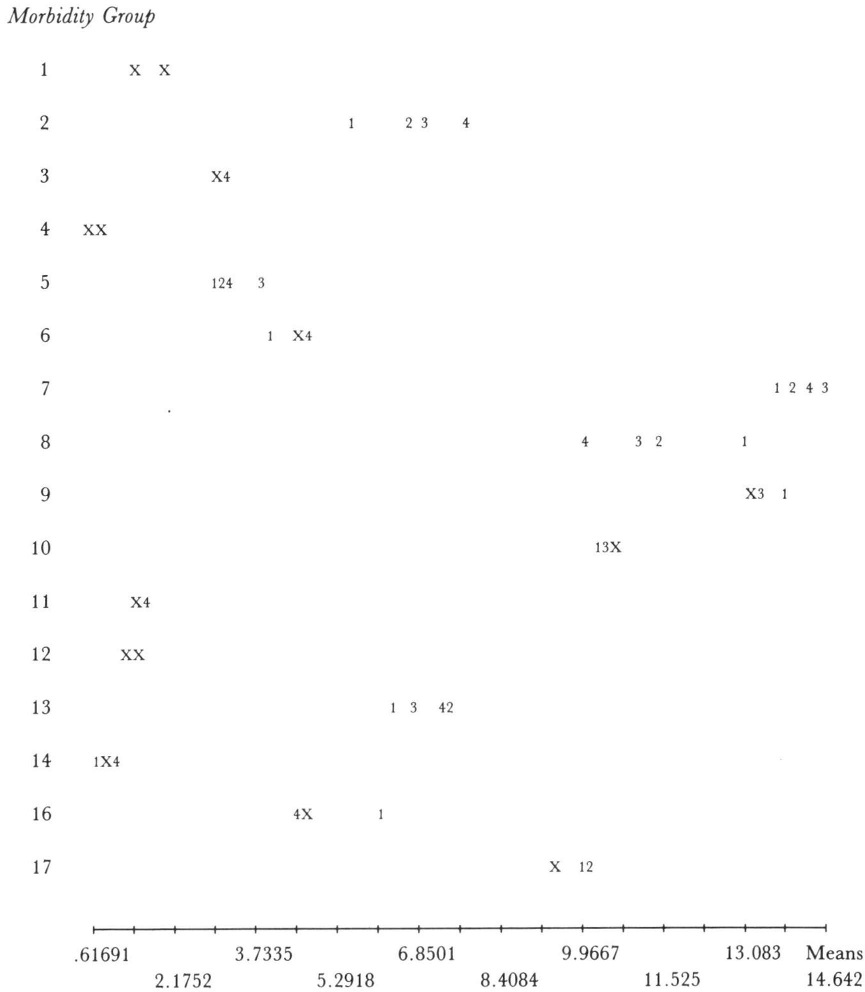

In Michigan, postal zip code areas are used. The age categories for 1980 are 0–14, 15–29, 30–44, 45–64, 65–74, and over 75 years. Substantial effort is made to gain accurate measurement of both discharges and populations of the micro areas. All discharges from community hospitals plus Veteran's Administration hospitals are recorded by individual abstract with demographics (age, sex, race, zip code),

Figure 3: Age-Adjusted Discharge Rates of Common, Medium, and Rare Discharge Diagnoses

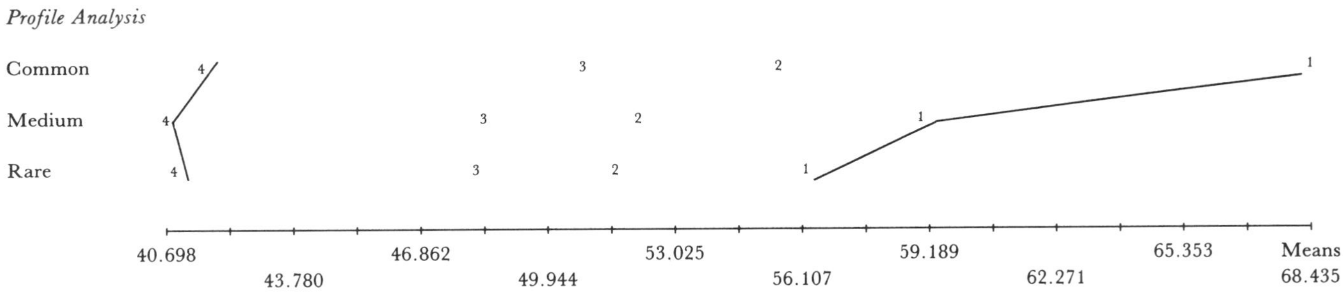

Figure 4: Age-Adjusted Discharge Rates of Short-, Medium-, and Long-Stay Diagnoses

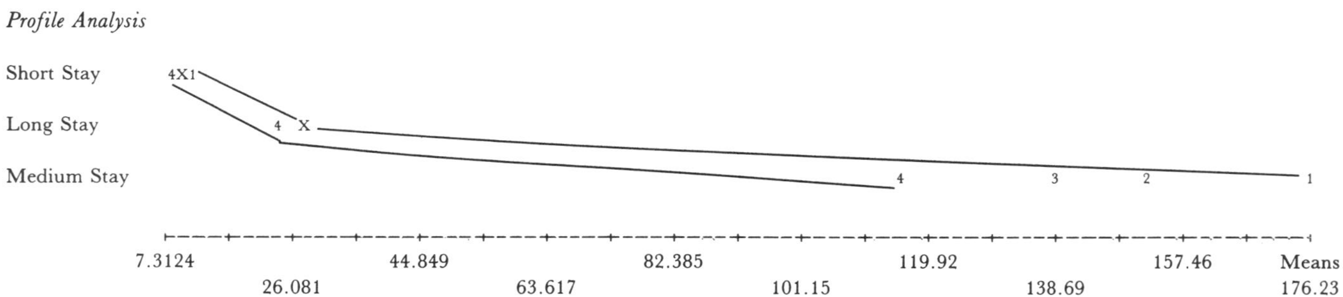

diagnostics (up to 14 diagnoses and up to 7 surgical procedures), and services (hospital, expected source of payment, admission status, and discharge status). Discharges from hospitals in northern Indiana and northwest Ohio supplement the Michigan data set. Rates for Michigan's upper peninsula (4 percent of the state population) are not reported because of lack of Wisconsin discharges. (Hospitalizations of residents of the lower peninsula in upper peninsula hospitals are included.) More remote travel is a source of error. We assume that it is randomly distributed among the communities. The zip code count of population for April 1, 1980, from the U.S. Bureau of Census is used in 1980. More complex inferential methods are used for other years.

The micro areas are grouped according to the hospital location preferred by the residents as measured by actual use. This was a two-step procedure. First, hospitals in the same town or in nearby locations were grouped together by a computer algorithm designed to identify hospitals with significant market overlap. Those groups were reviewed for reasonableness by panels of planners and administrators familiar with the area.

Second, each postal area is assigned to the hospital or group of hospitals having the largest single fraction (plurality) of its total use. These groups of zip code areas form the communities, or "clusters" in Michigan jargon. The clusters in Michigan are all formed of contiguous postal areas. Each has a hospital (or hospitals) in a centrally located postal area.

Application of these procedures led to the formation of 60 "clusters" in the lower peninsula, a population of 8.9 million persons in 1980. They range from 11,000 to 861,000 in population, and from 1 to 18 hospitals. The average cluster has 148,000 population and contains 3.75 hospitals. The clusters appear to be stable over time. Only 3 percent of the zip code areas shifted their plurality assignment between 1978 and 1980. Average market shares also remained the same, with two-thirds of the patients hospitalized in their cluster of residence. The maximum change in market share was only 6 percent.

Population-based rates are calculated for the communities by dividing the use (discharges or patient-days) *regardless of the hospital of occurrence* by the population on an age-specific basis, for each of several clinical services. Individual microlevel rates are of questionable reliability because of random postal coding errors and because variation in hospitalization may be significant from year to year, particularly at age- or disease-specific levels. At the cluster aggregation, coding errors tend to be less important. (Most errors are between zip codes which are both in the cluster.) Populations are large enough to generate several thousand admissions each year. Each community rate is standardized to the state population by multiplying the age-specific rates by the statewide age fraction of the population, and summing the product over all ages.

The ratio of the patient-days to the discharges is length of stay. The project produces not only specific measures of actual length of stay by various components of hospital population; it also produces expected lengths of stay, using the Commission of Professional Hospital Activities (CPHA) length-of-stay algorithm. The algorithm generates an expected length of stay for each "List A" group of related primary diagnoses and within the group for operated and nonoperated patients, each of five age categories of patients, and the presence or absence of additional diagnoses. Nearly 5,000 specific expected values are generated. This technique, used by CPHA for several years, has been judged similar to Diagnosis Related Group (DRG) standardization in its ability to explain length-of-stay variation (see *Nine Patient Classification Systems: Development, Description and Testing,* Hospital Research and Educational Trust, Chicago, 1982). The project improves slightly upon the CPHA method by limiting the days for calculating the expected stays to Michigan and making them comprehensive for all of the state discharges.

In cases where abstracts are missing according to the hospital's own count of discharges, existing records are replicated to restore the total. This process was used in only a dozen hospitals in 1980, when an unusually successful data collection effort was mounted. The replications reached three-fourths of the year's discharges for some small hospitals not routinely preparing discharge abstracts and for one larger hospital which moved in mid-year. In no case did the replicated cases exceed 2.5 percent of the community total.

Studies of the impact of Indiana and Ohio data show that clusters on state land borders require out-of-state data to be accurately measured. Studies of the impact of age and sex variation upon adjusted rates indicate that four categories of age are sufficient. Splitting the groups 15 years to 45 years and over 65 years generates a mean difference in the adjusted rate of 0.4 percent, with only 2 of 60 communities shifting more than 2 percent. Sex-specific contribution is even smaller. Given the difficulty of estimating age and sex categories in non-census years, such attempted precision could be dysfunctional.

The authors have unpublished papers supporting the calculations used, and available on request.

REFERENCES

1. Wennberg, J., and A. Gittelsohn. Small area variations in health care delivery. *Science* 182:1102–08, 1973.
2. Wennberg, J., et al. Health care delivery in Maine. *Journal of Maine Medical Association* 66:123ff, 255ff, 298ff, 1975.
3. Wennberg, J., and A. Gittelsohn. Variations in medical care among small areas. *Scientific American* 246(4):120–34, 1982.
4. Griffith, J. R., et al. Measuring community hospital services in Michigan. *Health Services Research* 16:135–59, 1982.
5. Mitchell, J. B., and J. Cromwell. Variation in surgical rates and the supply of surgeons. In D. L. Rothberg (ed.). *Regional Variation in Hospital Use*. Lexington, MA: Lexington Books, 1982.
6. Wennberg, J. E., and F. J. Fowler, Jr. A test of consumer contribution to small area variations in health care at delivery. *Journal of Maine Medical Association* 68:275, 1977.
7. McPherson, K., et al. Small variations in the use of common surgical procedures. *New England Journal of Medicine* 307:1310–14, November 18, 1982.
8. Roos, N. P., and L. L. Roos. Surgical rate variations—Do they reflect the health or socio-economic characteristics of the population? *Medical Care* 20:945–58, 1982.
9. Lembcke, P. Measuring the quality of medical care through vital statistics based on hospital service areas: Comparative study of appendectomy rates. *American Journal of Public Health* 42:276–86, March 1952.
10. Lembcke, P. Medical auditing by scientific methods. *Journal of the American Medical Association* 162, n. 7, October 13, 1956.
11. Roemer, M. I., and M. Shain. Hospital utilization under insurance (mimeograph). Ithaca, NY: Cornell University School of Business and Public Administration, 1959.
12. Roos, N. P. Hysterectomy: Variations in rates across small areas and across physicians' practices. *American Journal of Public Health* 74:327–35, 1984.
13. Rosenblatt, R. A., and I. S. Moscovice. The practice as gatekeeper determinants of physicians' hospitalization rates. *Medical Care* 22:150–59, 1984.
14. Wilson, P., and P. Tedeschi. Community correlates of hospital use. *Health Services Research* 19:333–55, Summer 1984.
15. Commission on Professional and Hospital Activities. Length of Stay in U.S. Hospitals: 1980. Ann Arbor, MI: The Commission, 1981.
16. Gibbons, J. D. *Non Parametric Statistical Inference*. New York: McGraw-Hill, 1971, pp. 250–56.
17. Harris, R. J. *A Primer of Multivariate Statistics*. New York: Academic Press, 1975, pp. 80–84.
18. Wennberg, J., et al. Will payment based on diagnosis-related groups control hospital costs? *New England Journal of Medicine* 311:295–300, August 2, 1984.

CHAPTER FOUR

Geographic Analysis of Health Services Use: Multidimensional Scaling

The analysis of health services problems using the tools and techniques of geography has a long history. Geographic analysis dates to the classic epidemiological inquiry of John Snow in 1855; however, researchers are sometimes slow to recognize the spatial components and characteristics of the issues and conditions they analyze. Medical and health services geographers have taken freely from the wide array of statistical techniques available, folding them into approaches to analysis and hypothesis testing in ways that have added the dimension of space to research problems. The article by Gesler and Meade is meant to represent this much broader set of spatial and geographic analysis methods.

In this article, the authors chose a planning problem that involves the description of rational service areas based on use patterns that may be discontinuous. The authors discuss how distance itself and general travel patterns may influence health care-seeking decisions and behavior. The implications of their findings are of interest to the planner, the regulator, and the marketer of health services.

Geographic analysis has been applied to many categories of problems where locational efficiency is the relevant goal. Another important area of concern to the medical and health services geographer is the development of service areas for impact studies, the tracing and tracking of disease patterns, and the discovery of health utilization and access inequities. The techniques often combine classical cartography—the construction of maps themselves—with scales and statisti-

interpretations of data, to illuminate a distribution or the dimen-
ɪns of a problem.

Locational and Population Factors in Health Care-Seeking Behavior in Savannah, Georgia

Wilbert M. Gesler and Melinda S. Meade

The use of regular sources of health care by a sample of residents of Chatham County, Georgia was examined through an analysis of the interactions among distance, sociodemographic, locational, and activity-space factors. Health care facilities were concentrated near downtown Savannah. Distance from home to regular source of care was a relatively more important factor for inner-city residents than for suburban or urban fringe residents. There were no clear differences by race, sex, age, occupation, or length of stay at present residence in the relative importance of distance. Strong associations were found between distance-to-care measures and measures of daily-activity spaces. Urban ecological structure appeared to play a more important role in health care-seeking behavior than did the personal characteristics of individuals in this small metropolitan area.

Health planners are vitally interested in examining the behavior of populations that are seeking health care. One approach to the study of this behavior is through spatial analysis. Spatial-analytic studies have focused on the relative location of and distance between consumers and providers, characteristics of these two groups, urban ecological structure, and the daily-activity spaces of consumers (Shannon, Bashshur, and Metzner 1969). Each of these factors has been shown to be of importance to people's accessibility to and utilization of health care resources. Of more interest is how the interaction of two or more of these factors influences health care-seeking behavior. Furthermore,

---

This article is supported by a grant from the National Science Foundation, NSF Award No. SES 8309557.

Address correspondence and requests for reprints to Wilbert M. Gesler, Ph.D., Associate Professor, Department of Geography, University of North Carolina, Chapel Hill, NC 27599. Melinda S. Meade, Ph.D. is Professor, Department of Geography, the University of North Carolina at Chapel Hill.

these factors will interact to affect health care-seeking behavior in different ways in different settings. The purpose of this article is to examine the roles of relative location, distance, population characteristics, daily-activity spaces, and interactions among them, as they pertain to regular sources of health care in a particular setting, Chatham County, Georgia, where the city of Savannah (1980 population, 141,390) is located.

Many health care studies (Weiss, Greenlick, and Jones 1971; Fuller 1974; McGuirk and Porell 1984; Shannon, Skinner, and Bashshur 1973) have shown distance and the distance decay effect to be of importance in consumer-provider contacts. Distance is only one of many factors involved, however. A wide range of studies have shown that distance interacts with other variables in contacts with physicians, hospitals, and other health care resources. Demographic and socioeconomic characteristics like age, sex, and occupation may affect travel distance (Haynes and Bentham 1982). In addition, distance behavior often depends on people's perceptions of disease itself (Girt 1973) and how it is diagnosed and treated (Mayer 1983). Transportation availability, and costs and facility characteristics also interact with distance (Joseph and Phillips 1984) in affecting people's use of health care.

Another consideration in consumer-provider access interaction is the relative location of these two groups (Weiss, Greenlick, and Jones 1971). Areas of residence of different types of people within cities and locations of service provision have been studied by urban geographers, city planners, and others. Simulations have shown that the spatial structure of urban areas is a significant factor in determining inequalities in access to services (McLafferty 1982). In many American cities, the percentage of the population that is black decreases and household income increases in step with movement from the central city to the suburbs. Also in many cities, hospitals and physicians tend to cluster in downtown areas, although they may also be found (especially in larger places) in suburban areas. These conditions hold for Savannah. Bashshur, Shannon, and Metzner (1971, 75) state that "[t]he historically central location of hospitals now produces distance problems for both ghetto blacks and suburban whites." In particular, although inner-city blacks are often close to health care resources, they may find difficulties in using them because of such problems as discrimination, inability to pay, and lack of transportation. Suburban whites, on the other hand, may have to travel longer distances to care.

People's degree of mobility—their daily-activity movements—also play a part in health-seeking behavior. The activity spaces of urban residents have been studied by several researchers (Horton and Reynolds 1971; Dangschat, Friedrichs, and Kiehl 1982; Wolpert 1965). For example, Shannon and Spurlock (1976) compared the activity spaces and travel patterns of 243 families living in Congress Heights, a community in Washington, D.C. They showed that different subgroups of this community carried out activities within different "ecological containers," exposing them to different health hazards or "environmental risk cells." They also found that for some subgroups little overlap appeared between daily-activity spaces and activity spaces related to health services. In a study in Flint, Michigan, Cromley and Shannon (1986) used the activity-space concept to analyze the movement patterns of a sample of independently living elderly people. After dividing the sample into several groups based on similarities among individual activity spaces, they summarized each group's aggregate activity space with standard deviational ellipses and suggested that ambulatory facilities should be located within these spaces.

One of the interesting questions that arises from health care studies that deal with distance is its *relative* importance. This can be measured in at least two ways. First, the contribution of distance to accessibility or utilization can be contrasted to other variables (for example, by using multiple regression and correlation techniques). One might conclude that distance is very important in its own right (McGuirk and Porell 1984); not as important as other variables (Weiss, Greenlick and Jones 1971); a surrogate for other variables (Shannon, Bashshur, and Metzner 1969); or a factor largely ignored or "overridden" in the case, say, of a very severe illness (Mering et al. 1976).

The second way to look at the relative importance of distance (the way used in this article) is to compare the health care sources actually contacted with all available alternatives. The notion of an intervening opportunity is important here (Morrill and Earickson 1968). If a person goes to the closest service possible, then distance is a relatively important factor for that person. If, on the other hand, a person bypasses intervening opportunities, then distance is not as important. A few studies have examined the relative importance of distance from this perspective. In a situation where there were three clinics to choose from, Weiss, Greenlick, and Jones (1971) found that as the distance from residence to nearest clinic increased, proportions of visits to the nearest clinic decreased—and that the percentage of visits to the nearest clinic declined with the age of the patient. In a study in Cleveland it was found that whites traveled longer distances to hospitals than blacks, but that the proportion of whites going to the nearest hospital was twice that of blacks (Bashshur, Shannon, and Metzner 1971). On average, blacks lived less than one mile from a hospital, but three-fourths of them traveled beyond the second-nearest hospital. Many people also traveled beyond the second-nearest hospital for religious reasons; this was true for 90 percent of the Jews studied, one-half of the Catholics, and two-thirds of the Protestants. Similar findings came out of an earlier study in Chicago (Morrill, Earickson, and Rees 1970), where many blacks avoided white physicians and white physicians abandoned black neighborhoods. Again, religious preferences took people beyond intervening opportunities. Spatial choice models are also based on a consideration of possible alternatives. A good example is the spatial demand model used by McGuirk and Porell (1984) in Allegheny County (site of Pittsburgh), Pennsylvania. They found (p. 84) that "distance and time factors strongly influence hospital choice, even in metropolitan areas where alternatives are widely available, and that their effects vary across service classifications and hospitals."

All of the foregoing factors, interacting to influence health-seeking behavior, led us to ask certain questions about our research into regular sources of care in Savannah. For example, would McLafferty's statement (1982, 353) that "[t]he very fact that high-income groups often live in low-density, peripheral areas suggests that distance and travel costs influence their activity patterns less than those of low-income groups," extend to Chatham County and historic Savannah? What other relationships among accessibility factors would be considered important in this unique setting?

METHODOLOGY

POPULATION SAMPLE AND DATA COLLECTION

The Savannah research focused on the effect of different environments on cardiovascular disease (CVD), and the study population was sampled accordingly. There were two principal considerations in selecting census tracts for study. The first was to stratify the choice of tracts by inner city, suburban, urban fringe, and planned industrial satellite in order to include the full range of environments. The second was to select tracts with high or low levels of CVD which were either well or poorly predicted by population and housing characteristics.

Data were available from the Savannah Community Cardiovascu-

Figure 1: Location of Survey Clusters in Chatham County, Georgia

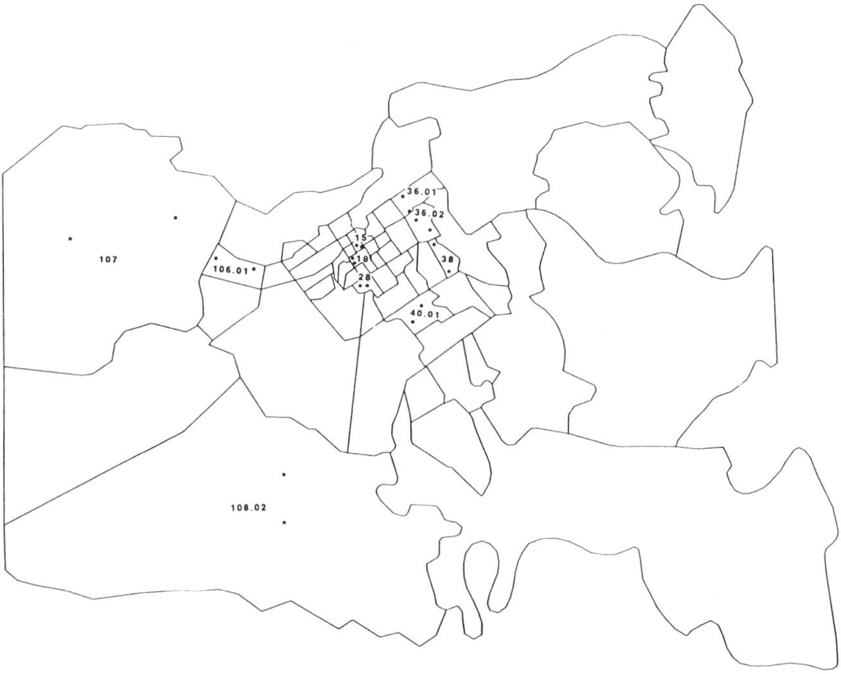

NOTE: NUMBERS SHOWN ARE CENSUS TRACTS

lar Council (CCC) on two indicators of CVD, blood pressures of all high school seniors from 1979 to 1982, and stroke mortality in the entire Chatham County population from 1978 to 1982. Census data for 1980 on socioeconomic and housing characteristics of the populations in the 62 census tracts of Chatham County were used in factor and discriminant analyses to determine their accuracy in predicting blood pressure and strokes in each tract. Ten census tracts were chosen for study (Figure 1).

Three tracts, 15, 18, and 28, were in the inner city (98 people, 23.5 percent of the respondents); four tracts, 36.01, 36.02, 38, and 40.01, were suburban (198 people, 47.5 percent); and two tracts, 107 and 108.02, were in the urban fringe (87 people, 20.9 percent). The tenth tract, 106.01, was essentially comprised of Garden City (34 people, 8.2 percent), a World War II-era planned industrial/port satellite community within a metropolitan area. Its distance from Savannah's

Table 1: Characteristics of the Sample Population

Category	*Subgroups*	*Number*	*Percent*
Race	Whites	239	57.3
	Blacks	178	42.7
Sex	Males	191	45.8
	Females	226	54.2
Age	12–24	102	24.5
	25–44	134	32.1
	45–64	122	29.3
	65–84	59	14.2
Occupation	Professional	31	7.4
	Managerial	30	7.2
	Clerks/Sales	47	11.3
	Skilled labor	44	10.6
	Unskilled labor	21	5.0
	Domestics	22	5.3
	Housewives	106	25.4
	Others*	116	27.8

*Students, retired, unemployed.

central business district (CBD) indicates that it is suburban, but its socioeconomic and housing characteristics suggest that it belongs to the inner-city category.

Within each census tract, two blocks were chosen at random; these formed the core of 20 sample clusters of 10 households each. Interviews were conducted over a six-week period in the summer of 1984, with a total of 417 respondents in the 200 households. Each person in each household who was 12 years old or older was interviewed. The data for this study come from these interviews.

Although certain population subgroups tended to live in some zones rather than others (for example, few blacks lived in urban fringe tracts), each of the four zones contained a mixture of races, sexes, ages, and occupations. Data on race, sex, age, and occupation are shown in Table 1. The amount of time respondents had lived at their present address was also recorded. (Mean time at current residence was 14.4 years.)

ACTIVITY SPACES AND RELATIVE DISTANCE INDEX

Respondents were asked where they went for their regular source of care. Out of a total sample of 417 people, 321 reported the name of a specific physician, clinic, or hospital emergency room. The locations of all regular health care sites reported were recorded (Figure 2). All

Figure 2: Location of Regular Sources of Care for Survey Respondents in Savannah, Georgia

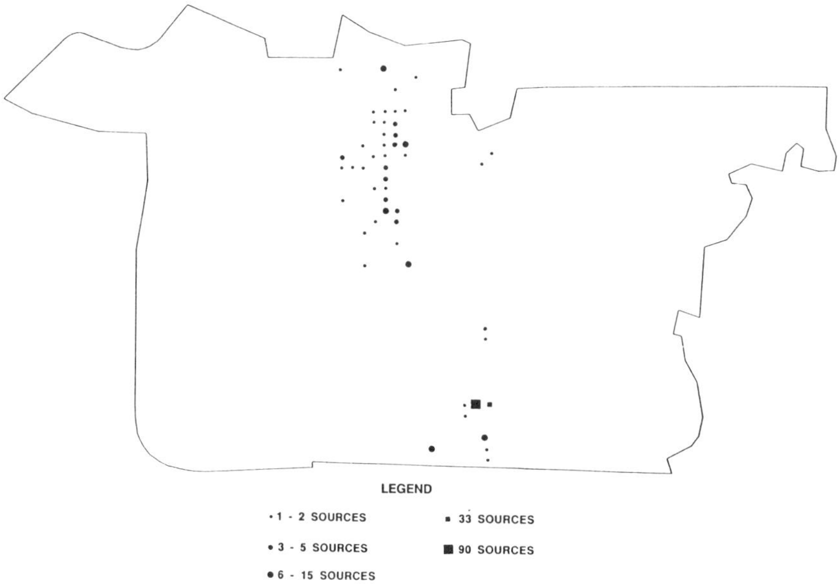

respondents were also asked the number of times during a month they had gone to work or school, had shopped for food or clothing, had attended church, had traveled to places for leisure activities, or had eaten out in restaurants. The amount of time people had spent at home was also noted. The locations of all activity sites were recorded, and activity frequencies—or duration in the case of work, school, and stays at home—were used as weights at each location. Locations and weights were then used together to construct two centrographic measures—the weighted mean center of activity spaces, and the size of standard deviational ellipses (SDEs) (Yuill 1971)—for each of the 20 study clusters. These same measures were also calculated to summarize the locations of regular sources of care. The SDE provides a two-dimensional graphic summary of spatial data points that is analogous to the standard deviation for one-dimensional data distributions.

A relative-distance index was calculated for individuals and groups (see Appendix for an explanation of this measure). In practice, the value of the index ranges from a negative number (-2 to -3) to a maximum of 1. A relatively large index indicates that distance is relatively important (Hightower 1965).

Three more distance variables were developed for each cluster: the Manhattan metric distance from home to the weighted mean center of all regular sources of care, the distance from home to the weighted mean center of activity spaces, and distance from activity-space center to the center of care.

RESULTS

DISTANCE TO CARE FOR POPULATION SUBGROUPS

Summary figures for the actual distances of various subgroups from their regular-care destinations are shown in Table 2. Hospitals and doctors are concentrated or clustered in two sections of Savannah. One cluster converges around the CBD (107 sources); and the other, located southeast of the CBD, centers on the two largest hospitals, Memorial and Candler (Figure 2). Forty-seven sources (14.6 percent of the total) were outside the city of Savannah but still in Chatham County. The location of these three clusters is a major reason why there is an increasing average actual distance from care as one moves from inner-city to suburban to Garden City to urban-fringe residential zones (Table 2). Blacks are closer to care than whites, partly because most blacks live in inner-city areas, and outer areas are populated mostly by whites. There is no difference between males and females in actual distance to care. Among the three lower age groups, a slight declining trend is shown in distance to regular care source. The oldest group was substantially closer to care. Actual distance to care for those in different occupations reflects the scatter of people with different job skills throughout the area.

Table 2 shows details of the values used to calculate the relative-distance index for regular care for various population subgroups (see Appendix for an explanation of the different distance measures). The average actual distance traveled for each subgroup has already been discussed. It is informative to examine minimum distances and hypothetical distances to determine if they followed the same trends among population subgroups as actual distances. In many cases (such as race), trends are the same but with some interesting anomalies (the minimum distance for suburban and Garden City subgroups, for example). All subgroups traveled substantially farther than the minimum distance for care. Actual and hypothetical distances were usually quite similar.

The last column, Index, shows the relative importance of the distance factor for the different groups of people. The absolute value of

Table 2: Relative-Distance Index for Regular Care for Population Subgroups

Group	N	*Actual Distance (Miles)*	*Minimum Distance (Miles)*	*Hypothetical Distance (Miles)*	*Index*
Zone					
Inner city	83	2.4	0.3	2.8	0.16
Suburban	155	3.8	1.5	4.0	0.06
Garden City	27	6.7	0.9	8.3	0.22
Urban fringe	56	13.7	4.4	14.0	0.03
Race					
White	173	6.8	2.2	7.2	0.09
Black	148	3.9	1.0	4.1	0.09
Sex					
Male	132	5.3	1.7	5.7	0.09
Female	189	5.5	1.6	5.8	0.09
Age					
12–24	68	6.1	2.0	5.9	-0.05
25–44	97	5.7	2.0	6.2	0.13
45–64	105	5.5	1.6	5.8	0.08
65–84	51	4.0	0.8	4.8	0.21
Occupation					
Professional	23	6.1	2.0	7.5	0.24
Managerial	24	5.1	1.6	5.7	0.15
Clerk	38	6.5	2.2	6.5	0.00
Skilled	26	5.2	2.0	5.3	0.03
Unskilled	16	6.6	2.6	7.5	0.19
Domestic	19	3.3	0.9	3.5	0.08
Housewife	88	5.5	1.5	5.7	0.05
Total	321	5.4	1.6	5.8	0.09

I is not large for any group; that is, there are no very large positive or negative values. For only one subgroup, the 12–24 year olds, was *I* found to be negative—that is, with actual distance greater than hypothetical distance.

The distance factor was more important for inner-city and Garden City residents than it was for suburban and urban-fringe people. There were no differences by race or sex in the distance index. Among age groups, the oldest respondents held distance to be most important; the 25–44 age group considered it next in importance; 45–64 year olds were next; the youngest group considered distance least important. The clearest differences in concern about distance to health care appeared among the occupational subgroups. In order of the decreasing importance distance held for them were professionals, unskilled

Table 3: Relative-Distance Index for Regular Care for Sample Population Clusters

Cluster	*Index*	*Cluster*	*Index*
15-1	-0.11	38-1	0.26
15-2	0.13	38-2	0.31
18-1	0.34	40.01-1	0.20
18-2	0.15	40.01-2	0.34
28-1	0.12	106.01-1	0.43
28-2	0.25	106.01-2	0.02
36.01-1	-0.09	107-1	0.02
36.01-2	-0.08	107-2	0.01
36.02-1	-0.05	108.02-1	0.05
36.02-2	-0.20	108.02-2	0.14

workers, managers, domestics, housewives, skilled workers, and clerks.

The findings just discussed require further elaboration and explanation. For example, it is somewhat surprising, given their relative locations and different socioeconomic status, to find that blacks and whites had a similar relative-distance index. This result can be illuminated by examining the relative-distance index comparisons among individuals and among household-survey clusters.

As one would expect, there is a great deal of variation in the index among the 321 individuals who had a regular source of care. In fact, *I* for individuals ranged from -2.48 to 1.00. The individual with the largest negative index lived 11.5 miles from his regular source of care, but the closest available facility was only 2.2 miles away and the hypothetical distance was 4.9 miles. For the six people with an index of 1.00, actual and minimum distances were the same.

Sample clusters comprised perhaps the most interesting level of analysis for the distance index (Table 3). Differences were striking. The clusters for which distance was most important were, in decreasing order, whites in Garden City (106.01-1), blacks in inner-city cluster 18-1 and whites in suburban cluster 40.01–2, whites in suburban cluster 38-2, whites in suburban cluster 40.01-2, blacks in suburban cluster 38-1, and blacks in inner-city cluster 28-2. Distance was least important for whites in suburban cluster 36.02-2, whites in inner-city cluster 15-1, whites in suburban cluster 36.01-1, and blacks in suburban cluster 36.01-2.

The results discussed in the preceding two paragraphs indicate that individual differences and the location of a cluster of households may be more important in determining health-seeking behavior than such population characteristics as race. The next part of the analysis concentrates on sample clusters.

DISTANCE, ACTIVITY SPACES, AND POPULATION CHARACTERISTICS FOR CLUSTERS

Spearman's rank-order correlations were computed among the following variables for clusters: the distance index, actual distance to care, distance from home to center of care, distance from home to center of activity space, distance of care center to activity-space center, size of cluster activity space, percent white, percent male, and mean age (Table 4). The distance measures involving home, care centers, and activity-space centers are highly positively correlated with each other and also with actual distance and activity-space size. It is clear that people living farther from health care (and downtown Savannah) travel greater distances both to medical and nonmedical activities, the latter of which are more "spread out." The relative-distance index is negatively correlated with these five variables, but only significantly so with the actual-distance variable. This indicates strongly that distance is a relatively unimportant factor for those who live farther from care.

A look at the scattergrams that plotted relative-distance index against the four distance variables reveals that the negative relationships held up well only for the 14 inner-city and suburban clusters. Whites in Garden City were an anomaly, with a very high index; this cluster is an outlier on all of the scattergrams. The remaining five clusters, blacks in Garden City and the four urban fringe clusters, display a slight positive correlation between index and the four distance variables. Removal of the Garden City and urban fringe clusters improved the correlation between index and actual distance considerably ($rs = -0.685$, $p = 0.007$), but changed the other index-distance correlations very little. The plot of index versus activity-space size showed no clear negative linear trend.

At the cluster level of analysis, race (measured as percent white) shows a significant positive correlation with actual distance, distance from home to care, and distance from home to activity-space center. Sex (percent male) is positively correlated with distance from home to activity-space center, ellipse size, and race. It is very likely that these results are an artifact of the location of the survey respondents. There were relatively high proportions of blacks and females in the inner city and relatively high proportions of whites and males farther out. In other words, the race and sex associations with distance and the index

Table 4: Spearman's Correlation Coefficients among Relative-Distance Index, Activity Distances, and Population Variables by Sample Population Clusters (*p*-values)

Variable	*Actual Distance*	*Home-Health Distance*	*Home-Activity Distance*	*Activity-Health Distance*	*Activity Ellipse Size*	*Percent White*	*Percent Male*	*Mean Age*
Distance index	-0.465 (0.039)	-0.300 (0.198)	-0.245 (0.300)	-0.202 (0.394)	-0.278 (0.237)	-0.071 (0.767)	-0.414 (0.069)	+0.209 (0.378)
Actual distance		+0.917 (0.000)	+0.821 (0.000)	+0.770 (0.000)	+0.698 (0.001)	+0.441 (0.052)	+0.292 (0.221)	+0.082 (0.731)
Home-health distance			+0.869 (0.000)	+0.877 (0.000)	+0.769 (0.000)	+0.514 (0.020)	+0.303 (0.194)	+0.153 (0.520)
Home-activity distance				+0.622 (0.003)	+0.896 (0.000)	+0.637 (0.003)	+0.438 (0.053)	+0.148 (0.533)
Activity-health distance					+0.532 (0.016)	+0.416 (0.068)	+0.049 (0.837)	+0.041 (0.865)
Activity ellipse size						+0.692 (0.001)	+0.548 (0.012)	+0.061 (0.799)
Percent white							+0.499 (0.025)	-0.183 (0.439)
Percent male								-0.286 (0.222)

Table 5: Relative-Distance Index for Population Subgroups by Residence Zone

	Residence Zone							
	Inner City		*Suburban*		*Garden City*		*Urban Fringe*	
Subgroup	N	*Index*	N	*Index*	N	*Index*	N	*Index*
Race								
White	9	-0.11	100	0.10	12	0.43	52	0.02
Black	47	0.20	82	-0.03	15	0.02	4	0.14
Sex								
Male	18	0.15	83	-0.02	9	0.34	22	0.08
Female	38	0.17	99	0.12	18	0.15	34	0.01
Age								
12-24	8	0.30	45	-0.18	2	0.00	13	-0.03
25-44	17	0.17	52	0.14	7	0.08	21	0.13
45-64	19	0.08	59	0.09	8	0.26	19	0.01
65-84	12	0.18	26	0.34	10	0.32	3	-0.14

found here may be a result of location with respect to the downtown area. The next question to test, then, was this: Within each zone, what happened to the relative-distance index when compared across population subgroups?

Table 5 shows the results of attempts to answer that question. Findings are inconsistent probably because, for one thing, some subgroups held few individuals. For whites in the inner city, all nine of them from a well-to-do block, distance was less important than it was for blacks in the inner city. In Garden City and the suburbs, distance was less important for blacks than for whites. Only four blacks had a regular source of care in the urban fringe clusters; distance was more important for them than for whites. There was no difference in index between males and females in the inner city. In the suburbs, distance was more important for females than for males; the reverse was true in Garden City and rural areas. Age patterns show considerable variation among the four zones. Occupation groups by zone were too small for meaningful analysis.

DISCUSSION

Any study of health care-seeking behavior must focus on some factors and omit others. For example, little mention was made here of the *type* of resources used for regular care (e.g., hospitals, physicians, clinics). This was not a serious problem, however, in the Savannah, Georgia context, because 260 of the 321 sources of regular care (81.0 percent) were of one type—the offices of private physicians. Thirty-six sources (11.2 percent) were public clinics and 13 (4.0 percent) were hospital emergency rooms; the remaining 12 sources (3.7 percent) were reported as "other." An analysis could have been performed for physician's offices alone, but the numbers of other types of regular sources were too few to produce meaningful results. Concentration on distance and relative distance meant that other barriers to health care, such as social or psychological distance between providers and consumers, were not examined. Further, the Chatham County study dealt with the usual source of care rather than all sources contacted or the frequency of contacts made.

This research joins a group of studies that have shown distance to be an important factor in making contacts with health care resources, but only in relation to several other factors. In this study, distance—mainly through the use of a relative-distance index—was used as an exploratory tool to examine relationships among these factors.

In its agreement with other health care research (e.g., Weiss, Greenlick, and Jones 1971), the study of the location of most health care opportunities in Savannah goes a long way toward explaining the travel behavior of people seeking medical help. As in many cities, hospitals, clinics, and doctor's offices are concentrated in or near the downtown area. Unlike many cities, however, Savannah has few medical facilities in the suburbs. This configuration appears to have its advantages. Inner-city residents, usually poor and with less access to private transportation, are closer to potential sources of care. Distance should be comparatively important to them and, at least in travel to regular care, it is. Distance is of less importance to people living farther from the downtown areas, perhaps because they can more easily afford to travel. Further, it was mentioned earlier that the poor in inner-city areas might forgo intervening opportunities because of discrimination or inability to pay (Bashshur, Shannon, and Metzner 1971; Morrill, Earickson, and Rees 1970). That may still be the case in Savannah. The data show that inner-city people went relatively more often to clinics and hospitals than to private doctors. However, since all of the types of facilities are very close to the households of inner-city residents, the fact that they bypass intervening opportunities makes little difference in travel distance. On the other hand, if, as indicated, the more well-to-do residents living farther from downtown were bypassing relatively more of the intervening opportunities, it would seem that they often ignored possible suburban or urban-fringe facilities to concentrate instead on the cluster of downtown places. These findings corroborate those of McLafferty (1982), mentioned at the close of the introductory section of this article.

At least four other considerations affect our interpretation of the relative difficulty between Savannah's inner-city and suburban-urban fringe people in overcoming distance to care. The first is that, although inner-city residents had shorter *distances* to travel, they might have taken a relatively long *time* to reach health care. Shannon, Skinner, and Bashshur (1973) found this to be true for visits to physicians and dentists in Cleveland, Ohio. They found a negative association between travel distance and travel time which could have been due to type of transportation used, waiting time for public transportation, the route traveled, and other factors. The second consideration has to do with multi-purpose trips. Comparison of activity spaces and health care-seeking spaces indicated some correspondence between the two. Thus, if people were in or near the sources of health care when at work or shopping, they could fairly easily include a health care visit in their daily round of activities. Perhaps this worked to the advantage of the more mobile suburbanites. Third, people who had lived in an area for a short time might have preferred to visit a doctor or clinic closer to their previous residence (Phillips 1979). Although our data could not be used to examine this point thoroughly, comparisons were made between the distance index and the length of time people had lived in their current residence. No significant associations were found between length of residence and index for all individuals considered together, across the 20 clusters, or within the four residence zones. The fourth point is simply that Savannah is a relatively small city—in population and square miles—and Chatham County is a relatively small metropolitan area. Most of the other studies cited in this article were carried out in larger places. Distance probably would not be as important a factor for Chatham County residents (even those on the urban fringe) as it would be for those living in a larger place.

An interesting finding in this study is that, although blacks were closer than whites to regular sources of care, there were no racial differences in relative-distance index. There were also no sex differences. The fact that both races and sexes (the latter more than the former) were represented to some degree in all parts of Chatham County accounts in part for this. There were differences between whites and blacks, males and females, in the four residential zones, but they tended to balance each other out.

It is important to note that many other studies—that did find population subgroup differences in access to care (e.g., Bashshur, Shannon, and Metzner 1971; Morrill, Earickson, and Rees 1970)—

were carried out before the full impact of the Medicare and Medicaid legislation of the 1960s had been measured. Indeed, some of these studies were partly responsible for the legislation itself. Reforms in health care may account somewhat for the lack of differences found between races, sexes, and ages in relation to distance to care in Chatham County in the 1980s. The lack of racial differences in the relative-distance index could be explained, at least in part, if it could be shown that Savannah, a city in the southern United States, was less segregated than other places where racial differences have affected accessibility. The evidence is mixed: a study of New Orleans, for example, showed that black domestics were often found to live in the same blocks as the whites they worked for (Lewis 1976). On the other hand, indexes of residential segregation for 109 selected cities, 1940–1970, showed that the southern cities sampled had populations more segregated than those of nonsouthern cities (Yeates and Garner 1980).

Distance was of least importance to the youngest age group studied (ages 12–24), partly because younger people made up greater proportions of the suburban and urban-fringe populations. Within zones, the association between age and index was mixed. (It should be noted that the need for health care and the type of health care sought differ by age group. Young people, for example, might be more willing than others to override distance to reach the health services they require.)

Not too much can be concluded from this research about the importance of distance for people in various occupations; no clear trend was apparent from less- to more-skilled jobs. In sum, the Savannah study did not strongly corroborate those studies that have shown demographic and socioeconomic variables to be associated with distance to health care (e.g., Haynes and Bentham 1982). Our findings are more consonant with those of Dangschat, Friedrichs, and Kiehl (1982) who found that population characteristics did not influence activity-space variables. That is, individual differences appeared to override general sociodemographic group classifications in activities that included health-seeking behavior.

As expected from the work of Horton and Reynolds (1971), Wolpert (1965), Shannon and Spurlock (1976), Cromley and Shannon (1986), and others, it was important to consider the daily-activity spaces of people in relation to their health care travel. The distance people traveled to their daily activities, such as jobs and shopping, and the size of their activity spaces were both related to the distance they traveled to regular sources of health care. The downtown focus both of health care and of other activities and the greater effort made by people who lived farther from downtown to reach these areas were all of importance here. Shannon, Bashshur, and Spurlock (1978) showed that in Washington, D.C., health-search spaces and daily-activity spaces showed varying degrees of correspondence for different groups. In Chatham County, inner-city spaces coincided more closely than did those of people living farther out, but even the suburban and urban-fringe spaces had a relatively close correspondence.

CONCLUSION

The main purpose of this article was to reexamine, in a unique setting, several of the factors that have been found to be associated with consumer-provider interactions in other health care studies. These factors include distance and relative distance to health care, differences among population subgroups in access to care, the relative locations of people and their sources of health care, and people's activity spaces. Findings from an examination of the interaction of these factors for individuals and various groups of people (based on population characteristics and geographic location) reveal several implications for health care planning. First, distance alone may have an important influence on accessibility since different subgroups of the population live at different distances from sources of health care. However, if one measures the relative distance to care (the distance people actually travel for care in relation to distances to all of the care site choices), these differences may become altered (as they did between age groups in this study) or may disappear (as they did between blacks and whites). It is clear that the distance variable should be treated with caution because it can be measured and interpreted in many different ways.

Second, the location of health care sources relative to the people who use them is important. Most of Savannah's health care facilities (hospitals, clinics, and physicians) are located either in the central business district or in a cluster somewhat southeast of the CBD. This means that people who live a greater distance from the center of Savannah have to travel farther for care. However, the relative-distance index showed that distance was of less importance to those who lived farther out, quite possibly because they could more easily afford travel than could inner-city people—who were closer to sources of health care. The planning implication here is the importance of maintaining health care facilities at close proximity to those people for whom distance holds a relatively important disadvantage.

Our work found, third, that differences among population subgroups (by race, sex, age, occupation, and length of residence) in accessibility to health care as measured by relative distance were not as pronounced as those found in other studies. There were no race, sex, and length-of-residence differences; age and occupational differences followed no clear pattern. Clear patterns of population subgroup differences also were not found when residential location (inner city, suburbs, urban fringe, and industrial satellite) was controlled for. It was suggested that reforms in health care delivery might be partly responsible for this finding. Perhaps health care planners should focus less on population subgroup differences and more on other types of differences. For instance, the Savannah study found very large individual differences among members of various population subgroups. Significant differences were also found among the 20 survey clusters, suggesting that specific geographic locations are important in health care-seeking behavior. These results point to the need for health care studies to turn from an emphasis on investigating population aggregates toward more microlevel examinations of people's behavior and specific geographic locales within large areas.

A fourth implication of this study is that each urban setting has unique characteristics and health provision must thus be based on local situations. A basic property of Savannah's urban ecology is the strong focus on its downtown area; medical facilities and activities such as shopping are centered there. Savannah is also a relatively small city, which may make access to care somewhat easier than in other places and would tend to eliminate accessibility differentials among population subgroups. It is also possible that Savannah has a comparatively low level of segregation, thus reducing racial differences in access in particular.

Fifth, the Savannah study showed that knowledge about the daily-activity spaces of people provides a valuable indicator for examining health care-seeking behavior. The study revealed that Chatham County residents focus their trips to work, shopping, and other activities toward the same general area where health care facilities are located. If people tend to use health care facilities near the places where they work or shop, then their distance from home to health care is not a very good measure of accessibility. The activity spaces were larger for people who lived farther away from the city center, a circumstance that helped to overcome the friction of distance for them. Clearly, it is advantageous to site health care resources within or close to the orbits of people's daily rounds.

APPENDIX

RELATIVE-DISTANCE INDEX

Three distances were calculated for each individual who reported using a regular source of care: (1) the actual, Manhattan metric, distance from a person's residence to the facility used for care (called *a* for actual distance); (2) the distance to the closest care facility, out of all places used, from the person's residence (called *m* for minimum distance); and (3) the average distance from the person's residence to all facilities used (called *h* for hypothetical distance). An index, *I*, was calculated for each individual from the formula $I = 1 - [(a - m)/(h - m)]$.

Consider what different values of *I* would indicate. (1) If distance was a relatively important factor, then distance would be minimized and *a* would be as close to *m* as possible. If this were the case, *I* would be close to a value of 1. (2) If distance was a relatively unimportant factor, to the extent that *a* was larger than *h*, then *I* would be negative. (3) Between the extremes of (1) and (2) would be the case where *a* is close to *h*; here *I* would approach 0 and distance would be of medium importance.

The index can be modified slightly to allow for group comparisons. The values *d(a)*, *d(m)*, and *d(h)* replace *a*, *m*, and *h*; all represent the average of the respective distances for the subgroup in question. The index then becomes: $I = 1 - \{[d(a) - d(m)]/[d(h) - d(m)]\}$.

REFERENCES

Bashshur, R. L., G. W. Shannon, and C. A. Metzner. "Some Ecological Differentials in the Use of Medical Services." *Health Services Research* 6(Spring 1971):61–75.

Cromley, E., and G. W. Shannon. "Locating Ambulatory Medical Care Facilities for the Elderly." *Health Services Research* 21(October 1986):499–514.

Dangschat, W. D., J. Friedrichs, and K. Kiehl. "Action Spaces of Urban Residents in an Empirical Study in the Region of Hamburg." *Environment and Planning A* 14, no. 9(1982):1155–74.

Fuller, G. "On the Spatial Diffusion of Fertility Decline: The Distance-to-Clinic Variable in a Chilean Community." *Economic Geography* 50, no. 4(1974):324–32.

Girt, J. L. "Distance to General Medical Practice and its Effect on Revealed Ill-Health in a Rural Environment." *Canadian Geographer* 17, no. 2(1973):154–66.

Haynes, R. M., and C. G. Bentham. "The Effects of Accessibility on General Practitioner Consultations, Out-Patient Attendances and In-Patient Admissions in Norfolk, England." *Social Science and Medicine* 16, no. 5(1982):561-69.

Hightower, H. C. "Recreation Activity Analysis: Towards a Spatial and Aspatial Methodology for Urban Planning." Ph.D. diss., Department of City and Regional Planning, University of North Carolina, Chapel Hill, 1965.

Horton, F. E., and D. R. Reynolds. "Effects of Urban Spatial Structure on Individual Behavior." *Economic Geography* 47, no. 1(1971):36-48.

Joseph, A. E., and D. R. Phillips. *Accessibility and Utilization: Geographical Perspectives on Health Care Delivery.* New York: Harper & Row, 1984.

Lewis, P. F. "New Orleans—The Making of an Urban Landscape." In *Contemporary Metropolitan America, Vol. 2*, edited by J. S. Adams, 97-217. Cambridge, MA: Ballinger, 1976.

Mayer, J. D. "The Distance Behavior of Hospital Patients: A Disaggregated Analysis." *Social Science and Medicine* 17, no. 12 (1983):819-27.

McGuirk, M. A., and F. W. Porell. "Spatial Patterns of Hospital Utilization: The Impact of Distance and Time." *Inquiry* 21, no. 1(1984):84-95.

McLafferty, S. "Urban Structure and Geographical Access to Public Services." *Annals of the Association of American Geographers* 72, no. 3(1982):347-54.

Mering, O. V., G. W. Shannon, W. Deal, and P. Fischer. "A Long Day's Journey to Health Care." *Human Organization* 35, no. 4 (1976):381-89.

Morrill, R. L., and R. J. Earickson. "Variation in the Character and Use of Chicago Area Hospitals." *Health Services Research* 3, no. 2(1968):224-38.

Morrill, R. L., R. J. Earickson, and P. Rees. "Factors Influencing Distance Traveled to Hospitals." *Economic Geography* 46, no. 2(1970):161-71.

Phillips, D. R. "Spatial Variations in Attendance at General Practitioner Services." *Social Science and Medicine* 13, no. 3(1979):169-81.

Shannon, G. W., and C. W. Spurlock. "Urban Ecological Containers, Environmental Risk Cells, and the Use of Medical Services." *Economic Geography* 52, no. 2(1976):171-80.

Shannon, G. W., R. L. Bashshur, and C. A. Metzner. "The Concept of Distance as a Factor in Accessibility and Utilization of Health Care." *Medical Care Review* 26, no. 2 (1969):143-61.

Shannon, G. W., R. L. Bashshur, and C. W. Spurlock. "The Search for Medical Care: An Explanation of Urban Black Behavior." *International Journal of Health Services* 8, no. 3(1978):519-30.

Shannon, G. W., J. L. Skinner, and R. L. Bashshur. "Time and Distance: The Journey for Medical Care." *International Journal of Health Services* 3, no. 2(1973):237-44.

Weiss, J. E., M. R. Greenlick, and J. F. Jones. "Determinants of Medical Care Utilization: The Impact of Spatial Factors." *Inquiry* 8, no. 1 (1971):50-57.

Wolpert, J. "Behavioral Aspects of the Decision to Migrate." *Papers of the Regional Science Association* 15(1965):159-69.

Yeates, M., and B. Garner. *The North American City.* New York: Harper & Row, 1980.

Yuill, R. S. "The Standard Deviational Ellipse: An Updated Tool for Spatial Description." *Geografiska Annaler* 53B(1971):28-39.

Section Two

Modeling Health Care Use and System Performance

CHAPTER FIVE

Time-Series Regression in Quasi-Experimental Evaluation Design

There are many pitfalls to avoid in evaluating the effect of an intervention. Observed changes in the group receiving or exposed to the intervention may be due to historical trends, to random or periodic movement, or to selection bias—the experimental unit may have been improving without the intervention or may not be typical of the designated universe. Interventions designed to reduce infant mortality, for example, can be analyzed in time-series regression models corrected for autocorrelation, thus avoiding many of these problems. In the case of infant mortality, relatively accurate data exist over time, allowing the researcher insight into possible selection biases and into trends over time. Prior rates of infant mortality usually are excellent predictors of current rates; therefore, accurate models can be built.

However, the researcher, if restricted to a quasi-experimental design, as in this case, needs to establish control groups to ensure that other historical trends do not account for observed improvement. Since the Rural Infant Care Program was designed to be implemented in areas that had unusually high rates of infant mortality, but with the possibility of improvement in the medical treatment available for these newborns, great care was taken to set up comparison groups that would control for selection problems, historical trends, and the impact of other programs.

Time-series analyses were done in two ways: using linear (assuming constant arithmetic change) and log-linear (assuming a constant proportional change) dependent variables—infant mortality rates by year. A preintervention change in rates in 1970 was controlled for. Results are reported for each site. Unusual findings are examined in detail. The time-series regression models produce parameter estimates indicating that neonatal mortality rates were indeed reduced by the intervention. The authors thus conclude that, even without mitigating the poverty and isolation that define communities with high infant mortality rates, improvements to the medical care system can decrease infant mortality rates.

Reducing Infant Mortality in Rural America: Evaluation of the Rural Infant Care Program

Steven L. Gortmaker, Colleen J. G. Clark, Stanley N. Graven, Arthur M. Sobol, and Arline Geronimus

The Rural Infant Care Program (RICP), initiated in 1979, was developed to improve perinatal health care in ten rural sites with histories of high infant mortality rates. Time-series regression models indicate that neonatal mortality rates were reduced, following program initiation, by 2.6 per 1,000 live births (p = *.0002); black neonatal mortality rates were reduced by an estimated 4.5 per 1,000* (p = *.0004). Three sets of comparison areas exhibited no significant changes in rates. Postneonatal mortality rates did not increase in the target areas following initiation of RICP, indicating that deaths were not merely being postponed. Nine of ten individual sites showed reductions in infant mortality following program initiation. Birthweight-specific mortality data indicated that the decline was due mainly to reductions in neonatal mortality among low-birthweight infants. No reductions in the incidence of low birthweight were observed in the target areas. Substantial gaps in the delivery of prenatal care remained due to the continuing poverty of the population and the resultant lack of financial coverage for health services. We conclude that improved perinatal medical care can reduce infant mortality in poor rural areas to average levels experienced in the United States, and that the high rates still observed in some rural counties are unnecessary.*

Although infant mortality rates in the United States have been decreasing from year to year, this country still has higher rates than most other

---

Supported By Grant #05146 from the Robert Wood Johnson Foundation.

Address correspondence and requests for reprints to Steven Gortmaker, Ph.D., Associate Professor and Acting Chairman, Department of Behavioral Sciences, Harvard School of Public Health, 677 Huntington Avenue, Boston, MA 02115. Arthur M. Sobol, A.M. and Arline Geronimus, D.Sc. are from the Department of Behavioral Sciences, Harvard School of Public Health; Stanley N. Graven, M.D. is Professor and Chairman, Department of Community and Family Health, College of Public Health, University of South Florida; and Colleen J. G. Clark, M.P.H. is a Dr.P.H. student in the Division of Epidemiology, Columbia University School of Public Health.

industrialized nations [1]. Within the United States, rates experienced in some social groups and geographic areas are remarkably high [2–5]. During the period 1976–1980, 10 percent of all counties in the United States had infant mortality rates which were above 20.0 per 1,000 live births; 54 of these counties were significantly greater than 20.0 at $p < .05$ (see Figure 1). While these were generally rural counties, the cities of St. Louis, New Orleans, Baltimore, and Washington, DC were also included. This level of mortality is comparable to that reported for Costa Rica (20.2), Cuba (19.6), Poland (21.3), and Bulgaria (20.2) in 1980 [1].

This study describes the results of an experiment designed to reduce excess rates of infant mortality in ten rural areas of the United States. The Rural Infant Care Program (RICP), first announced by the Robert Wood Johnson Foundation in 1979, has been a cooperative effort among medical schools, state health departments, and local professionals in nine states.

One of the explanations for persistently high infant mortality rates in isolated rural areas of the United States focuses on the population characteristics of these counties. The argument is that infant mortality is high in poor, underinsured, isolated populations with low levels of education and inadequate housing, and that the persistence of high infant mortality rates in these areas can be attributed to the continuing poverty and isolation of the population. The implication of this argument is that only fundamental improvement in the local social and economic environment will reduce infant mortality rates. A different argument is that high levels of infant mortality are not due solely to characteristics of the population, but can be attributed as well to deficiencies in the medical care system.

The RICP was designed to test the efficacy of interventions which assumed that this second hypothesis was true. The RICP acknowledged that characteristics of the population increased their risk of infant mortality, but that ameliorating deficient social conditions would be an extremely difficult task. It assumed, however, that improvements in the perinatal system itself could be made more easily—and faster—and that these changes would reduce infant mortality even in the face of local poverty.

It was hypothesized that bringing together local providers and appropriate personnel from medical schools and state health departments would result in improvements in prenatal primary care, better identification of high-risk pregnancies, and increased referrals to tertiary centers, and that infant deaths could be prevented if the delivery of neonatal intensive care services to low-birthweight infants was improved. Numerous studies have documented the improved survival of very low birthweight infants born in tertiary centers [6–8]—hence the importance of regionalization of perinatal care [9, 10].

To evaluate the effects of the RICP, time-series of vital statistics data were examined before and after initiation of the interventions. Three different comparison areas were constructed as part of this evaluation. Time-series data from the comparison areas were used to control for alternative explanations that might account for the decreases in infant mortality observed in the target areas following program initiation.

An important alternative hypothesis to be tested was whether changes in infant mortality in the target areas were not the result of the RICP, but rather were due to general socioenvironmental changes, including the Improved Pregnancy Outcome (IPO) projects funded by the Office of Maternal and Child Health. These IPO programs carried out a wide variety of activities aimed at reducing infant mortality through improved regionalization of perinatal services, including strengthening central state administration of maternal and child health services, funding demonstration projects, promoting provider education, advancing regionalization of perinatal services, improving data/information systems, and developing advisory/advocacy groups. A number of these goals were also objectives of the RICP. IPO projects, however, were for the most part focused on statewide activities; much of the funding went to central state administration. Federal IPO funding totaled $50 million during the years 1976–1985 [11].

METHODS

SELECTION OF RURAL INFANT CARE PROGRAM SITES

Ten sites were targeted for programs receiving grants under the RICP. The sites consist of one or more counties lying within rural areas of nine states, and collectively average 23,000 births per year (see Figure 1). Twenty-six medical schools submitted preliminary proposals and 17 were site visited. The funded sites were selected by an advisory committee which considered extent of the need (i.e., excess infant mortality), project conception, and leadership commitment from the medical school. All sites had to have an infant mortality rate in 1977 above their respective state rate for that year, and a minimum of 1,000 births per year. In addition, all funded sites were located in states with IPO projects. Sociodemographic and health status characteristics of the tar-

Figure 1: RICP Target Counties (Shaded Black), and Other Counties of the United States (Slanted Lines) with Infant Mortality Rates Greater than 20 per 1,000 During 1976–1980 ($p < .05$)

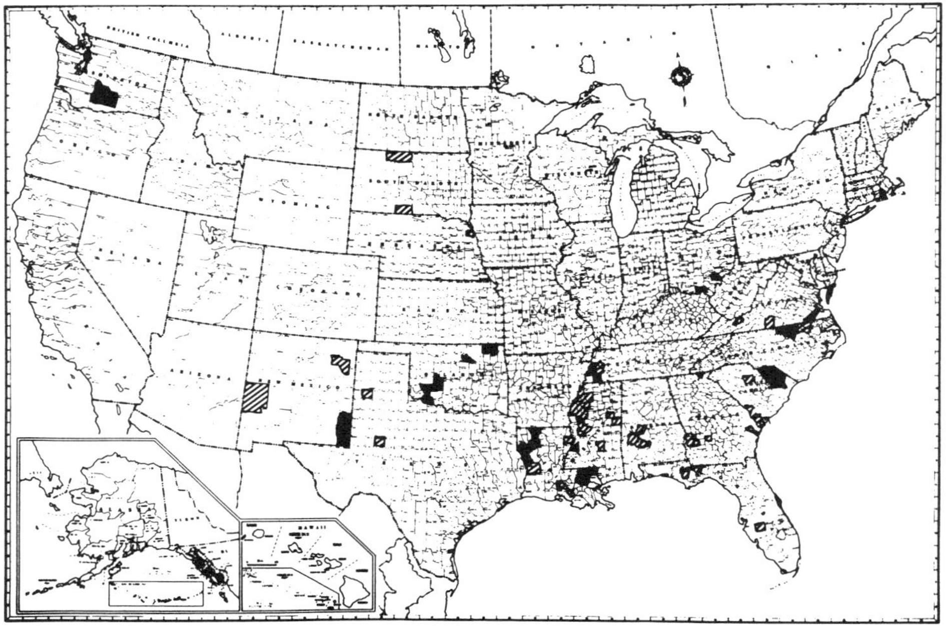

RICP Target Areas

Counties with Infant Mortality Rates Greater than 20 per 1,000 in 1976–1980

get areas are described in Table 1, along with data concerning three sets of comparison areas described below in the Evaluation Design section, and data for all rural and urban counties of the United States. The RICP target areas had infant mortality rates above national averages during the past two decades, had more than twice the percentage of black births when compared with other rural counties of the United States, and had substantially higher rates of poverty. An average of 50 percent of blacks were living in poverty in the target areas in 1980.

DESCRIPTION OF PROGRAM INTERVENTIONS

The RICP provided special funding and assistance to ten medical schools in an attempt to improve the delivery of health services to mothers and infants in the targeted rural areas. The projects were generally funded for four years, from about 1980 to 1984. Average funding was $700,000 per site for a four-year period; some sites spread the funds out over five years. Projects were organized by faculty at the participating medical schools. RICP funds were used to pay for support staff working in the target areas, faculty salaries, computing, administrative and secretarial services, and travel to and from the target areas. For the average site, about one-third of the RICP budget was used to pay for health personnel operating in the target areas. One-quarter of the typical RICP project budget paid for faculty salaries.

It is important to note that, in general, RICP funds were not used to pay for primary health services or hospital bills. The goal was to utilize existing resources as well as to develop new resources to pay for the delivery of health services to pregnant women and infants so that the projects could be sustained after funds from the Robert Wood Johnson Foundation were expended.

The ten sites focused on improving a wide range of perinatal services in the target areas. Typical activities undertaken within each site ranged from documentation of the community's infant mortality problem to specific plans for increasing access to prenatal care, improving transport of sick neonates, upgrading professional skills in isolated rural hospitals, and increasing referrals of high-risk pregnancies to tertiary centers. Because precise interventions were not specified in the program requirements, actions reflected local needs as well as resources and constraints, and varied among the ten sites. Data collected during yearly monitoring site visits show that activities in all the following areas occurred in all sites:

Problem Identification. Identification of excess levels of infant mortality was generally accomplished by the medical school project investi-

Table 1: Characteristics of RICP Target Counties, non-RICP Comparison IPO(76) and IPO(78) Matched Comparison Counties, and Other Rural and Urban Counties in the United States

Characteristics	*RICP Target Counties*	*Comp. Counties IPO(76)*	*Comp. Counties IPO(78)*	*Non-RICP Comp. Counties*	*Rural U.S. Counties*	*Urban U.S. Counties*
Number of counties	37	37	37	602	2,618	459
Births (average per year, 1971–1977)	21,590	19,457	12,781*	612,968	1,060,526	2,198,454
Mean infant mortality rate (per 1,000 live births)						
1966–1970	28.9	28.9	27.6	24.2	23.2	20.5
1956–1960	38.9	35.7	36.2	29.9	28.0	25.2
Infant mortality rate (1974–1978)						
White	17.2	16.2	17.8	13.8	14.0	13.0
Nonwhite	29.9	28.6	32.2	23.3	24.8	22.4
Overall	21.7	20.3	19.3	16.0	15.6	14.9
Percentage nonwhite births (1975–1978)	38.4	30.0	10.8*	17.5	15.3	20.6
Mean percent of families below poverty level, 1979						
Nonwhite	50.3	51.6	47.0	36.5	29.6	24.2
White	16.4	18.7	24.7*	15.4	15.7	7.8
Mean unemployment rate, persons 16 + years old (1979)	7.8	8.6	7.2	8.0	7.5	7.2
Percent designated as medically underserved areas, 1979 (all of county)	89	97	95	59	54	5
Number of pediatricians, OB/GYNs per 100,000 (1979)	4.6	6.1	4.7	8.5	4.9	19.7
Number of physicians per 100,000 population (1979)	63.0	63.5	59.5	81.2	68.2	164.2

*Difference between matched and target counties significant at $p < .05$.

gators during the application phase in 1979; continuing surveillance occurred throughout the project. A couple of target areas were altered by substituting one county for another because local health care providers expressed little interest in the problem or because infant mortality was not substantial. All other areas were kept intact, even in the face of hostility from local physicians.

Program Meetings in the Target Areas. These usually consisted of meetings with local physicians, hospital administrators, and public health department professionals. Participants included representatives from the medical school that organized the project, the state health department, and, periodically, from visiting members of the RICP advisory committee. Meetings in the target area began during the application phase (1979), and continued throughout the program. On average, more than one meeting per week took place in each site once funding began. The initial meetings were mostly informational; data indicating higher than average infant mortality rates had to be confirmed, and local resources and needs assessed. Important contacts, however, were often made at this stage, as local physicians gathered to discuss perinatal issues, including individual cases, and often for the first time met doctors from the tertiary centers.

A significant issue in target communities was the delivery of care to the indigent; state Medicaid guidelines vary widely among states, and other reimbursement policies (e.g., those covering handicapped children, neonatal intensive care, maternal and neonatal transport by ambulance or aircraft) were just as variable and complicated. In many target areas, substantial numbers of pregnant women had no financial coverage for services—these included members of families living in poverty that were not eligible for Medicaid benefits. In addition, local hospitals, clinics, welfare agencies, and other institutions all had past experiences and practices that needed to be understood, even if they were not agreed with. It was reiterated to the local physicians again and again that regionalization of perinatal care did not mean taking business away from local physicians; often, in fact, only very expensive cases were taken off the hands of local practitioners as more appropriate care was delivered at tertiary centers [9].

In some areas, members of the local medical community were quickly organized to assess the local situation and work toward solutions. Conversely, in other areas there were denials that any infant mortality problem existed. In these areas, a search usually ensued for professionals who expressed an interest in the problem.

Service Expansion in Target Areas. Nine of the ten sites expanded prenatal care services via clinics, which were usually located in public health departments. Some of these expanded services were paid via RICP funds, although most were paid from other sources. Three projects hired on-site health professionals, including nurses, certified nurse midwives, a pediatric nurse practitioner, and community coordinators for the delivery of perinatal services. Some sites hired nurses and physicians to staff clinics in a "circuit-riding" fashion. Other sites reallocated existing resources. Most sites developed high-risk obstetric and pediatric clinics. The high-risk obstetric clinics were developed to identify high-risk pregnancies (e.g., women with diabetes), so that they could be referred to specialty care when appropriate. A few sites expanded well-child clinics, and three sites began programs utilizing lay home visitors. All sites organized inservice training for staffs of the local target area hospitals; some hospitals were upgraded from Level I to Level II or II + [12]. In a number of sites, deliveries in some Level I hospitals were discouraged.

Development of Regionalization. Two different models of regionalization were developed: for those medical schools within commuting distance of the target area, emphasis was placed upon identification of high-risk pregnancies and maternal and neonatal transport to Level III centers [12], along with the upgrading of local hospitals. For sites at a considerable distance from a tertiary center, where delivery at the tertiary center was less feasible, the focus became the upgrading of local facilities and staff skills, with transports taking place when appropriate. The upgrading of staff skills at local hospitals included additional training in important areas such as resuscitation and stabilization of newborns.

Specific initiatives facilitated referrals to tertiary centers. One site had a residency program where local providers could work in the Level III NICU. In other sites, workable channels of communication between tertiary center and local health providers were established for the first time. The financial issues related to referrals were complex, and work was needed at a variety of levels to arrive at solutions.

Community Advisory Groups. These proved difficult to organize, although useful meetings took place between health professionals and community leaders.

EVALUATION DESIGN

The RICP was a quasi-experimental [13] demonstration project; the interventions were implemented within ten sites, and three sets of comparison areas were selected. The main goal of the RICP was to reduce infant mortality rates in the target counties, exceeding rate declines that would have been expected in the absence of the program. Vital statistics data were available to incorporate into an interrupted-time-series design with comparison series [13]. The assumption was that effectiveness of the RICP interventions would be reflected in a sharp and continuing change in vital statistics indicators in the target areas, and that no such change would be observed in the comparison series.

We followed this design using three comparison series to control for threats to the validity of our inferences concerning effectiveness of the RICP [13].

1. *The non-RICP comparison areas* consist of all counties which are not target areas in states with RICP programs. These areas were *not* chosen to be similar to the RICP target areas—in fact, they had infant mortality rates substantially lower than the target area rates before the interventions began. They included both urban and rural areas. These areas as an aggregate experienced rates of infant mortality which were "average," and which can be viewed as rates which the RICP target areas were aspiring to attain. The extent to which the RICP areas could lower their infant mortality rates to these average levels could be regarded as one criterion of success, because the target areas were initially defined by virtue of their excess levels of infant mortality relative to rates reported for their state. Furthermore, the non-RICP comparison series allowed us to test for the possible confounding influence of more general improvements in infant mortality taking place at the same time as the RICP interventions.

The other two sets of comparison areas were selected to be as similar as possible to the RICP target areas in their infant mortality experience, as well as with respect to other socioeconomic and health system characteristics. These comparison areas were selected to control for two types of possibly biasing influences. First, by selecting areas with similar past histories of elevated rates of infant mortality, we could control for any regression effects due to the selection of extreme values. These matched comparison areas also allowed us to estimate the effect of the RICP, controlling for the impact of the federal IPO program as well as for any other historical influences that might have worked to lower infant mortality in poor, rural areas during this time period. We expected that no significant changes would occur in mortality observed in these comparison time-series following either initiation of the IPO projects or initiation of the RICP.

2. *The second comparison series, IPO(76)*, consists of matched areas from states eligible to participate in the RICP which did not receive RICP grants, but which did receive IPO funds beginning in 1976.

(The states are Alabama, Arkansas, Mississippi, South Dakota, and West Virginia.) Empirical analyses indicated that an area's past history of infant mortality was the best predictor of future infant mortality; other sociodemographic data did not significantly add explanatory power. Thus, we relied upon past time-series of infant mortality rates (averages for 1956–1960, 1966–1970, and 1971–1975) in selecting matched comparisons using multivariate minimum-distance matching [14]. A computerized national data base of information at the county level was used to select the most closely matched areas.

3. *The third comparison series, IPO(78)*, consists of matched rural areas in states which received IPO funds beginning in 1978. These states are Kentucky, Missouri, and Texas. Average rates for the years 1956–1960, 1966–1970, 1971–1975 and 1973–1977 were used in the matching process.

Social, economic, and health characteristics of the comparison areas are displayed in Table 1. There were generally small and statistically insignificant differences between target and IPO(76) areas. The IPO(78) comparisons were collectively smaller in size, a smaller proportion of births were black, and a greater percentage of whites lived in poverty. These differences reflect the unusual nature of the target counties—few other U.S. areas were comparable in all respects.

DESCRIPTION OF DATA

Infant mortality and natality data include vital statistics from the National Center for Health Statistics (NCHS), state health department data tapes, and published and unpublished state vital statistics. Checks for consistency of NCHS and state data found no significant differences. Infant death and birth certificate data were available for all target areas for all years 1956–1984. Because almost all of the nonwhite births in the target areas were black, we refer to these infants as blacks.

Linked birth and death certificate data were available for six of the sites for 1976–1984 (76 percent of target-area births). Linked data for Louisiana were unavailable for 1980 and 1982, and were imputed based upon the remaining data (averages for the years 1979 and 1981 were used to replace the missing data for this state); separate analyses restricted to the complete data showed no substantial differences. Population data were from the 1980 U.S. Census, physician data came from American Medical Association files, and designations of medically underserved areas were obtained from the Bureau of Health Professions Area Resource File. An index of the adequacy of prenatal care was constructed, based on birth certificate data concerning the number and timing of prenatal visits and length of gestation [15, 16].

DATA ANALYSIS

Time-series regression models were fit; they assume that, in the absence of the RICP, the target areas would have experienced infant mortality rates during the years 1979–1982 which could be predicted based on their 1964–1978 experience. Because many of the series exhibited a change in trend or level in 1970, segmented regression models were specified [17]. Regression coefficients were estimated assuming first-order autocorrelated errors; this approach takes into account interdependencies observed between rates in adjacent years [18–19].

The regression models fit in Table 2 and Table 3 are of the form:

$$MR_t = a_0 + b_1 (YEAR) + b_2 (INT)(YEAR) + b_3 (INT) + b_4 (RICP) + e_t$$

where:

MR_t = a mortality rate during year t.
$YEAR$ = a linear trend term.
INT = 1 if $YEAR > 1970$; $INT = 0$ otherwise.
$RICP$ = 1 if $YEAR > 1978$; $RICP = 0$ otherwise.
a_0 = a constant.
b_i = regression coefficients.
e_t = an error term.

The regression models fitted in Tables 2 and 3 control for preintervention trends in mortality, and allow for preintervention changes in level and slope in 1970. The effect of the RICP was modeled as a change in level beginning in 1979; this fit better than modeling the effect as a change in slope in 1979. *t*-Tests were used to estimate statistical significance of coefficients; coefficients were dropped in a step-down manner if $p < .05$. Slope and level changes in 1970 were not required for models of neonatal mortality in non-RICP counties. R^2 statistics ranged from .95 to .99, indicating that the models fit the data well. The excellent fit of the models to the data indicated that regression to the mean cannot be considered a plausible explanation for the observed changes in infant mortality rates—the fit was simply too precise. Underlying binomial variation was assumed for the estimation of significance levels in Figure 1.

Log-linear models were also fitted to the time-series data by making the dependent variable in the models the natural logarithm of the

Table 2: Coefficient Estimates from Linear and Log-Linear Regression Models Predicting Neonatal and Postneonatal Mortality in RICP Target Counties 1964–1984

Target Area Outcome	*Linear Regression Coefficient Estimate/ Change in Level of Mortality per 1,000 live births**	p-*Value*	*First-Order Autocorrelation of Error Term*	R^2 *(Adjusted)*	*Transformed Log-Linear Coefficient Estimate/ Annual Percent Change in Mortality*	p-*Value*	*First-Order Autocorrelation of Error Term*	R^2 *(Adjusted)*
Neonatal mortality	-2.64	.0002	-.50	.99	-21.9%	.0001	-.54	.99
Postneonatal mortality	0.13	.8559	-.03	.95	1.4%	.8951	.01	.91
Nonwhite neonatal	-4.51	.0004	-.17	.97	-25.7%	.0002	-.12	.97
Nonwhite postneonatal mortality	0.38	.8146	-.23	.95	1.8%	.8743	-.32	.95

*The regression models controlled for a linear trend in mortality over time, a change in the level of mortality in 1970, and a change in the slope in 1970 in the target areas.

Table 3: Coefficient Estimates from Regression Models Predicting Infant Mortality in the RICP Target Areas, non-RICP Comparison Areas, IPO(76), and IPO(78) Comparison Areas, 1964–1968 (See Text for Discussion of Equation)

Area and Year Intervention is Assumed to Start	*Linear Regression Coefficient Estimate*	p-*Value*	*First-Order Autocorrelation of Error Term*	R^2 *(Adjusted)*	*Transformed Log-Linear Regression Estimate**	p-*Value*	*First-Order Autocorrelation of Error Term*	R^2 *(Adjusted)*
Target areas/1979	-2.73	.0014	-.51	.99	-14.8%	.0111	-.29	.99
Target areas/1980	-2.01	.0300	-.59	.97	-13.9%	.0111	-.58	.99
Non-RICP comparison areas/1979	0.09	.8707	.29	.99	-0.6%	.7941	.08	.99
IPO(76)								
Comparison area/1976	-0.68	.4033	-.44	.98	+ 1.9%	.6521	-.41	.98
IPO(78)								
Comparison area/1978	-0.99	.4946	-.18	.96	-7.1%	.3523	-.15	.95

*The regression estimates have been translated into estimated annual percent change in mortality rates: $100(e^B - 1)$.

mortality rate. The linear models assume a constant arithmetic change in mortality rates; the log-linear model assumes a constant proportional change; $100(e^b - 1)$ is an estimate of the percent change in the mortality rate [20]. The R^2 statistics from these models were quite similar to those from the linear models but, in general, fit the models of neonatal mortality a bit better, as evidenced by higher *t*-statistics.

RESULTS

Figures 2 and 3 are plots over time of neonatal and postneonatal mortality in the RICP target areas compared to the experience of non-RICP areas in the nine RICP states. These plots reveal a sharp drop in target-area neonatal mortality beginning in 1979, the year in which the program was announced, target areas defined, problems identified, and proposals submitted. (The 95 percent confidence interval around the 1979 rate is 9.3–11.9 per 1,000.) By 1982–1984, the neonatal rate in the target areas was very close to the non-RICP rate—the closest

Figure 2: Trends in Neonatal Mortality in the RICP Target Areas, Compared with non-RICP Areas During the Years 1964–1984

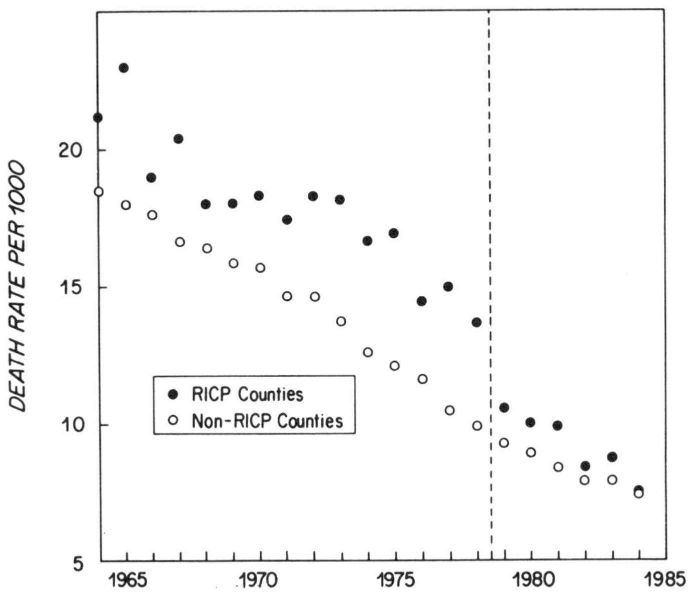

Figure 3: Trends in Postneonatal Mortality in the RICP Target Areas, Compared with non-RICP Areas During the Years 1964–1984

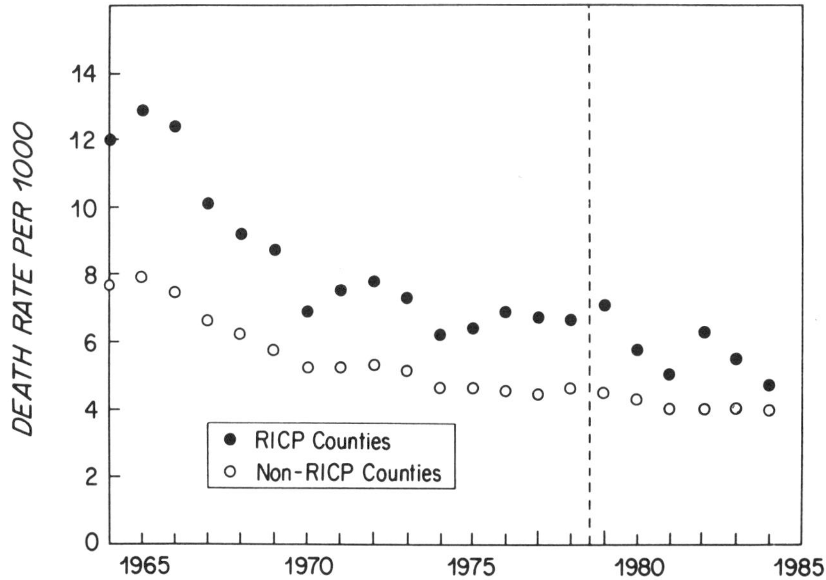

these rates had been in the past 18 years. The time-series regression models indicate (Table 2) a decline in neonatal mortality attributable to the RICP of 2.6 per 1,000 during the period 1979–1984 ($p = .0002$). Log-linear models indicate a decline of 22 percent ($p = .0001$). No statistically significant change in postneonatal mortality was associated with the RICP, indicating that neonatal deaths were not merely being postponed to the postneonatal period [21].

The estimated effects of the RICP were pronounced among black infants, who constitute 36 percent of all RICP births. Figure 4 describes changes in neonatal mortality among black births in the target areas compared to black births in non-RICP counties. Sharp decreases in neonatal mortality rates appear in 1979, and the rates then stay close to the non-RICP rates during 1979–1984. Time-series regression models indicate (Table 2) significant decreases among blacks in neonatal mortality—a decrease of 4.5 per 1,000 ($p = .0004$)—but not in postneonatal mortality, beginning in 1979. Log-linear models indicate a 25 percent decrease in black neonatal mortality ($p = .0002$).

Regression models fitted to overall infant mortality rates in the target areas (total neonatal and postneonatal mortality) indicate a statistically significant decrease of 2.7 per 1,000 ($p = .0014$) (Table 3), indicating that approximately 360 infant lives were saved during the period 1979–1984. Regression models fit to the black infant mortality rates indicate a decrease of 4.2 per 1,000 ($p = .02$). The log-linear regression models showed a 15 percent decrease in overall infant mortality ($p = .0011$) and a 17 percent decrease in black infant mortality ($p = .01$) following the intervention.

Time-series regression models were fit to mortality data from each site. Nine sites reduced infant mortality rates following initiation of the RICP; three of the reductions were statistically significant ($p < .05$), while the average reduction was 2.9 per 1,000. One site showed a significant rise in infant mortality. Eight sites demonstrated decreases in neonatal mortality, with four being statistically significant ($p < .05$). The average reduction in neonatal mortality was 3.1 per 1,000.

No Changes in Comparison Series

During this same time period, there was no evidence of similar sharp statewide reductions in infant mortality rates, that is, no statistically significant change observed in the non-RICP comparison series (see Table 3). Neither the IPO(76) nor the IPO(78) comparison series demonstrated a change in infant mortality following initiation of the IPO projects in 1976 and 1978. This evidence indicates little effect of the IPO projects in these poor rural areas, as well as no significant "regression to the mean" effect (Table 3).

The sharp reductions in target area rates that began in 1979 support the argument that the RICP was influencing mortality independently of IPO projects, since the IPO projects were initiated during the period 1976–1979. However, the decreases in infant mortality observed in the target areas could have been contingent upon previous IPO funding—in all RICP states, IPO projects began before the RICP (four of the IPO projects began in 1977, three in 1978, and two in 1979) [11]. Therefore, the changes in mortality observed in the RICP project area could be due in part to the influence of the IPO projects in these states. We have no way, however, of estimating simultaneously the effects of both the RICP and IPO in the target areas.

While these analyses do not indicate effects of the IPO projects in these states in changing mortality in the comparison areas, these findings should be recognized as very limited in their applicability to the entire IPO program, which operated in more states than those discussed here and included many more areas [22, 23].

Figure 4: Trends in Black Neonatal Mortality in the RICP Target Areas, Compared with non-RICP Areas During the Years 1964–1984

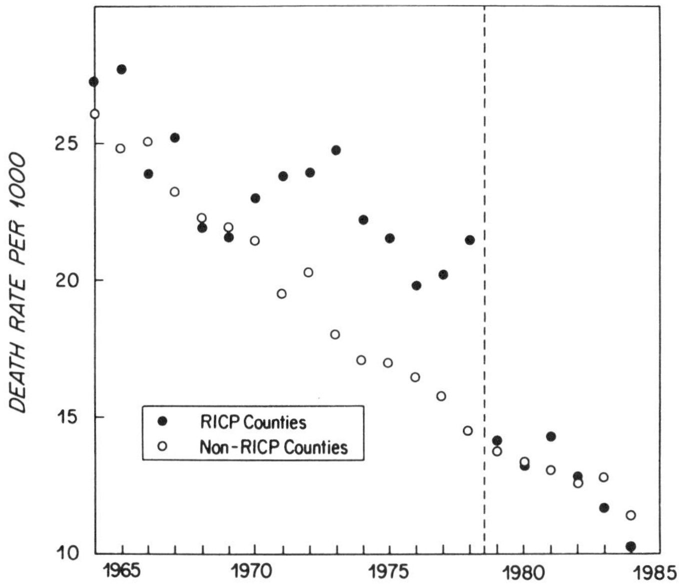

Changing Birthweight-Specific Mortality and Process Measures

Further insight into these infant mortality reductions was gained by examining linked birth and death certificate data from the six sites where data were available. These six sites accounted for 76 percent of RICP births and were generally representative of all the target areas. Five of the six demonstrated reductions in infant mortality—one experienced an increase. Of the sites effecting decreases in mortality, one was located at a considerable distance from a Level III tertiary center, and the rest were within commuting distance.

Data from these sites are displayed in Table 4. During 1976–1978, rates of neonatal mortality for births of less than 2,500 grams (LBW) in the target areas were substantially higher (by 14 percent) than the rate in non-RICP counties, but were virtually the same during 1979–1982. Similar comments apply to the rates of neonatal mortality among very low birthweight (VLBW) infants. Significant reductions in neonatal mortality among births of greater than 2,500 grams also occurred.

Table 4: Mortality and Process Measures in Six Rural Infant Care Sites with Linked Infant Birth and Death Certificate Data During Preintervention (1976–78) and Postintervention (1979–82) Periods

	*Six Target Areas**			*Non-RICP Comparison Areas*		
Indicator	*1976–78*	*1979–82*	*% Change*	*1976–78*	*1979–82*	*% Change*
Neonatal mortality (rate per 1000)	14.1	9.6	-32%	10.3	8.3	-19%
Neonatal mortality among <2500-gram births (per 1000)	116	84.1	-28%	99.7	83.0	-17%
Neonatal mortality among >2500-gram births (per 1000)	3.8	2.5	-34%	2.7	2.2	-19%
Neonatal mortality among <1500-gram births (per 1000)	517	384	-26%	463	387	-16%
Percent low birthweight	9.2	8.7	-5%	7.8	7.6	—
Percent very low birthweight	1.5	1.5	—	1.3	1.3	—
Percent of <1500-gram births born in Level III hospital	24%	42%	+43%	36%	47%	+23%
Percent of births with inadequate prenatal care	23%	18%	-22%	14%	10%	-29%
Number of births	49,307	68,997		867,953	1,270,708	

*Linked data are from Louisiana, Washington, Tennessee, North Carolina, and South Carolina. Target areas in these states account for 76 percent of RICP births.

However, because most neonatal deaths occur among LBW infants, reductions in mortality among LBW infants were responsible for most of the decrease in infant mortality in the target areas.

These changes in birthweight-specific mortality are probably the result of improvements in the delivery of services at all types of hospitals: this would include better maternal and neonatal transfers to Level III tertiary centers as well as improved practices at local target-area hospitals. The inservice training which took place at target-area hospitals included important topics such as resuscitation and stabilization: skill in these practices literally means life or death to newborns. We did not have data available on the interhospital transfer of newborns, and thus could not estimate how these practices may have improved following the RICP.

One indicator of the successful implementation of regionalized perinatal care is the percentage of very low birthweight infants from a given geographic area who are born in Level III hospitals [8]. As illustrated in Table 4, these percentages increased substantially in the target areas after initiation of the RICP. In 1976, only 18 percent of VLBW infants in the six target areas were born in tertiary centers, compared to a rate of 33 percent among non-RICP area residents in the same states. By 1982, the percent of target-area VLBW infants born in tertiary centers (51 percent) was similar to that found in the non-RICP areas (51 percent).

Data concerning neonatal transfers were not available on a systematic basis from the sites, although we have anecdotal evidence that better referrals of sick infants to the tertiary centers were taking place after the RICP was initiated.

Two RICP sites were located at considerable distances from Level III centers, and referrals were thus difficult. Both sites,however, demonstrated reductions in infant mortality ($p < .02$ and .08). Process data were available from one: while the percent of VLBW infants born in Level III centers did not change (the proportion remained at less than 10 percent), the percent of VLBW births taking place in Level I hospitals declined from more than 30 percent in 1978 to less than 10 percent in 1982.

The percentage of births with inadequate prenatal care decreased in the six target areas beginning in 1979. For each of the preintervention years, 1976–1978, the percent of target-area births with inadequate prenatal care was 23 percent. This was higher than the percent observed (15 percent) in the non-RICP areas during this same time period. The percentage of births with inadequate prenatal care decreased following initiation of the RICP, and averaged 18 percent over the period 1979–1982. However, a similar decrease occurred in the non-RICP areas, and hence the gap was not narrowed after initiation of the program.

The one site which did not effect decreases in infant mortality (a statistically significant increase occurred) also did not achieve gains in these other process and outcome measures. During the preintervention period, VLBW infants in this target area were born in Level III centers at a rate (47 percent) exceeding that for infants in non-RICP areas in the state (28 percent) and at a level far above that seen in other RICP sites. This site had thus already achieved some of the gains in infant survival associated with regionalization of perinatal services. Neonatal mortality among target area LBW infants was similar to levels in non-RICP counties both before and after the RICP was initiated. This site was also notable in that little contact with local physicians was sustained, and most project energy was focused on the computerization of health department patient data. It is also interesting to note that this site is located in the same state as another unsuccessful rural regionalized perinatal care program [24].

The incidence of LBW or VLBW infants did not decrease in any of the six sites during the period 1976–1982. The persistence of a higher than average rate of LBW infants in the sites represents an important issue to be addressed in the future.

DISCUSSION

HOW EFFECTIVE WAS THE RICP?

The Rural Infant Care Program focused on improving systems of perinatal care. A difficulty in interpreting the outcome data is that sharp changes in mortality first appeared in 1979—the year target areas were identified, but before funding from the Robert Wood Johnson Foundation was actually disbursed. Some facts concerning the timing of the RICP are clear: in 1978, the program did not exist and no associated activity was taking place in the sites. In 1979, a wide variety of activities were taking place within sites as target areas were identified, proposals were written, and preliminary agreements were made. Sites actually began receiving funds from the Robert Wood Johnson Foundation in 1980.

The changes in infant mortality observed in 1979 could conceivably be attributed to three different sources. The first of these is random variation: if the 1979 data are taken as a single postintervention data point, there is no statistically significant decrease in infant mortality when linear time-series regression models are fitted ($p = .10$). However, there is a statistically significant decrease ($p = .01$) when the better fitting log-linear models are estimated. Furthermore, decreases in infant mortality rates in 1979 occurred in six of the ten individual sites. Thus, the decrease in 1979 cannot be easily attributed to chance variation. It is important to note, however, that the 95 percent confidence interval around the 1979 percentage decrease is wide (3–20 percent).

The contribution of the RICP to 1979 declines in infant mortality becomes plausible when certain characteristics of the sites are recalled.

The target areas have small populations with an average of 2,200 births per year. In most sites only a few physicians are responsible for the delivery of obstetric and pediatric care. By targeting an area, with medical school and state health department representatives making visits to local health care providers, most of the local perinatal care system quickly became involved. We would argue that target area health care providers were the recipients of an intervention as soon as this communication and visitation commenced. The RICP program was formally announced in July 1979, and proposals which identified target areas were received from eight of the successful medical schools by October 1979. We believe the RICP began to have an effect during 1979, by initiating these actions.

To support this argument, we note that a critical variable in the recent nationwide reduction of infant mortality rates has been neonatal intensive care [6, 7]. In many of the target areas, good referral networks with tertiary centers did not exist prior to the RICP. These services could be immediately improved by face-to-face communication on a single visit between referring and tertiary physician during the grant application process. These initial contacts also placed community health professionals "under surveillance." Previous studies have noted rapid changes in practice following identification of local medical problems [25, 26].

A third argument concerning the decrease observed in 1979 is that the sites were selected to some extent because they already had part of the intervention in place. This argument would assert that the rather immediate effect of the program in 1979 should be attributed to the selection of relatively well organized sites for participation in the program. We have no way of knowing the relative contributions of the RICP versus this "selection process" to the decreases in infant mortality observed in 1979. However, one way to control for "selection" is to take 1980 as the starting date. The log-linear models reported in Table 3 indicate that if the starting date is assumed to be 1979, target-area infant mortality rates are reduced by 14.8 percent (p = .0011), after taking into account the preexisting downward trend in infant mortality rates. If 1980 is taken as the starting date, the percent reduction is an estimated 13.9 percent (p = .0011). Thus, substantial effects are noted even if we make these adjustments.

Regardless of the extent to which we attribute all or part of the observed reductions in infant mortality to the influence of the RICP, the data indicate quite clearly that infant mortality rates in poor, isolated rural areas with substantial minority populations can be changed to average levels experienced in the United States. Furthermore, these changes can be induced rather rapidly through changes in the delivery of health care.

GENERALIZABILITY OF RESULTS

To what other geographic areas can we generalize the results of the RICP? One valid way of generalizing the results of the intervention would be to apply them to other target areas selected in a manner similar to that employed by the RICP. States, for example, could make resources available to develop improved services in rural areas following a similar selection process. Sites would not be selected at random, but would be selected, instead, if a project with a reasonable chance of success was developed as a proposal. The results of the RICP evaluation thus indicate the sorts of changes in infant mortality that could be expected as outcomes in a similar program.

If random assignment of geographic areas to treatment and control areas had been employed with the RICP, we would expect smaller estimates of effectiveness than those estimated for the RICP, because presumably there would have been a substantial number of geographic areas where neither local providers, medical schools, nor state health departments were interested in the problem. If we would like to generalize the results of the RICP to this wider group of sites, we need to eliminate the "selection bias" that brought particular sites into the program. We have already discussed the selection issue and have found that controlling for these by assuming that the programs began in 1980 does produce a slightly smaller estimate of effect—the decreases in mortality, however, remain substantial and statistically significant.

IMPLICATIONS

This evaluation of the Rural Infant Care Program indicates that it is possible to identify rural areas with persistently high rates of infant mortality and to initiate programs that reduce it. The evidence presented here of effectiveness of the RICP points to the usefulness of targeted monitoring programs within states. State and local perinatal commissions, for example, can be organized with this purpose in mind.

The outcome data indicate that the RICP affected a wide variety of measures. Mortality rates experienced by LBW and VLBW infants were excessive in the target areas before the RICP began, and decreased to average levels following the intervention. There was also evidence for substantial increases in maternal transports and referrals to Level III tertiary centers from the rural target areas, as well as for more appropriate use of Level II hospitals. Improvements in the delivery of prenatal care also followed the introduction of the RICP, but similar magnitudes of change were observed in the non-RICP comparison areas. No changes were observed in rates of LBW or VLBW in the target areas.

This differential effectiveness was not unexpected: previous research has demonstrated the highly effective nature of technology developed to improve infant survival following birth, while evidence for the effective reduction of the incidence of low birthweight is much less impressive [27].

We were not able to collect data for a cost-benefit analysis in the present study; however, two recent studies—one in Rhode Island [28] and another in Ontario, Canada [29]—provide evidence of the positive cost benefit of providing neonatal intensive care to VLBW infants.

It is important to keep in mind that the RICP was not designed as a financing program. While some of the RICP funds were earmarked for service delivery, most effort was directed toward developing improved systems of care and finding other funding sources, so that improvements would persist beyond the end of RICP funding. In all the RICP target areas, the prevalent poverty of the population and the generally inadequate financial coverage of health services for pregnant women created continual crises in the delivery of care, even after the RICP was initiated. One locally successful financing program was developed in the New Mexico target area: county funds were used to pay for prenatal and hospital care of women not covered by other programs. This program was unusual, however, and to this day substantial gaps remain in the financial coverage of health care for pregnant women in the RICP target areas.

The successful implementation of programs like RICP requires current and accurate data. While designations of medically underserved areas are made regularly by the federal government, these designations are focused more on lack of health professionals, and less on mortality data [30] which, in any case, are always a few years old. In addition, certain important vital statistics data, such as linked birth certificate-death certificate data, are only available via states. State health departments typically note areas with higher than average levels of infant mortality, although these listings often involve only one year of data. More detailed designations currently appear as piecemeal research; Williams et al., for example [31], describe an approach to identifying areas of excessive perinatal mortality in California. State vital statistics systems could extend their data analysis beyond meeting reporting requirements and producing yearly reports.

Better documentation of geographic areas with persistently high infant mortality and inadequate regionalization of perinatal care, however, is only a first step. Resources are needed to deliver comprehensive prenatal services to all pregnant women, or identifiable high-risk pregnancies will be missed. Referral networks need to be established with tertiary centers, and inservice training should be provided where needed. The RICP demonstrated the value of local initiative in addressing these problems and showed that effective cooperation can be achieved among local physicians and nurses, hospital administrators, local health departments, state health departments, and tertiary hospitals. Even among extremely isolated and disadvantaged population groups, and in different geographic areas, important progress was made in combating infant mortality without waiting for improvements in underlying socioeconomic problems.

Significant health problems persist in these population groups, reflecting persistent economic difficulties in the target areas, including continuing gaps in the financing of health services. Postneonatal mortality has remained excessive, rates of low birthweight in the target areas are higher than average, and black infant mortality is still much higher than white infant mortality. Thus, as recently noted in a study of one urban area, the improved delivery of neonatal intensive care technology will not necessarily eliminate all disparities in infant mortality [32].

ACKNOWLEDGMENTS

The directors of all ten RICP sites provided invaluable assistance in obtaining data. These included: H. E. Thompson, M.D., Louisiana State University School of Medicine-Shreveport; H. W. K. Batson, M.D., Tulane University School of Medicine; L. R. Berger, M.D., M.P.H., University of New Mexico School of Medicine; F. Jelovsek, M.D., M.S., Duke University School of Medicine; R. W. O'Shaughnessy, M.D., Ohio State University College of Medicine; W. M. Crosby, M.D., University of Oklahoma College of Medicine; H. Heins, M.D., M.P.H., Medical University of South Carolina, College of Medicine; P. J. Sweeney, M.D., M.P.H., University of Tennessee Center for Health Sciences; R. L. Anderson, M.D., Eastern Virginia Medical Authority; and W. L. Shaul, M.D., University of Washington School of Medicine. Roger Banks helped immensely in gathering data. State health departments kindly provided access to birth certificate and death record information. Members of the Rural

Infant Care Program Advisory Committee offered much valuable advice: Kenneth G. Johnson, M.D. (Chairman), Solan Chao, M.D., Henry W. Foster, M.D., Maxine D. Hayes, M.D., Henry Heinz, M.D., Perry Henderson, M.D., Vince Hutchins, M.D., Richard D. Krugman, M.D., George Lythcott, M.D., Marie Meglen, M.S., C.N.M., Irwin R. Merkatz, M.D., William Moore, M.D., George E. Pickett, M.D., and George Ryan, M.D. The comments of numerous anonymous reviewers are appreciated.

REFERENCES

1. *Demographic Yearbook, 1983.* New York: United Nations, 1985.
2. Shapiro, S., E. R. Schlesinger, and R. E. L. Nesbitt, Jr. *Infant, Perinatal, Maternal and Childhood Mortality in the United States.* Cambridge, MA: Harvard University Press, 1968.
3. Gortmaker, S. L. Poverty and infant mortality in the United States. *American Sociological Review* 44:280–97, April 1979.
4. Kleinman, J. C., J. J. Feldman, and R. H. Mugge. Geographic variations in infant mortality. *Public Health Reports* 91(5):423–32, 1976.
5. Kleinman, J. C., and S. S. Kessel. The Recent Decline in Infant Mortality. In: *Health United States, 1980.* Department of Health and Human Services, National Center for Health Statistics, Washington, DC: Government Printing Office, 1980.
6. Lee, K. S., et al. Neonatal mortality: An analysis of the recent improvement in the United States. *American Journal of Public Health* 70:15–21, 1980.
7. Phillip, A. S., et al. Neonatal mortality risk for the eighties: The importance of birth weight/gestational age categories. *Pediatrics* 68:122–30, 1981.
8. Gortmaker, S. L., et al. The survival of very low-birth-weight infants by level of hospital of birth: A population study of perinatal systems in four states. *American Journal of Obstetrics and Gynecology* 152(4):517–24, 1985.
9. Merkatz, I. R., and J. G. Johnson. Regionalization of perinatal care for the United States. *Clinics in Perinatology* 3(2):271–76, September 1976.
10. McCormick, M. C., S. Shapiro, and B. H. Starfield. The regionalization of perinatal services: Summary evaluation of a national demonstration program. *Journal of the American Medical Association* 253(6):799–804, 1985.
11. Goldenberg, R. L., and J. Koski. The Improved Pregnancy Outcome Project: An Analysis of the Impact of a Federal Program on Infant Mortality. Department of Health and Human Services, Office of Maternal and Child Health, Washington, DC, 1984.
12. National Foundation Committee on Perinatal Health. *Toward Improving the Outcome of Pregnancy: Recommendations for the Regional Development of Maternal and Perinatal Health Services.* White Plains, NY: National Foundation-March of Dimes, 1976.

13. Campbell, D. T., and J. C. Stanley. *Experimental and Quasi-Experimental Designs for Research*. Chicago: Rand McNally and Company, 1971.
14. Anderson, S., et al. *Statistical Methods for Comparative Studies*. New York: John Wiley and Sons, 1980, pp. 99–102.
15. Institute of Medicine. *Infant Death: An Analysis by Maternal Risk and Health Care*. Washington, DC: National Academy of Sciences, 1973.
16. Gortmaker, S. L. The effects of prenatal care upon the health of the newborn. *American Journal of Public Health* 69:653–60, 1979.
17. Gillings, D., D. Makuc, and E. Siegel. Analysis of interrupted time series mortality trends: An example to evaluate regionalized perinatal care. *American Journal of Public Health* 71(1):38–46, January 1981.
18. *SAS/ETS User's Guide, 1982 Edition*. Cary, NC: SAS Institute, Inc., 1982.
19. Goldberger, A. S. *Econometric Theory*. New York: John Wiley and Sons, 1964.
20. Kleinman, J. C. State trends in infant mortality, 1968–84. *American Journal of Public Health* 76(6):681–87, 1986.
21. Hack, C. H., et al. Changing trends of neonatal and postneonatal deaths in very-low-birth-weight infants. *American Journal of Obstetrics and Gynecology* 137:797–800, 1980.
22. Strobino, D. M. (Editorial): Is it possible to evaluate the IPO Project? *American Journal of Public Health* 74(6):541–42, 1984.
23. Peoples, M. D., R. C. Grimson, and G. L. Daugherty. Evaluation of the effects of the North Carolina Improved Pregnancy Outcome Project: Implications for state-level decision-making. *American Journal of Public Health* 74(6):549–54, 1984.
24. Siegal, E., et al. A controlled evaluation of rural regionalized perinatal care: Impact on morbidity and mortality. *American Journal of Public Health* 75(3):246–53, 1985.
25. Dyck, F. J. Effect of surveillance on the number of hysterectomies in Saskatchewan. *New England Journal of Medicine* 296:1325, 1977.
26. Wennberg, J. E., et al. Changes in tonsillectomy rates associated with feedback and review. *Pediatrics* 59:821, 1979.
27. McCormick, M. C. The contribution of low birth weight to infant mortality and childhood morbidity. *New England Journal of Medicine* 312:82–90, 1985.
28. Walker, D. J. B., B. R. Vohr, and W. Oh. Economic analysis of regionalized neonatal care for very low-birth-weight infants in the state of Rhode Island. *Pediatrics* 76(1):69–74, 1985.
29. Boyle, M. H., et al. Economic evaluation of neonatal intensive care of very-low-birth-weight infants. *New England Journal of Medicine* 308: 1330–37, 1984.
30. Lee, R. C. Designation of health manpower shortage areas for use by public health service programs. *Public Health Reports* 94(1):48–59, 1979.
31. Williams, R. L., et al. Monitoring perinatal mortality rates: California, 1970 to 1976. *American Journal of Obstetrics and Gynecology* 136(5):559–68, 1980.
32. Wise, P. H., et al. Racial and socioeconomic disparities in childhood mortality in Boston. *New England Journal of Medicine* 313:360–66, 1985.

CHAPTER SIX

Structural Equations and Path Analysis Approaches to Analytical Model Building

Certain behavioral dimensions such as stress or social support, which play a major role in either health behavior or occupational behavior, present large difficulties for the health services researcher. While many different items and scales are extant in the literature for measuring these variables, there is no consensus on which is "the best"; indeed, measures may differ depending on the hypotheses being investigated.

Building models to represent complex interactions is the business of quantitative health services research. Often the models employed are implicit, represented only by the choice of variables. The model is assumed to "fit" the situation. In the next article, Pamela Toft and James Anderson have explicitly defined and tested a model to explain nurse satisfaction and absenteeism. They carefully distinguish between exogenous and endogenous variables, describe scale derivations where applicable and, with structural equation modeling techniques using a sample of nurses and hospital units, estimate the parameters of a path-analytic model.

In order to validate the model, the authors designed an intervention to affect role conflict, role ambiguity, and stress. After implementation, they readministered relevant instruments. They then looked at changes in the coefficients representing direct and indirect effects, finding reduced absenteeism and apportioning the causation to endogenous variables. The authors also report on their use of computer simulations to estimate the impact of different changes. The tables used to present their results are complete and relatively easy to interpret. The model presented in this article builds on earlier behavioral and organizational research; it is to be hoped that future research will incorporate its findings.

Organizational Stress in the Hospital: Development of a Model for Diagnosis and Prediction

Pamela A. Toft and James G. Anderson

A model of organizational stress in the hospital was developed and tested. The model utilized measures of organizational climate, supervisory practices, and work group relations as predictors of the amount of role conflict and ambiguity that nurses perceived in providing patient care. Role conflict and ambiguity were treated as variables that intervene between organizational variables and the level of stress that the nursing staff experienced. Nursing stress was viewed as a direct cause of job dissatisfaction and as an indirect cause of absenteeism among the nursing staff. Data from 158 registered nurses, licensed practical nurses, and nursing assistants on seven nursing units in a 1,160-bed private teaching hospital were used to estimate the parameters of a structural equation model. The model was used to predict the results of a survey feedback project designed to change the supervisory style used on the units. Pre- and posttest data from four surgical units were used to validate the model. The findings suggest that, as predicted, supervisory practices that led to more open expression of views and joint problem solving resulted in reduced role conflict, ambiguity, and stress; increased job satisfaction; and lower levels of absenteeism among the nursing staff.

INTRODUCTION

Results from an earlier study of the causes and effects of nursing stress suggest that factors inherent in the nursing role that result in role conflict and ambiguity are important determinants of stress [1]. This article extends the earlier model of stress to explicitly include role

---

Pamela A. Toft, Ph.D. is Senior Vice President, Division of Human Resources, Organization Development and Customer Services, Methodist Hospital of Indiana, Inc., 1701 N. Senate Boulevard, P.O. Box 1367, Indianapolis, IN 46206. James G. Anderson, Ph.D. is Professor of Sociology, Department of Sociology and Anthropology, Purdue University, and is affiliated with the Division of Academic Affairs, Methodist Hospital of Indiana, Inc. Address correspondence and requests for reprints to Dr. Toft.

conflict and ambiguity and their organizational determinants—organizational climate, supervisory style, and work group relations [2–4].

Role perceptions, specifically, role conflict and ambiguity, are introduced as variables that intervene between organizational variables and the level of stress that the nursing staff experiences in providing patient care [5–7]. Nursing stress is viewed as a direct cause of job dissatisfaction and as an indirect cause of absenteeism among the nursing staff [8]. This expanded model is depicted in Figure 1. Theory and research that support the hypothesized causal relations among the variables are discussed in the next section.

A structural equation model was constructed from questionnaire data obtained from the nursing staff as part of an organizational development program in a large private community teaching hospital. Computer simulation experiments were performed with this model to predict the probable outcome of feedback sessions on three experimental units. This program was designed to change the supervisory style used on the units. The actual model and the empirical results of the simulation experiments are presented in the results section. Finally, pre- and posttest data from three experimental and one control hospital unit are used to validate the model.

A Hypothetical Model of Organizational Stress

Research based largely on Likert's model of human organizations [9] suggests several important social-psychological factors that characterize the influence process in multilevel institutions such as hospitals—namely, organizational climate, supervisory style, and work group relations. Empirical studies based on longitudinal data support the causal sequence shown among these variables in Figure 1 [3–4].

ORGANIZATIONAL CLIMATE

Organizational climate refers to conditions created for work groups by others higher up in the organizational hierarchy. These conditions provide the environment in which work groups operate. Organizational climate determines to a substantial degree the leadership behavior of work group supervisors [3–4]. For example, an organizational climate characterized by a deemphasis on hierarchy, conflict resolution

Figure 1: Model of Organizational Stress in the Hospital

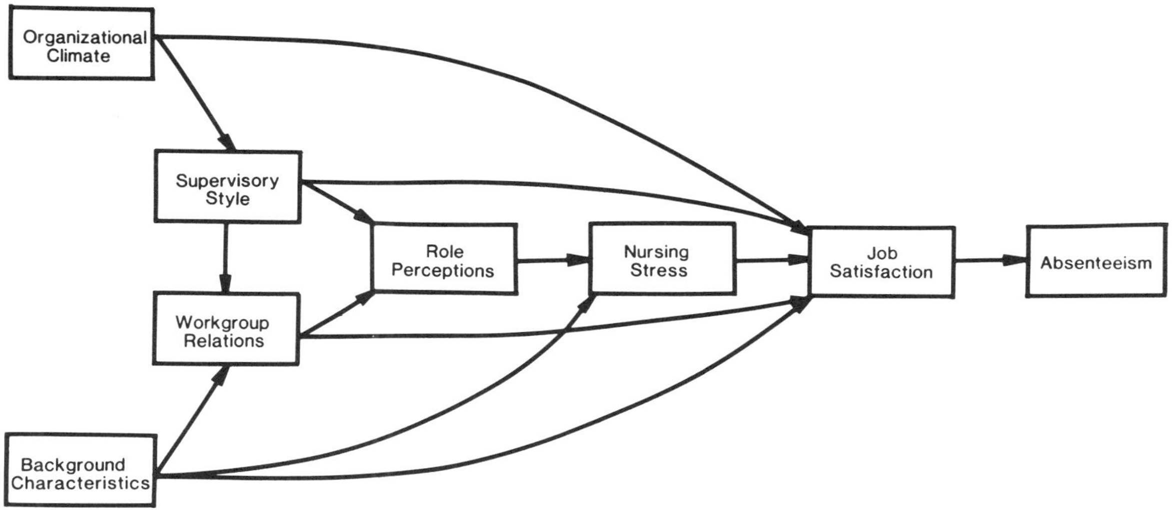

through direct confrontation, joint problem solving, and open communication results in an open supervisory style [10].

The organizational climate also directly affects staff role perceptions and job satisfaction [11]. For example, a number of studies have indicated that when nursing staff perceive conflicts between the two lines of authority that make up the organizational structure of the hospital, they experience role conflict and ambiguity [12–15] as well as job dissatisfaction [16].

SUPERVISORY STYLE

Research suggests that the behavior of supervisors has important effects on work group relations as well as on subordinate motivation, satisfaction, and performance. Bowers and Seashore's study [17] found that the best predictor of peer support, goal emphasis, and work facilitation was the corresponding behavior of the group's supervisor. Oaklander and Fleishman [18] came to a similar conclusion regarding the effects of supervision on work group relations in a study of 118 supervisors in three hospitals. They found significantly less interpersonal conflict and hostility and fewer noncooperative relationships among nursing personnel in groups where the supervisor allowed subordinates greater participation in decision making and encouraged two-way communication.

Further, evidence from a number of studies indicates that supervisory behavior, such as assigning tasks, specifying procedures, and clarifying expectations, creates a structure for subordinates that results in a reduction in role ambiguity and an increase in job satisfaction among high occupational level employees [6, 19, 20]. At the same time, behavior that creates a supportive work environment has been found to be associated consistently with high levels of subordinate satisfaction and performance [7, 21]. Such an environment involves support, openness, trust, friendliness, and advance notice of organizational changes that affect subordinates.

WORK GROUP RELATIONS

Most of the actual tasks performed by the nursing staff in providing patient care are part of a team effort. In part, this reflects increased technological sophistication and specialization [15, 22]; in part, it represents institutionalized defenses against the stress and anxiety resulting from frequent staff exposure to life-threatening situations requiring fast, appropriate decisions [1, 23]. Consequently, the model hypothesizes that nursing staff who perceive their work group as open, supportive, cohesive, and able to resolve conflict satisfactorily, will experience less role conflict and ambiguity and will be more satisfied with their work.

ROLE PERCEPTIONS

Role conflict arises from different expectations regarding an individual's behavior, whereas role ambiguity occurs when an individual is unclear about what is expected of him/her and unsure of the responses to his/her behavior. Role theory predicts (and studies in many types of complex organizations confirm) that role conflict and ambiguity result in stress, job dissatisfaction, and decreased levels of performance [1, 5, 6, 7, 24]. Consequently, the model hypothesizes that role conflict and role ambiguity affect job satisfaction directly as well as indirectly by resulting in increased stress among the nursing staff [25, 26].

NURSING STRESS

The model predicts that staff who frequently experience stressful situations in the performance of their nursing duties will be the most dissatisfied with their work. This relationship has been demonstrated with data from a national survey of large scale organizations [5] as well as from the results of a study of nursing units in a large private teaching hospital [1, 27].

JOB SATISFACTION AND ABSENTEEISM

Virtually all major reviews of the literature have found a consistent, significant relationship between job dissatisfaction and absenteeism [8]. Consequently, the model postulates that absenteeism will result when high levels of job dissatisfaction exist among the staff.

BACKGROUND CHARACTERISTICS

A number of characteristics of individuals have been found to be related to stress. A study by Gray-Toft and Anderson [1] found that registered nurses experience significantly more stress than licensed practical nurses and nursing assistants due to differences in the roles that they perform. Consequently, the model postulates that RNs will experience the most role conflict, ambiguity, and stress—NAs the least.

Personality characteristics have also been found to account for differences among the individuals in the amount of role conflict, role ambiguity, and stress they experience in organizations [1, 5]. Consequently, the model hypothesizes that staff members with high levels of trait anxiety will experience more role conflict, ambiguity, and stress in performing their duties.

METHODOLOGY

DATA COLLECTION

Several instruments were developed to measure the variables that comprise the model. These are described below.

Organizational Questionnaire

An organizational questionnaire modeled after the Michigan Organizational Assessment Questionnaire [28] was developed to measure staff perceptions of organizational climate, supervisory style, work group relations, role conflict and ambiguity, job satisfaction, and background characteristics. The majority of the items were based on information obtained through interviews with vice-presidents, clinical directors of nursing, supervisors, and staff on seven nursing units, although some items from the Michigan instrument were used as well. The questionnaire was modular and scales were derived from separate factor analyses of sets of items designed to measure each of the constructs included in the model. The number of items that make up each scale, sample items, and reliability coefficients are shown in Table 1.

Job Description Index

An additional measure of job satisfaction was used to validate the model's predictions. The Job Description Index [29] provides five subscales that measure satisfaction with different aspects of the work environment. The satisfaction with supervision subscale was used for this study.

Nursing Stress Scale

An expanded version of the Nursing Stress Scale developed by Gray-Toft and Anderson [30] was used to measure stress. The scale consisted of 46 nursing situations that commonly occur in hospital units. Staff were asked to indicate on a four-point scale how frequently they found each situation stressful. Factor analysis was used to create eight subscales as well as a total stress score which was used in this analysis.

Table 1: Scales with Sample Items and Reliability Coefficients

Scale	Number of Items	Reliability Coefficient*
Organizational Climate—Hospital Administration	7	.78
Indicate the extent to which you feel the following statements are true of the hospital as a place to work:		
613 Differences and disagreement between units or departments are accepted and worked through		
619 Hospital Administration has clear-cut goals and objectives		
Organizational Climate—Communication	6	.78
617 When decisions are being made, the persons affected are asked for their ideas		
618 I am able to challenge a decision of my immediate supervisor		
Supervisory Style	3	.91
Indicate whether you agree or disagree with each of the statements as a description of your direct supervisor.		
412 Is willing to listen and consider my ideas		
416 Makes sure subordinates have clear goals to achieve		
417 Is available when I need him/her		
433 Maintains high standards of performance		
Work Group Relations	10	.89
How much do you agree or disagree with each statement about your work group? In general . . .		
312 Conflicts are brought out into the open in my work group		
313 I can find support in my work group when I am under stress		
317 If we have a decision to make, everyone is involved in making it		
Role Conflict	4	.71
How much do you agree or disagree with each statement as a description of your job?		
115 On my job I can't satisfy everybody at the same time		
123 I have so much work that I can't do everything well		
Role Ambiguity	5	.64
119 I seldom know whether I'm doing my job well or poorly		
120 On my job I do not know exactly what is expected of me		

Continued

Table 1: Continued

Scale	*Number of Items*	*Reliability Coefficient**
Nursing Stress Scale	46	.92
Indicate how often each situation is stressful for you:		
10 The death of a patient, including suicide		
11 Conflict with a physician		
27 Feeling inadequately prepared to help with the emotional needs of a patient		
Job Satisfaction—Extrinsic Satisfaction	3	.71
Indicate how satisfied you are with each of the following aspects of your job:		
224 The fringe benefits you receive		
231 The amount of pay you get		
Job Satisfaction—Intrinsic Satisfaction	7	.83
225 The friendliness and supportiveness of the people you work with		
230 The opportunity you have to help people		
232 The opportunity you have to take part in making decisions		
Job Satisfaction—Supervision	18	.67
Place a "Y" beside an item if the item describes your job; an "N" if it does not; a "?" if you cannot decide. My supervisor:		
– Asks my advice		
– Hard to please		
– Tells me where I stand		
Absenteeism	1	–
The number of times a staff member was absent from work during a 9-month period divided by 9		
Training	1	–
This variable was coded as follows:		
3 – Nursing Assistant		
4 – Licensed Practical Nurse		
5 – Registered Nurse		
IPAT Anxiety Scale	40	.92
Total Raw Score		

*Coefficient Alpha.

Sample items as well as a reliability coefficient for the total scale are shown in Table 1.

Institute for Personality and Ability Testing (IPAT) Anxiety Scale

The IPAT Anxiety Scale was used to measure trait anxiety [31]. This instrument consists of 40 questionnaire items.

Absenteeism

Absenteeism was obtained from nursing administration records. Since the records do not include detailed reasons for an absence, the measures used to test the model include all absences from work for any reason, including sickness, personal reasons, and unexcused absences.

SAMPLE

These instruments were administered to the two clinical directors of nursing and to all supervisors and full-time nursing staff on four surgical units and three psychiatric units in a 1,160-bed private teaching hospital in the Midwest. Clinical directors and unit supervisors were excluded from this analysis so that the model could include a measure of staff perceptions of supervisory behavior. Unit secretaries, too, were excluded, because this group of employees is not responsible for direct patient care and many of the items on the Nursing Stress Scale were thus inappropriate. The final sample used to estimate the parameters of the model shown in Figure 1 consisted of 159 registered nurses, licensed practical nurses, and nursing assistants.

MULTIVARIATE ANALYSIS

A structural equation model was constructed to examine the hypotheses concerning the causes and effects of organizational stress [32]. Hypothesized relationships are represented by arrows linking groups of variables in Figure 1. The organizational climate variables and background characteristics at the left of the diagram are considered to be exogenous since they are relatively enduring characteristics of the organization and of individual staff members, even though they may change over longer periods of time. Anxiety is considered to be largely a trait measure and, thus, exogenous. All of the other variables in the model are considered to be endogenous, jointly dependent upon one another and on the exogenous variables, and subject to short-term change.

Table 2: Intercorrelations, Means, and Standard Deviations (N = 158)

	Administration	*Communication*	*Training*	*Anxiety Score*	*Supervisory Style*
Hospital administration		0.63	-0.23	-0.07	0.21
Communication			-0.03	0.05	0.33
Training				-0.05	-0.01
Anxiety score					-0.03
Supervisory style					
Workgroup relations					
Role conflict					
Role ambiguity					
Nursing stress					
Extrinsic satisfaction					
Intrinsic satisfaction					
Mean	2.80	2.53	5.13	27.79	3.51
Standard deviation	0.57	0.64	0.85	11.86	0.56

The model is recursive; consequently, the regression coefficients of the structural equations were estimated by ordinary least squares. The intercorrelation matrix for the variables included in the model is shown in Table 2. Standardized partial regression and multiple correlation coefficients are presented in Table 3. All coefficients were significant at the .05 level or above. The effects of model variables are decomposed into their direct and indirect components in Table 4 [33].

A number of computer simulation experiments were performed with the model [34]. These experiments were used to predict the outcome of survey feedback sessions [35] with the nursing staff of three surgical units. These sessions were designed to change the behavior of nursing supervisors in order to permit greater staff participation in decision making.

Table 2: Continued

Workgroup Relations	*Role Conflict*	*Role Ambiguity*	*Nursing Stress*	*Extrinsic Satisfaction*	*Intrinsic Satisfaction*	*Absenteeism*
0.14	-0.25	-0.24	-0.19	0.21	0.31	0.07
0.28	-0.16	-0.26	-0.13	0.26	0.51	-0.03
-0.13	0.23	0.20	0.38	0.18	0.12	-0.15
-0.02	0.20	0.15	0.32	-0.12	-0.13	0.04
0.64	-0.09	-0.36	-0.15	0.22	0.52	-0.13
	-0.14	-0.39	-0.13	0.12	0.49	-0.18
		0.34	0.34	-0.19	-0.26	0.04
			0.36	-0.06	-0.40	0.03
				-0.15	-0.26	0.03
					0.50	-0.09
						-0.09
3.13	3.03	2.50	0.96	3.31	3.42	4.19
0.65	0.68	0.57	0.33	0.74	0.63	4.24

VALIDATION OF THE MODEL

To validate the model's predictions, three surgical units were selected as experimental units and one unit as a control. Nursing supervisors on the experimental units were provided with comparisons of their self-ratings and staff ratings concerning their style of supervision. Feedback sessions were also held with the supervisor and staff of each shift to discuss the survey findings and problems that they wished to address.

At the conclusion of these sessions, several of the instruments used to measure work group relations, role conflict and ambiguity, nursing stress, and satisfaction with supervision were readministered to staff on the experimental and control units. In addition, nursing administration records were used to compute individual absentee rates for 9 months previous to the project and for 9 months after the feedback sessions had been discontinued.

Table 3: Structural Equations for the Model of Organizational Stress Standardized Regression and Multiple Correlation Coefficients

	Predetermined Variables			
	Organizational Climate		*Background Characteristics*	
Dependent Variable	*Administration*	*Communication*	*Training*	*Anxiety Score*
Supervisory style		0.335		
Workgroup relations			-0.125	
Role conflict	-0.194		0.194	0.194
Role ambiguity		-0.151	0.176	0.158
Nursing stress			0.320	0.274
Extrinsic satisfaction		0.216	0.291	
Intrinsic satisfaction		0.329	0.277	
Absenteeism				

FINDINGS

Results of this study confirm the findings of other studies that suggest that role conflict, role ambiguity, and stress are inherent in the nursing role [1, 12, 36, 37]. Table 4 indicates that level of training, and consequent responsibility for patient care, is a significant determinant of each of these variables which directly affect job satisfaction and indirectly affect absenteeism. At the same time, the findings suggest that one of the major psychological functions that organizational practices, supervision, and work groups perform in hospitals is the reduction of role conflict, role ambiguity, and stress.

The model indicates that administrative efforts to establish goals, to plan and coordinate, and to resolve interdepartmental conflicts result in increased job satisfaction and reduced absenteeism primarily by reducing the level of role conflict that staff experience. The Hospital Administration variable has a direct, negative effect on role conflict in

Table 3: Continued

Endogenous Variables							
		Role Perceptions			*Job Satisfaction*		*Multiple Correlation Coefficient*
Supervisory Style	*Workgroup Relations*	*Conflict*	*Ambiguity*	*Nursing Stress*	*Extrinsic*	*Intrinsic*	
							0.335
0.636							0.649
							0.363
-0.163	-0.218						0.492
		0.146	0.206				0.577
		-0.162		-0.181			0.409
0.199	0.260	-0.138		-0.214			0.724
					-0.054	-0.067	0.105

Table 4. House and Rizzo [7] found that similar practices in a manufacturing company led to a reduction in role ambiguity. These different results suggest that the effect of organizational practices may be somewhat dependent upon the nature of the work and the type of employee. In organizations where much of the work is carried out by professionals and is of a nonroutine nature, traditional management functions such as goal setting, planning, and coordinating may lead to a reduction in conflict by clarifying jurisdictions and overall goals, but may have little effect on the ambiguous nature of the tasks and roles performed by professional employees.

In contrast, efforts to involve staff in decision making reduce the amount of role ambiguity that staff experience, and thus lead to increased job satisfaction and reduced absenteeism. Table 4 indicates that representation, consultation, and involvement of staff in decision making (communication) directly and indirectly led to a significant reduction in role ambiguity among the nursing staff. In addition to their direct effects, these organizational practices result in a more

Table 4: Interpretation of the Direct and Indirect Effects of Variables in the Model of Organization Stress

Dependent Variable	*Predetermined Variables*	*Total Effect*	*Direct Effect*	*Indirect Effects Via*						
				Supervision Style	*Workgroup Relations*	*Role Conflict*	*Role Ambiguity*	*Nursing Stress*	*Extrinsic Satisfaction*	*Intrinsic Satisfaction*
Supervisory style	Communication	0.335	0.335	—	—	—	—	—	—	—
Workgroup relations	Training	-0.125	-0.125	—	—	—	—	—	—	—
	Communication	0.213	—	0.213	—	—	—	—	—	—
	Supervision	0.636	0.636	—	—	—	—	—	—	—
Role conflict	Training	0.194	—	—	—	—	—	—	—	—
	Anxiety	0.194	—	—	—	—	—	—	—	—
	Administration	-0.194	—	—	—	—	—	—	—	—
Role ambiguity	Training	0.203	0.176	—	0.027	—	—	—	—	—
	Anxiety	0.158	0.158	—	—	—	—	—	—	—
	Communication	-0.251	-0.151	-0.100	—	—	—	—	—	—
	Supervision	-0.302	-0.163	—	-0.139	—	—	—	—	—
	Work group	-0.218	-0.218	—	—	—	—	—	—	—
Nursing stress	Training	0.384	0.320	—	—	0.028	0.036	—	—	—
	Anxiety	0.335	0.274	—	—	0.028	0.033	—	—	—
	Role conflict	0.146	0.146	—	—	—	—	—	—	—
	Role ambiguity	0.206	0.206	—	—	—	—	—	—	—
Extrinsic satisfaction	Training	0.191	0.291	—	—	-0.036	-0.006	-0.058	—	—
	Anxiety	-0.088	—	—	—	-0.036	-0.002	-0.050	—	—
	Administration	0.036	—	—	—	0.036	—	—	—	—
	Communication	0.220	0.216	0.004	—	—	—	—	—	—
	Supervision	0.005	—	—	0.005	—	—	—	—	—
	Work group	0.008	—	—	—	—	0.008	—	—	—
	Role conflict	-0.188	-0.162	—	—	—	—	-0.026	—	—
	Role ambiguity	-0.037	—	—	—	—	—	-0.037	—	—
	Nursing stress	-0.181	-0.181	—	—	—	—	—	—	—

Intrinsic satisfaction	Training	0.136	0.277	–	-0.033	-0.033	-0.007	-0.068	–	–
	Anxiety	-0.099	–	–	–	-0.033	-0.007	-0.059	–	–
	Administration	0.034	–	–	–	0.034	–	–	–	–
	Communication	0.415	0.329	0.086	–	–	–	–	–	–
	Supervision	0.377	0.199	–	0.171	–	0.007	–	–	–
	Work group	0.263	0.260	–	–	–	0.003	–	–	–
	Role conflict	-0.169	-0.138	–	–	–	–	-0.031	–	–
	Role ambiguity	-0.044	–	–	–	–	–	-0.044	–	–
	Nursing stress	-0.214	-0.214	–	–	–	–	–	–	–
Absenteeism	Training	-0.022	–	–	0.002	0.0017	0.007	0.007	-0.016	-0.019
	Anxiety	0.011	–	–	–	0.0037	0.007	0.007	–	–
	Administration	-0.005	–	–	–	-0.005	–	–	–	–
	Communication	-0.040	–	-0.006	–	–	–	–	-0.012	-0.022
	Supervision	-0.025	–	–	-0.012	–	-0.005	–	–	-0.013
	Work group	-0.035	–	–	–	–	-0.018	–	–	-0.017
	Role conflict	0.021	–	–	–	–	–	0.003	0.009	0.009
	Role ambiguity	0.005	–	–	–	–	–	0.005	–	–
	Nursing stress	0.024	–	–	–	–	–	–	0.010	0.014
	Extrinsic satisfaction	-0.054	-0.054	–	–	–	–	–	–	–
	Intrinsic satisfaction	-0.067	-0.067	–	–	–	–	–	–	–

open, supportive style of supervision and more supportive work group relations that further attenuate role ambiguity.

A second important finding is the relationship between supervision and role ambiguity. Supportive supervision leads to a reduction in role ambiguity. In contrast, House and Rizzo [7] found that a reduction in role conflict among employees of a manufacturing company resulted from similar supervisory practices. This may indicate that, like organizational climate, the effects of supervisory practices may depend somewhat on the type of employee and the nature of his/her work. In health service organizations such as hospitals, where employees must exercise judgment and make critical decisions—in some instances under life-threatening circumstances, one of the major functions of a supervisor may be the reduction of role ambiguity for staff.

Another important finding is the effect of the supervisor's behavior on work group relations. The model indicates that supportive supervisory behavior results in more open, supportive relations among co-workers. Such work group relations in turn lead to a significant reduction in role ambiguity among nurses. Menzies [23] has also noted the importance of group defense mechanisms in alleviating stress among nurses in a teaching hospital.

As predicted by role theory [5], the level of stress that nurses experience in performing their duties is largely determined by the amount of role conflict and role ambiguity they perceive. Table 4 indicates significant direct effects of these two variables on stress. In addition, higher levels of training and trait anxiety, in part, result in more stress for nurses by exposing them to more role conflict and ambiguity.

The results indicate that job satisfaction is significantly reduced when staff experience high levels of role conflict, ambiguity, and stress in carrying out nursing tasks. This confirms the findings of a national study of employees which found that a lack of clarification of the scope and responsibilities of their jobs led to increased tension and anxiety, and decreased job satisfaction and productivity among 35 percent of the sample [5].

The model also confirms a finding of the earlier study of nursing stress [1]. When stress and other factors affecting job satisfaction are controlled, RNs are the most satisfied with their work. The direct effects of training on Extrinsic and Intrinsic Job Satisfaction (Table 4) are both positive. The indirect effects, however, are negative, indicating that the higher levels of role conflict, ambiguity, and stress that RNs experience significantly reduce their satisfaction with their work.

Satisfaction with both the extrinsic and intrinsic aspects of nursing is enhanced significantly by the direct involvement of staff in decision making. The direct effects of the communication variable on both measures of job satisfaction are large and positive. In addition, Table 4 indicates that open, supportive supervision and work group relations have significant positive effects on satisfaction with the intrinsic nature of the nurse's hospital role.

As predicted, absenteeism is largely a function of job satisfaction. As satisfaction increases, absenteeism declines, a finding that has been confirmed by a series of studies [8]. The indirect effects in Table 4 indicate that role conflict and stress result in higher rates of absenteeism primarily through their negative effects on job satisfaction. Conversely, organizational efforts that lead to greater participation in decision making, and more supportive supervision and work group relations result in a decrease in absenteeism by improving job satisfaction.

SOME EXPLORATORY ANALYSES WITH THE ORGANIZATIONAL STRESS MODEL

Further insights into the dynamics of the model of organizational stress can be obtained from computer simulation experiments with the structural equation model shown in Table 3 [34]. Such experiments permit predictions of the effects of organizational practices designed to create a more open, supportive, participative work environment. Table 5 shows the results of three computer simulation experiments.

The first policy that was simulated had to do with changes by the hospital administration involving goal setting, planning, coordinating, and adoption of innovative techniques. The first three columns indicate the predicted effects of these changes. The effects appear to be quite small. A decrease in role conflict was predicted as well as a very small increase in job satisfaction. The model predicted that little or no change in absenteeism would result from these organizational changes.

The model was also used to predict the effects of policies or procedures that would result in greater representation and participation by nursing staff in decision making. It was predicted that one unit increase on the communication variable would result in more open, supportive supervision and work group relations. A decrease in the amount of role ambiguity and stress that staff experience in providing patient care was also predicted. The analysis indicates that, as a result, job satisfaction would increase and absentee rates would decrease.

Table 5: Results of Computer Simulation Experiments Using the Model of Organizational Stress

Aspect of the Organization Affected	*Effects of a One Unit Change in*								
	Hospital Administration			*Communication*			*Supervisory Style*		
	Direct	*Indirect*	*Total*	*Direct*	*Indirect*	*Total*	*Direct*	*Indirect*	*Total*
Supervisory style	0	0	0	0.34	0	0.34	—	—	—
Workgroup relations	0	0	0	0	0.21	0.21	0.64	0	0.64
Role conflict	-0.19	0	-0.19	0	0	0	0	0	0
Role ambiguity	0	0	0	-0.15	-0.10	-0.25	-0.16	-0.14	-0.30
Nursing stress	0	-0.03	-0.03	0	-0.05	-0.05	0	-0.06	-0.06
Extrinsic satisfaction	0	0.04	0.04	0.22	0.01	0.23	0	0.01	0.01
Intrinsic satisfaction	0	0.03	0.03	0.33	0.13	0.46	0.20	0.18	0.38
Absenteeism	0	-0.004	-0.004	0	-0.04	-0.04	0	-0.03	-0.03

Finally, the effects of a change in supervisory behavior were analyzed. It was predicted that more openness and supportiveness among supervisors would have a significant positive effect on work group relations. The model predicts that a significant reduction in role ambiguity would occur as well as in stress. At the same time, there would be a significant increase in job satisfaction resulting in decreased absenteeism among the nursing staff.

VALIDATION OF THE MODEL OF ORGANIZATIONAL STRESS

Pre- and posttest data from a survey feedback project [35] on four surgical units were used to validate the model's predictions. After the pretest data were collected, feedback sessions were held with nursing supervisors and with staff on the three experimental units. These sessions were designed to encourage a more open, supportive, participatory style of supervision on these units. After the project was completed, posttest data were collected from the three experimental units and one control unit. The results are shown in Table 6.

As predicted by the model, role conflict, role ambiguity, and nursing stress significantly declined on the experimental units. Satisfaction with supervision increased significantly. The absentee rate on the experimental units declined while absenteeism on the control unit increased, although neither difference was statistically significant.

DISCUSSION

The model that was developed in this study provides important insights into the nature of organizational stress in hospitals. The results clearly indicate that role conflict and ambiguity are important intervening variables that mediate the effects of organizational variables on stress, job satisfaction, and absenteeism among the hospital nursing staff. In general, the findings suggest that staff are more satisfied and perform more effectively when administrative and supervisory practices result in an environment that permits an open expression of views and joint problem solving. Such an organizational environment leads to more open and supportive relations among co-workers, which in turn reduces role ambiguity affecting stress, job satisfaction, and absenteeism.

The findings of this study extend the results of earlier studies

Table 6: Effects of Survey Feedback to Change Supervisory Style on Hospital Surgical Units

Aspects of the Organization Affected	*Experimental Units* N = *84*			*Control Unit* N = *30*		
	Pretest Mean	*Posttest Mean*	t-*Value*	*Pretest Mean*	*Posttest Mean*	t-*Value*
Workgroup relations	3.15	3.06	0.90	2.80	2.71	0.45
Role conflict	3.22	3.00	3.29*	3.08	2.75	3.02†
Role ambiguity	2.60	2.46	2.20†	2.55	2.35	1.35
Nursing stress	0.98	0.79	4.40*	0.85	0.73	1.44
Job satisfaction supervision	2.03	2.23	-2.20‡	1.86	2.06	-1.61
Absenteeism	0.54	0.46	0.94	0.45	0.59	-1.54

*$p < .001$.
†$p < .01$.
‡$p < .05$.

concerning the effects of organizational climate and supervision [10, 38]. Other studies have noted that supportive supervisory practices affect subordinate job satisfaction and performance by reducing role ambiguity [7, 19, 20]. The effect of such practices on work group relations and the latter's subsequent effect on satisfaction have not been demonstrated before, however.

What is more, this study suggests a number of dynamic relationships among organizational characteristics of the hospital and nursing role perceptions that have not been noted before. An important finding is that organizational practices and supervisory behavior can be used to reduce role conflict and role ambiguity among the nursing staff, two major causes of stress, job dissatisfaction, and absenteeism.

While the elements included in the model represent many important aspects of the hospital's organizational structure, many variables are missing, as indicated by the moderate magnitude of the multiple correlation coefficients associated with the structural equations. Notably lacking are variables that describe the nature of nursing tasks and individual and group differences in values and skills. In general, the factors included in the model represent aggregations of many aspects of the organization. Such aggregation, however, makes it possible to perform analyses and make predictions concerning organizational changes—as has been done in this study. The expansion of this model to include a wider variety of variables holds promise for a significant increase in our understanding of how the hospital's organizational structure affects the ability of its staff to perform their functions.

REFERENCES

1. Gray-Toft, P. A., and J. G. Anderson. Stress among hospital nursing staff: Its causes and effects. *Social Science and Medicine* 15A:639-47, September 1981.
2. Bowers, D. G. *System 4: The Ideas of Rensis Likert*. Ann Arbor, MI: University of Michigan Press, 1975.
3. Franklin, J. L. Down the organization: Influence processes across levels of hierarchy. *Administrative Science Quarterly* 20:153-64, June 1975.
4. Franklin, J. L. Relations among four social-psychological aspects of organizations. *Administrative Science Quarterly* 20:422-33, September 1975.
5. Kahn, R. L., E. M. Wolfe, R. P. Quinn, J. D. Snoek, and R. A. Rosenthal. *Organizational Stress: Studies in Role Conflict and Ambiguity*. New York: John Wiley, 1964.
6. Rizzo, J. R., R. J. House, and S. I. Lirtzman. Role conflict and ambiguity in complex organizations. *Administrative Science Quarterly* 15:150-63, June 1970.
7. House, R. J., and J. R. Rizzo. Role conflict and ambiguity as critical variables in a model of organizational behavior. *Organizational Behavior and Human Performance* 7:467-505, June 1972.
8. Locke, E. A. The nature and causes of job satisfaction. In M. D. Dunnette (ed.). *Handbook of Industrial and Organizational Psychology*. Chicago: Rand McNally, 1976, pp. 1297-1349.
9. Likert, R. *The Human Organization*. New York: McGraw-Hill, 1967.
10. Payne, R., and D. S. Pugh. Organizational structure and climate. In M. D. Dunnette (ed.). *Handbook of Industrial and Organizational Psychology*, Chicago: Rand McNally, 1976, pp. 1125-73.
11. James, L. R., and A. P. Jones. Organizational climate: A review of theory and research. *Psychological Bulletin*, 12:1096-1112, December 1974.
12. Corwin, R. The professional employee: A study of conflict in nursing roles. *American Journal of Sociology* 66:604-15, May 1961.
13. Coser, R. L. Authority and decision making in a hospital: A comparative analysis. *American Sociological Review* 23:56-63, February 1958.
14. Georgopolous, B., and F. Mann. *The Community General Hospital*. New York: Macmillan, 1962.
15. Mauksch, H. O. The organizational context of nursing practice. In F. Davis (ed.). *The Nursing Profession: Five Sociological Essays*. New York: John Wiley, 1969, pp. 109-37.
16. Pearlin, L. I. Alienation from work: A study of nursing personnel. *American Sociological Review* 27:314-26, June 1962.
17. Bowers, D. G., and S. E. Seashore. Predicting organizational effectiveness with a four-factor theory of leadership. *Administrative Science Quarterly* 11:238-63, September 1966.

18. Oaklander, H., and E. Fleishman. Patterns of leadership related to organizational stress in hospital settings. *Administrative Science Quarterly* 16:520-32, March 1964.
19. House, R. J. A path goal theory of leader effectiveness. *Administrative Science Quarterly* 16:321-38, September 1971.
20. Valenzi, E., and G. Dessler. Relationships of leader behavior, subordinate role ambiguity and subordinate job satisfaction. *Academy of Management Journal* 21:671-78, December 1978.
21. Filley, A. C., and R. J. House. *Managerial Process and Organizational Behavior*. Glenview, IL: Scott Foresman, 1969.
22. Perrow, C. Hospitals: Technology, structure and goals. In J. G. March (ed.). *Handbook of Organizations*. Chicago: Rand McNally, 1965, pp. 910-71.
23. Menzies, I. E. P. A case-study in the functioning of social systems as a defense against anxiety. *Human Relations* 13:95-121, May 1960.
24. Smith, E. E. The effects of clear and unclear role expectations on group productivity and defensiveness. *Journal of Abnormal and Social Psychology* 55:213-17, September 1957.
25. Calhoun, G. Hospitals are high-stress employers. *Hospitals* 54:171-76, June 1980.
26. Cartwright, L. K. Sources and effects of stress in health careers. In G. C. Stone, F. Cohen, and N. E. Adler (eds.). *Health Psychology*, San Francisco: Jossey-Bass, 1979, pp. 419-45.
27. Gray-Toft, P. A. Effectiveness of a counseling support program for hospice nurses. *Journal of Counseling Psychology* 27:346-54, July 1980.
28. Cammann, C., M. Fichman, G. D. Jenkins, Jr., and J. R. Klesh. The Michigan Organizational Questionnaire. Unpublished manuscript. Institute for Social Research, University of Michigan, Ann Arbor, MI, 1980.
29. Smith, P. C., L. M. Kendall, and C. L. Hulin. *The Measurement of Satisfaction in Work and Retirement*. Chicago: Rand McNally, 1969.
30. Gray-Toft, P. A., and J. G. Anderson. The nursing stress scale: Development of an instrument. *Journal of Behavioral Assessment* 3:11-23, Spring 1981.
31. Krug, S. E., I. H. Scheier, and R. B. Chattell. *Handbook for the IPAT Anxiety Scale*. Champaign, IL: Institute for Personality and Ability Testing, 1976.
32. Duncan, O. D. *Introduction to Structural Equation Models*. New York: Academic Press, 1975.
33. Alwin, D. F., and R. M. Hauser. The decomposition of effects in path analysis. *American Sociological Review* 40:37-47, February 1975.
34. Anderson, J. G. A social indicator model of a health services system. *Social Forces* 55:661-87, December 1977.
35. Bowers, D. G., and J. L. Franklin. *Survey-Guided Development I: Data-Based Organizational Change*. La Jolla, CA: University Associates, 1977.
36. Thorner, I. Nursing: The functional significance of an institutional pattern. *American Sociological Review* 20:531-38, October 1955.
37. Johnson, M. M., and H. W. Martin. A sociological analysis of the nurse role. In J. K. Skipper and R. C. Leonard (eds.). *Social Interaction and Patient Care*. Philadelphia: Lippincott, 1965, pp. 29-39.
38. Barrow, J. C. The variables of leadership: A review and conceptual framework. *Academy of Management Review* 2:231-51, April 1977.

CHAPTER SEVEN

Stepwise Regression and Discriminant Function Analysis

Given the rapid spread of new health plans in the market for health services, consumers are often faced with what is essentially a choice between two alternatives—to continue their current insurance arrangements or to elect to join a new and different health insurance program or provider organization. Their prior coverage may have coexisted with other alternative arrangements, but the introduction of a new plan into a market gives them the chance to change to that plan. Those who opt for a change, and their characteristics, represent important questions for planners and managers of programs. These researchers answer these questions by analyzing the differences between the people who changed and those who did not.

The article by Grazier, Richardson, Martin, and Diehr develops models using multivariate discriminant function analysis that distinguish between switchers and nonswitchers from two existing programs, a health maintenance organization and a standard indemnity plan. The discriminant analytical model they chose is appropriate to the bivariate choice option because it does not posit a dependent-independent variable arrangement. Rather, the task is to characterize, descriptively, what is known about two existing conditions. They are casting the analytical problem as one of interpretation of choices made, rather than classification, given a set of characteristics of a number of objects or individuals. In both of these uses of discriminant analysis, the model specification follows the lead of canonical correlation analysis where causation and dependence are not considered important.

The use of discriminant function analysis is currently less common than that of other analytic techniques that examine multiple variables and their relationship to two mutually exclusive groups of objects, units, or people. An alternative for this example might be analysis of variance (ANOVA) or multivariate analysis of variance (MANOVA) or a logistic regression model with a bivariate dependent variable. However, the assumptions of discriminant function analysis meet the characteristics of this problem most appropriately. The two groups are mutually exclusive and do not represent any hierarchy or measure (high, low) on a scale, and the choice they make is truly bivariate and does not follow a logistic probability curve.

The results of discriminant function analysis are presented in a straightforward fashion as the percentage of individuals in the two groups who are properly or improperly classified. The canonical correlation coefficients are less clearly presented in their application to the problem at hand; they represent the contribution of each of the variables to the model's overall discriminant power. The reader can obtain an appreciation of the relative clarity with which the interpretation of results using these two techniques can be communicated.

Factors Affecting Choice of Health Care Plans

Kyle L. Grazier, William C. Richardson, Diane P. Martin, and Paula Diehr

The research reported here examined the factors which affected the decision to remain with either Blue Cross of Washington and Alaska or Group·Health Cooperative of Puget Sound, or to change to an independent practice association (IPA) in which the primary care physicians control all care. The natural setting allowed examination of (1) the characteristics of families with experience in structurally different plans; (2) a decision not influenced by premium differentials; (3) the importance of the role of usual provider; and (4) a family-based decision using multivariate techniques. An expected utility model implied that factors affecting preferences included (1) future need for medical care; (2) access to care; (3) financial resources to meet the need for care; and (4) previous level of experience with plan and provider. Analysis of interview and medical record abstract data from 1,497 families revealed the importance of maintaining a satisfactory relationship with the usual sources of care in the decision to change plans. Adverse selection into the new IPA as measured by health status and previous utilization of medical services was not noted.

In recent years, families have been faced with new models of delivery and financing of health care. Independent practice plans, closed-panel

---

Supported in part by Grants 18-P-97144/0 from the Health Care Financing Administration, United States Department of Health and Human Services; W. K. Kellogg Foundation; the National Health Care Management Center of The University of Pennsylvania; University of California, Berkeley, Biomedical Research Support Grant #1-445910-32064-7; and The University of California, Berkeley, Grossman Fund.

Address correspondence and requests for reprints to Kyle L. Grazier, Dr.P.H., Assistant Professor, School of Health Policy and Administration, University of California, Berkeley, 416 Warren Hall, Berkeley, CA 94720. William C. Richardson, Ph.D. is Executive Vice President and Professor, Pennsylvania State University, University Park. Diane P. Martin, Ph.D. and Paula Diehr, Ph.D. are affiliated with the School of Public Health and Community Medicine, University of Washington, Seattle, where Dr. Martin is an Associate Professor of Public Health and Community Medicine and Dr. Diehr is a Professor of Biostatistics.

group practice plans, and other types of innovative health care systems incorporate financing with provision of services, the intent being to limit enrollee risk and contain costs. This innovation increases the significance of the consumer's decision about which "insurer" to choose, since the outcome determines not only the family's potential financial investment in its health but also its access to care.

The success of these new options depends on their ability to attract enrollees from other plans, since the vast majority of employed people in the United States already have health insurance [1]. Whether families change to the new plans or remain with the old depends on attributes of the consumers, particularities of the plans, and effectiveness of the marketing programs. Past experience with other plans, sociodemographic characteristics of the enrollees, and past and expected need for health care might all contribute to a family's decision. In addition is the willingness to accept change or innovation—whether the consumer is willing to experiment with a new plan as well as a new *type* of plan.

Given the unpredictability of the need for services and the rising costs of medical care, ensuring access to health care and insuring against the possibility of financial devastation from illness is considered by many consumers to be an imperative. In settings where health insurance is a benefit of employment, the decision to select a particular type of plan involves assessment of a plan's benefit structure, its accessibility to particular care features, expediency of reimbursement, and anticipated out-of-pocket costs to the family.

For those consumers not familiar with the structural or organizational differences and therefore unaware of the implications of their choice, a well-informed decision on health care coverage will require a new and considerable effort. Whether a new plan can attract consumers is an issue of marketing strategy. A plan must be competitive with regard to benefits, costs, and access to care, but it must also attract a clientele which appreciates the value of preventing excessive use of the plan, thereby keeping down costs that the plan itself would incur.

A new health care plan considering entry into a market must assess the financial feasibility of its survival among already-insured enrollees given the interest and effort required by the prospective enrollee to change to a new plan. In order to assess the economic feasibility of survival in such an environment, the new plan must be able to identify the type of subscriber it would attract. To determine the effort required of the subscriber in changing plans, the plan must be able to identify factors believed to be important to the potential enrollee.

This study was designed to determine the factors which affected families' decisions to remain either with a comprehensive fee-for-service plan, Blue Cross of Washington and Alaska, or with a closed-panel group practice plan, Group Health Cooperative of Puget Sound; or, alternatively, to switch to a new primary care network plan, United Healthcare. United Healthcare was first offered to Washington State employees in King County in July 1978. The entire premium for United Healthcare as well as for the first two plans was paid by the state.

The new, individual-practice plan option, organized and sponsored by Safeco Insurance Company, was referred to as a primary care network plan: all care to enrollees was provided or approved by a primary care physician selected by the enrollee in advance. This physician also managed the financing of all care through a fund established by the plan for each enrollee, to cover all primary and specialist in- and outpatient care [2]. There was no deductible or coinsurance; most "claims" to United Healthcare were submitted by the physician. The new plan offered organizational and structural alternatives to the other options.

Blue Cross is a fee-for-service indemnity plan for nonhospital services and a service benefit plan with respect to hospital services, which has been available to this population in some form since the early 1970s. The plan has reimbursed most expenses incurred for inpatient and outpatient care provided by all traditional health care practitioners with a $50 deductible ($150/family) per calendar year and 10 percent copayment (for the next $1,950 in claims per year).

Group Health Cooperative of Puget Sound is a large (300,000-member) closed-panel, consumer-owned group practice prepayment plan with several facilities in the Seattle area which provide inpatient and outpatient care, as well as telephone service. Only care provided by or otherwise approved by its employee practitioners is covered by the plan. There is no deductible for most services, and a two dollar copayment is required on prescriptions.

The study population is comprised of Washington State employees, including those in higher education, who live in King County (which includes Seattle). This population is not new to the concept of health insurance (in its broadest sense) nor, since it is served by Group Health Cooperative, are its members unaccustomed to structural diversity in the manner in which health care is delivered and financed. In addition, Washington State employees have experienced traditional indemnity-type coverage as well as service benefit plans.

This setting for the introduction of a new type of plan offers a test of acceptance and survival in a well-developed and experienced market. It also allows examination of the key differences between those enrollees who demonstrate their interest in the new plan by switching plans and those who do not. The study's uniqueness lies in the circumstances under which critical variables which are suspected to influence the decision to change plans—or not—can be examined.

Because this article looks at a family's change from a comprehensive fee-for-service plan or a prepaid group practice to an independent practice plan, the study differs from earlier research which mainly concerned only traditional versus prepaid insurance plans. Earlier work included the effect of differences in comprehensiveness of benefits, while in this study benefits are similar among the three options. Although there are limitations in the application of earlier findings to this setting, we have drawn on the concepts of risk vulnerability, accessibility, and patient satisfaction with provider.

The literature on choice of plan leads us to examine factors such as: existence of a usual provider as a measure of accessibility; family characteristics which reflect stage of development as an indicator of medical risk, risk perception, or need; and family income and family size (per capita income) as an indicator of risk of financial loss due to illness. The model we propose relies on these factors as well as others believed important in this particular setting: the presence and extent of other insurance coverage in the family; the physical *and* mental health of the enrollees; the length of experience with Group Health Cooperative and Blue Cross; family members' relationships with usual sources of care (i.e., recency of use, satisfaction with provider, ability to continue that relationship under a new plan); time-based accessibility to care; and actual use of health services during the 6-month period immediately preceding the choice. All of these indicators are evaluated in a framework which assumes that the decision maker acts as if to maximize his or her expected utility.

Sample and Data Sources

The population of interest consisted of individuals who were employed by a Washington higher education or other state agency; who resided in King County, which includes the city of Seattle; who had a health plan effective date prior to May 1, 1978; and who were active employees on December 31, 1978. These criteria eliminated from the population employees who were not eligible to switch coverage in the May 1978 open enrollment period, during which Blue Cross, Group Health

Cooperative, and United Healthcare were offered as the health plan alternatives. Employees excluded from the population were those newly hired, employed less than 2 months, or retired. Thus, the four groups of interest were:

1. Enrollees who chose to remain with Blue Cross (BC)
2. Enrollees who chose to remain with Group Health Cooperative (GHC)
3. United Healthcare enrollees previously with Blue Cross (BC-UHC)
4. United Healthcare enrollees previously with Group Health Cooperative (GHC-UHC).

A family unit was defined for these analyses as a subscriber and all family members covered by a state health plan. Table 1 presents a classification of the eligible population of family units and the sample included in the study. A total sample of 1,936 families was chosen [3].

Contact with the families found 85.4 percent to be eligible for this study. Major reasons for ineligibility were termination of state employment by the time of interview, residence outside of King County, and retirement from state employment. Eleven subscribers or half of one percent of the sample could not be contacted, resulting in an overall eligible sample of 1,654 subscribers. Of those eligible for the study, 94.9 percent agreed to participate.

Since our model assumes that the sample represents those families who had a choice of health plans, only those families who reported knowledge of open enrollment are considered. The analysis used 1,497 families.

Data sources included a household interview which averaged an hour in length and, in order to address explicitly the question of potential adverse selection into UHC, abstracts of BC claims and GHC medical records.

Interviewing completed between April 1979 and January 1980, collected variables on need for care, accessibility, financial capacity to cover the costs of illness, experience with plans, and satisfaction with plans. Interviewing just prior to the July decision was preferable; however, this was not administratively feasible. As a result, the time between enrollee decision and data collection varied from 10 to 20 months. This length of time increases the possibility of simultaneous equation bias in the coefficients for the independent variables. These possible biases must be recognized in any conclusions drawn from the analysis.

Table 1: Population and Sample Distribution of Health Plan Subscribers

	GROUP									
	BC		*GHC*		*BC-UHC*		*GHC-UHC*		*TOTAL*	
	N	%	N	%	N	%	N	%	N	%
Eligible population of family unit	8,148	—	7,619	—	676	—	192	—	16,330	—
Sample, family units (as percent of population)	722	9.00	518	7.00	504	75.00	192	100.00	1,654	85.40
Ineligibles	75	10.40	82	15.80	81	16.10	33	17.20	271	14.00
No contact	7	0.97	2	0.39	1	0.20	1	0.52	11	0.57
Respondent families (as percent of eligibles)	599	93.50	413	95.20	407	96.40	151	95.60	1,570	94.90
Respondent families eligible for decision* (as percent of respondents)	554	92.00	385	93.00	407	100.00	151	100.00	1,497	95.00

*The final group used for analysis eliminated 73 families who reported no knowledge of the 1978 open enrollment period.

Extensive utilization data were retrieved from BC claims files and GHC medical records for the *6-month period prior to* the introduction of UHC (January 1978 through June 1978). Charges were difficult to compare across the three plans, because Group Health has no charges, and Blue Cross and United Healthcare may have used different pricing systems. To obtain comparable measures of the volume of services used in each plan, California Relative Value Scale units (CRVS) were used. This scale assigns a number of units to each procedure performed, in six categories: medical, anesthesia, surgical, x-ray, laboratory, and administrative. These units are consistent within categories, but not across categories. In addition, the value of a unit depends on whether the service is performed on an inpatient or an outpatient basis. Blue Cross charge data were used to estimate the average charge *per CRVS unit*. For example, one outpatient unit of medical service is worth (on average) $2.61 but one unit of anesthesia is worth $27.03; if the anesthesia is administered during an outpatient procedure, a unit of anesthesia is worth $36.93.

To achieve a single measure of the volume of services for each person, we assigned CRVS units to each procedure, weighted them, and summed them for each person. Details of the data collection methods, coding, and weighting procedures used are described elsewhere or are available from the authors [4, 5].

METHODS OF ANALYSIS

The objectives of the analysis were to examine the factors believed important in the consumers' choice and to assess the extent of adverse selection of enrollees. Thus, the analysis is composed of two major stages, one in which factors believed to influence the decision were subjected to bivariate and multivariate analysis, and another in which these associations were tested while controlling for prior utilization.

The dependent variable, switching or not switching to UHC, represents some measure of utility of the family's choice. The use of regression analysis allows prediction of ordering of preferences for switching or not switching. There are two basic assumptions in the choice of models. First, the approach assumes that all subjects have the same "tastes" or criteria for a desirable outcome. For example, families desire low costs of health care, high quality, accessible services, adequate plan coverage, etc. This assumption permits one to consider together all members of either Blue Cross or Group Health Cooperative in developing estimates of the model. The second assumption is that the decision maker acts to make the best use of available resources.

Since many variables were collected at the individual level and the family level, several family-based indicators for each variable were compared to determine which were most closely correlated with the switching decision: family average, the family member with the most extreme response, or the subscriber's response. For example, physical health status measured by the health perception question was defined in three ways: the average family health status, health perception of the least healthy family member, and the subscriber's report of his/her own health status.

For each variable, bivariate testing was performed to determine which variables when taken alone were significantly related to choice. To reduce the number of variables, a stepwise linear regression analysis was performed for each of the four sets of variables to derive a smaller set of variables which could predict choice. All of these analyses were performed separately for BC and GHC. A multivariate model to predict choice was then constructed by taking the strongest correlates of choice from each subset and entering them in a linear discriminant analysis. Variables predicting previous use and some sociodemographic variables were also included in the model.

FINDINGS

FACTORS INFLUENCING CHOICE

Blue Cross enrollees were more than three times as likely to switch to UHC than were GHC enrollees (8.3 percent compared to 2.5 percent).

The *need for care* set of variables included a family's life stage, mental and physical health status, and whether anyone in the family was under medical care during the 1978 open enrollment period. In addition, the subscriber's age, sex, race, and education were included in this set (as well as in the financial set) to evaluate their contribution to the subjective assessments of need.

The Blue Cross and Group Health Cooperative groups were at approximately the same stage in the family life cycle; however, bivariate analysis reveals that Group Health Cooperative families at a lower-risk life stage were more likely to switch to United Healthcare while Blue Cross families at a higher-risk life stage were more likely to switch. The family life stage measure was not significant for the Group Health Cooperative estimation but did contribute to the Blue Cross estimation.

With respect to the physical health status variables, a substantial majority of families reported their health as good or excellent, and with fewer than two chronic conditions among members. The physical health status measures were very similar between the Blue Cross and Group Health Cooperative groups and did not appear to affect the change-of-plan decision.

Mental health status, measured by the frequency of certain positive and negative feelings, was significantly related to choice of plan only for the Group Health Cooperative switchers and nonswitchers [6, 7]. All groups reported relatively high levels of mental health, regardless of the scale used.

Still considering need for care, a subscriber's age and sex were correlated with choice of plan differently for Blue Cross and Group Health Cooperative. Group Health Cooperative families with female subscribers were more likely to change to United Healthcare. Blue Cross families with younger subscribers were more likely to change to the new plan.

The *access to care* variables included presence of usual providers and their use by the subscriber and family; satisfaction with usual sources; whether providers were on the UHC list; and appointment, travel, and waiting times. The familys' relationships with their usual sources of care and time-based measures of accessibility of care, i.e., appointment acquisition time, travel time to the provider's office, and waiting time in the office, were significantly related to choice. Relationships with usual sources of care were studied not only in terms of their presence or absence for all family members as well as for the subscriber, but also with respect to recent use of the provider by the subscriber or "all, some, or no" family members. Blue Cross switchers and nonswitchers were also asked to report whether the usual sources for the family were on the United Healthcare list of participating physicians, thus allowing a family to continue relationships despite changing health care plans. In addition, the value of a family's average satisfaction with usual sources, the value represented by the least satisfied member, and the influence of the subscriber's satisfaction with his or her usual sources were studied. Both the family's average time-measure variables and the greatest time reported by a family member were tested.

Only 4.8 percent of the Blue Cross families and 1.9 percent of the Group Health Cooperative families had no usual sources of care for any family member. All family members had usual sources in 86 percent of the Blue Cross switcher and nonswitcher families, and in 93 percent of the Group Health Cooperative families. There were not, however, significant differences in source of care between switchers and nonswitchers in either of the plans. Recent use of a usual source by subscriber differed significantly between switchers and nonswitchers in both groups: Blue Cross subscribers who switched were *more* likely to have had recent use, while Group Health Cooperative subscribers who switched were *less* likely to have had recent use.

All measures of satisfaction with the usual sources of care (family average, least satisfied family member, and subscriber's satisfaction) appeared to play a much larger role in Group Health Cooperative decision making than in the switching decision for Blue Cross enrollees. Switchers from Group Health Cooperative were more likely to be more dissatisfied with their usual source, regardless of how satisfaction was measured, than Blue Cross switchers, who differed significantly from nonswitchers only in the level of subscriber's satisfaction: switchers were more likely to have a dissatisfied subscriber.

Accessibility of care for Blue Cross switchers and nonswitchers was characterized differently from that of the Group Health Cooperative groups. With regard to the Blue Cross groups, the greater proportion of family members with usual sources on the UHC list of participating physicians, the more likely the family was to switch to United Healthcare. Over 85 percent of the Blue Cross switchers, as compared to less than 12 percent of the nonswitchers, had one or more usual providers on the UHC list.

Significant differences also appeared in the various time-based accessibility measures when considered alone. There were significant group differences related to appointment acquisition time between Blue Cross switchers and nonswitchers—nonswitchers reported longer acquisition times than switchers. For Group Health Cooperative groups, reports of time spent waiting in the provider's office were significantly different for switchers and nonswitchers—switchers reported significantly longer waits than nonswitchers. Travel time was not a significant issue to any of the groups; the mean travel time was approximately 20 minutes.

Variables measuring *financial capability* to cover the costs of care included measures of income (gross family and per capita family); subscriber's occupation, education, race, age, and sex (as measures of potential earning power and thus financial risk); and the extent of other health care coverage (private and state) in the family, while employed by the state or not, for all family members, for each and all of the 3 years prior to the 1978 open enrollment.

Once again the variables which were related to choice of plan differed between the Blue Cross and Group Health Cooperative groups. Reported gross and per capita income were not significantly different for Group Health Cooperative switchers and nonswitchers. However, there were significant differences in both gross income and per capita income between the Blue Cross groups, with per capita income (while controlling for the other variables) clearly related to the decision to switch. Both gross and per capita incomes were less for those switching to United Healthcare than for those remaining with Blue Cross. Blue Cross nonswitchers reported an average gross annual income of $26,000 compared to $22,500 for switchers; mean per capita income for Blue Cross nonswitchers was $12,800 compared to $11,600 for switchers.

In both Blue Cross and Group Health Cooperative, switching families were significantly more likely to have subscribers with nonprofessional, nonmanagerial occupations.

The existence of other health care coverage in a family prior to open enrollment differed in its importance between Blue Cross and Group Health switchers. Blue Cross switchers were less likely to have had other insurance coverage, while Group Health Cooperative switchers were more likely than nonswitchers to have had other coverage.

Variables used to measure *experience and satisfaction with previous plans* consisted of measures of exposure to the health care plans, both while employed by the state or elsewhere; reports of problems either with plan administration and/or with any provider while covered by the plans; reports of out-of-pocket costs for health care from January to June 1978, and of satisfaction with that amount; and frequency with which a family changed state health care plans during the time from July 1975 to June 1978 (prior to the July 1978 switch). These different measures allowed investigation of many aspects of experience with plans which deliver services as well as finance care. It was also important to measure past exposure to the Group Health Cooperative plan by Blue Cross enrollees and vice versa, since willingness to enroll in a new plan with some of the similarities of both Blue Cross and Group Health Cooperative may be influenced by even limited exposure to a variety of other plans.

This particular measure of exposure to the "other" plan (Blue Cross enrollees having experienced GHC coverage and vice versa) proved to be significantly different between switchers and nonswitchers from each plan even when length of state employment was controlled. Switchers from both plans reported greater exposure to the other plans than nonswitchers.

It is interesting to note the differing emphasis on problems with providers reported by the Group Health Cooperative groups, and problems with plan administration reported by the Blue Cross groups. Significantly more problems with providers were reported by GHC switchers to United Healthcare. Similarly, Blue Cross switchers reported significantly more problems with plan administration than nonswitchers.

There are interesting differences both between plans and within plans. Blue Cross switchers and nonswitchers reported approximately equal out-of-pocket costs for care, averaging $121 for nonswitchers and $128 for switchers. These amounts probably reflect the fact that Blue Cross has a $50 deductible per person up to three persons per family per calendar year, in addition to a 10 percent copayment. The amounts reported were for the first half of the deductible period. In contrast, Group Health Cooperative nonswitchers reported an average of $22 spent during this same period for care, while switchers reported a mean of $51 for care. This significant ($p < .001$) difference between Group Health Cooperative switchers and nonswitchers is also reflected in the measure of costs as percentage of income, with switchers having values slightly greater than twice those of nonswitchers. Out-of-pocket costs at Group Health Cooperative stem from care received outside the system or from charges for eyeglasses, maternity care costs, or charges for mental health visits beyond the ten allowed per year.

The variable created to measure the frequency of a family's switching state health plans during the 3 years pre-1978 was found to be significant only in the Blue Cross analysis, with switchers to United Healthcare having been more likely than Blue Cross nonswitchers to have changed state plans at least once during the preceding 3 years.

COMPREHENSIVE MODELS OF CHOICE

A model including all factors related to switching was estimated using the technique described earlier. Table 2 presents the Blue Cross discriminant analysis results. All variables of the Blue Cross model were statistically significant to at least the $p < .01$ level, with the exception of the measure for plan administration problems and per capita income ($.05 < p < .06$). By far the strongest variable when other variables are held constant is that which measured the proportion of family members with usual sources of care on the United Healthcare list. The relative size of the standardized canonical discriminant function coefficient indicates its importance to the model. As indicated by the earlier results, families with younger female subscribers were more likely to switch, as were families with lower per capita incomes. This may be an

Table 2: Blue Cross Discriminant Analysis Results

Standardized Canonical Discriminant Function Coefficients

Characteristic	*Coefficients*	p ≤
Need		
Subscriber's age	-0.2013	.001
Under medical care during June 1978	-0.1397	.007
Access		
Proportion of family with usual source of care on UHC PCP list	0.9229	.001
Experience		
Months of BC coverage July 1977–June 1978	-0.1877	.003
Satisfaction with out-of-pocket costs	0.2385	.001
Report of problems with plan administration	0.1044	.056
Length of state employment July 1975–June 1978	0.1545	.012
Number of switches in state plan 1975–1978	0.1285	.009
Financial		
Subscriber's sex	0.1436	.006
Per capita income	-0.0892	.059

*Classification Results (Percent)**

	Predicted Group	
Actual Group	Nonswitchers	Switchers
Nonswitchers	80.6	19.4
Switchers	19.9	80.1

Correctly Classified: 80.39
Significance < .001
R^2 = .369

*The default rule used assumed that the product of prior probabilities and costs of misclassification cancel one another.

indication of the higher health risk as well as economic vulnerability described by previous research. The absence of a deductible in a plan which allows maintenance of usual providers could be especially appealing to young families and single-parent families.

The less exposure to the Blue Cross plan during the year before the switch, the more likely a family would switch to United Healthcare. This may reflect unwillingness to learn a new system once another has been mastered. But the direction of the coefficient on the variable, length of state employment, confuses the issue: the longer one worked for the state the more likely the family would switch to the new plan. This may be due to the manner in which the variable was measured—recent history of employment rather than total years of employment with the state. It might also be due to interaction. While no two-way interaction was found, some higher-order interaction which has not been identified may exist.

Being under medical care during open enrollment was more likely in nonswitchers than switchers. When we control for all variables, those families with a member under care during the decision period were less likely to change to United Healthcare. It is not known (1) who in the family was under care; (2) whether the person's usual source was a primary care provider or a specialist; or (3) if the provider was a primary care practitioner, whether the physician was on the UHC list. One could speculate that the care was from a specialist and, therefore, that changing to a plan which required approval for that care would not be attractive to the decision maker. One might also suggest that this reflects greater identification with a plan, comfort with a provider, or merely experience in using a plan.

Those families reporting dissatisfaction with out-of-pocket costs and plan administration were more likely to change to the new plan. Concern about costs is consistent with the fact that lower-income families changed plans. The paperwork involved in filing claims for reimbursement as well as delays in reimbursement are complaints common with dissatisfied enrollees in traditional indemnity plans, including Blue Cross.

The model shown in Table 2 explains 36.8 percent of the variance in choice of plan. The final set of variables correctly classified 80.4 percent of the Blue Cross cases.

Table 3 presents the Group Health Cooperative final discriminant function estimates. The estimates for the Group Health Cooperative model once again reveal an access variable as the strongest predictor of switching when all other variables are held constant. The less satisfied any family member was with his or her usual provider, the more likely the family was to switch to United Healthcare. The other two accessibility measures, recent use of usual source by subscriber, and the interaction of recent use and lowest family satisfaction with provider did not contribute significantly to the equation.

Subscribers who switched from Group Health Cooperative were more likely to be female, as were the Blue Cross switchers. When all other variables are held constant, the direction of the effect of subscriber's age on the equation changes from the bivariate result: families with older subscribers were more likely to change to United Healthcare than to remain with Group Health Cooperative.

Subscriber's occupation was significant in the equation; subscribers with professional and managerial occupations were more likely to remain with Group Health Cooperative than to switch. The discrim-

Table 3: Group Health Cooperative Discriminant Analysis Results

Standardized Canonical Discriminant Function Coefficients

Characteristic	*Coefficients*	p ≤
Need		
Subscriber's sex	0.1371	.063
Mental health: Lowest negative feelings	0.0886	.170
Access		
Least satisfaction with usual source	1.0558	.001
Recent use of usual source by subscriber	-0.0664	.360
Interaction of above access measures	-0.3599	.150
Experience		
Report of problems with provider	0.1992	.020
Months of GHC coverage from any source 1975–1978	-0.3443	.001
Financial		
Subscriber's age	0.1823	.028
Subscriber's occupation	0.2631	.001
Sum of the means of other family 1975–1978	0.1098	.120

*Classification Results (Percent)**

	Predicted Group	
Actual Group	Nonswitchers	Switchers
Nonswitchers	83.8	16.2
Switchers	30.0	70.0

Correctly Classified: 79.91
Significance $< .001$
R^2 $= .297$

*The default rule used assumed that the product of prior probabilities and costs of misclassification cancel one another.

inant function coefficient revealed the relatively high importance of the variable to the switching decision.

The *experience with plan* variables, satisfaction with providers and length of exposure to Group Health Cooperative, were both significant when the effects of the other variables were held constant. Families with less exposure to the Group Health Cooperative plan but higher dissatisfaction with providers while covered were more likely to change to United Healthcare.

This set of measures explained 29.7 percent of the variance in switching plans. The variables correctly classified 79.9 percent of all Group Health Cooperative cases.

To determine the generalizability of switching rules developed, we applied the GHC rule to the BC data and vice versa to see how well each rule would perform in predicting switchers in the other provider system.

We deleted the variables in the rules which were specific to the plans and recreated the rules with the remaining variables. When the BC rule was applied to the GHC families, there was a reasonable amount of separation between the switchers and the nonswitchers. Thus, the BC rule can be said to generalize to quite a different setting (the prepaid group practice), although the amount of separation between switchers and nonswitchers in the new setting is not large.

When the GHC rule was applied to the BC families, however, there was, in effect, no separation between the BC switchers and the BC nonswitchers. Thus, the GHC rule does not seem at all applicable to the BC family data.

This suggests that there are general reasons for switching, as exemplified by the BC rule, as well as plan-specific rules, as exemplified by the GHC case.

THE EFFECT OF PRIOR UTILIZATION

It is evident from the preceding analyses that the health status of an individual in a family, or of the family on average, is not a consequential factor in the choice of plans. The only one of the several components of health status which was at all correlated with switching—although possibly spurious—was a dimension of mental health for GHC families. It will be recalled that there was some tendency for families with members having positive mental health to switch to UHC.

Another way of assessing selection bias in choice of plan is to evaluate actual utilization behavior of potential switchers. Prior utilization can be viewed as a composite measure of health status on one hand and of a tendency to use health services on the other. The insurance industry has commonly used this approach in its experience rating of groups.

Abstracts of BC claims and GHC medical records were compiled for all utilization of inpatient and outpatient services for all family members from January to June 1978, 6 months prior to open enrollments. Both for the BC sample and the GHC sample, the analysis used as prior utilization variables the 12 family-average measures encompassing inpatient and outpatient use separately: total use, medical use, laboratory use, radiology use, surgery use, and hospital-related physician visit use. The remaining three utilization variables were: family average-total hospital visit use, family average-total surgery use, and family average-total use.

Considering first the BC discriminant analysis, three variables entered the equation: family size (to calculate family averages), total outpatient use, and total hospital visits. Larger families were more likely to switch from BC to UHC. The effects of the utilization variables, however, were mixed. Lower total outpatient use was associated with switching, while the reverse was true for total hospital visits. The contribution of either or both of these variables to predicting switching, however, was negligible. For example, the total variance explained (R^2) for the equation without prior utilization, as specified in the earlier section (Table 2), was approximately .36. The change in R^2 as a result of adding the two utilization variables was .008.

Finally, for BC, the contribution of average family total prior utilization, controlling for the variables shown in Table 2, was considered. This variable (average family total prior utilization) was forced into the basic equation. Again the increase in R^2 was negligible ($\triangle R^2 = .002$). The variable was not statistically significant ($p = .085$), and the relationship between total utilization and switching to UHC was negative; that is, UHC experienced favorable selection.

Turning to GHC, only family average total surgery use entered the equation. The increase in R^2 was .007 on a total explained variance (from Table 3) of approximately .30. The relationship between surgical utilization prior to open enrollment and the decision to switch to UHC was negative. That is, UHC experienced favorable selection, however slight. As with the BC sample, we considered total prior utilization alone, controlling for the variables from Table 3. No relationship was found between switching to UHC and total prior utilization ($p = .20$).

Thus, we conclude that evaluation of actual utilization behavior of potential switchers during the 6-month period preceding choice of plan shows no adverse selection into UHC from either Blue Cross or Group Health Cooperative. This result is consistent with the absence of a relationship between the health status measures and switching reported above.

DISCUSSION

Because the two groups were analyzed separately, only a general comparison of Blue Cross and Group Health Cooperative results is possible. Nonetheless, there are certain similarities and differences.

The less time a family had been exposed to either Blue Cross or Group Health Cooperative, the more likely it was to leave that plan and try United Healthcare. Families who had had a plan for a long time may have felt comfortable with the workings of their plan, believing that the costs involved in making a change outweighed the benefits.

BC and GHC families with female subscribers were more likely to change to United Healthcare. This may reflect the general dissatisfaction some women felt with health care in general and may have been an attempt to find a "better" system. In terms of benefit coverage for women, United Healthcare was the only one of the three plans which covered the complete costs of voluntary sterilization, contraceptive devices, and spontaneous or elective abortions. While the utilization data showed no evidence of adverse selection into UHC overall, specific areas such as these may have attracted a disproportionate number of potential users of these services.

The importance to these families of satisfaction—with plan administration, providers, and costs—was striking in its significance to the decision and in the differing emphasis placed on it by switchers from Blue Cross versus those from Group Health Cooperative. Perhaps because Blue Cross enrollees could maintain a satisfactory relationship with their provider even if they switched, report of dissatisfaction with plan administration was much more common from Blue Cross enrollees than from Group Health enrollees and much more common from Blue Cross switchers than nonswitchers. In contrast, perhaps because Group Health Cooperative enrollees see plan administration *as* delivery of services, complaints about GHC providers were much more common among Group Health Cooperative switchers than nonswitchers.

The phenomenon of the usual provider, traditional in the American medical system, appears to maintain its importance to these groups of enrollees. The major predictor of switching in the Blue Cross sample was presence of the family's usual sources on the United Healthcare list. The single most important predictor of switching from Group Health Cooperative was level of satisfaction with the family's usual source of care.

Only a few studies that have used multivariate techniques to analyze the decision to change plans are available for comparison with our results. These studies have been thorough and well documented: Berki et al. [8], Ashcraft [9], and Scitovsky et al. [10]. Although study designs are similar, it should be noted that there were premium differentials in the setting studied by Scitovsky et al., and that the studies dealt with enrollees who may or may not have had experience with another plan.

The study by Berki et al. is the only one of the three studies amenable to comparison with the Blue Cross switcher/nonswitcher analysis. In the Berki et al. analysis, usual source of care (in this case, type of provider) was not significant in the Blue Cross/open-panel plan decision. Berki et al. also found family life stage to be a critical predictor in this decision; however, family life stage was not significant; only subscriber age (a component of family life stage) lent support to their findings. Blue Cross switchers to United Healthcare were found in our research to be younger, consistent with Berki's finding that the younger family stages were more likely to choose the open-panel plan.

One result of this research in comparison with that of Berki et al. is the lack of support in our findings for the health risk hypothesis but some support for the financial risk hypotheses, as evidenced by the income differences in the BC model. Berki et al. found higher numbers of chronic conditions and higher per capita incomes in such switchers, thus supporting both hypotheses.

Some components of all three studies are applicable to comparison with the results of the Group Health Cooperative analysis. In the Group Health Cooperative analysis, findings, consistent with Scitovsky's were found with regard to switchers having had less time with their former plans and with regard to lack of support for the health-risk hypothesis. Unlike the lack of association for GHC found in this study, Berki et al., Ashcraft, and Scitovsky et al. all found support for the financial-risk hypothesis insofar as switchers were found to have higher gross family incomes (Scitovsky et al.) or higher per capita incomes (Berki et al. and Ashcraft). Again, however, no support for the health-risk hypothesis was found in this research or in the research of these other authors.

In conclusion, while families from Blue Cross and Group Health Cooperative differ sociodemographically and have had experience with divergent systems of financing and delivering health care, the observed preference for a primary care network plan was apparently affected by considerations related to accessibility of care.

APPENDIX

GROUP MEANS FOR VARIABLES USED IN ANALYSIS

VARIABLE	GROUP BC	BC-UHC	GHC	GHC-UHC
Need for Care				
Family life state	4.58†	5.04	4.69*	4.54
Family age	38.29*	36.28	32.58	31.64
Physical Health Status				
Health status: Family average (1 = excellent → 4 = poor)	1.59	1.62	1.57	1.60
Health status: Least healthy person (1 = excellent → 4 = poor)	1.76	1.81	1.75	1.80
Number of chronic conditions: Family average	1.33	1.37	1.29	1.29
Number of chronic conditions: Least healthy person	1.83	1.86	1.79	1.81
Conditions under care: Family average	1.39	1.63	1.57	1.18
Conditions under care: Least healthy person	1.08	1.14	1.05	1.17
Mental Health Status				
Mental health: Least healthy adult (1 = healthy → 7 = unhealthy)	2.19	2.26	2.28	2.43
Highest on positive-feeling scale	10.48	10.46	10.38	10.39
Lowest on positive-feeling scale	9.68	9.60	9.56	9.65
(For both positive scales: 3 = unhealthy → 12 = healthy)				
Highest on negative-feeling scale	11.45	11.67	11.72	12.20
Lowest on negative-feeling scale	9.90	10.20	10.39*	11.00
(For both negative scales: 6 = healthy → 24 = unhealthy)				
Subscriber's education in years	15.99*	5.51	15.79‡	14.79
Average adult's education	15.66	15.36	15.63‡	14.69
Subscriber's age	44.84*	43.40	39.82	38.05

Continued

APPENDIX: Continued

VARIABLE	*GROUP*			
	BC	*BC-UHC*	*GHC*	*GHC-UHC*
Subscriber's sex (1 = male, 2 = female)	1.48*	1.57	1.49*	1.61
Subscriber's race (1 = white, 2-4 = nonwhite)	1.20	1.28	1.40	1.33
Under medical care during June 1978 (0 = no, 1 = yes)	0.32	0.36	0.29	0.31
Access to Care				
Presence of usual sources of care in family (0 = none have usc, 1 = some have usc, 2 = all have usc)	1.79	1.83	1.93	1.87
Subscriber has usual sources of care (0 = no, 1 = yes)	0.67*	0.77	0.79	0.82
Recent use of usual sources by family members (0 = no usc, 1 = none used, 2 = some used, 3 = all used)	2.46†	2.62	2.54	2.55
Subscriber has recent use of usual sources (1 = no use, 2 = use)	1.67‡	1.81	1.81‡	1.59
Family's sources on UHC list (1 = no sources on list, 2 = some sources on list, 3 = all sources on list)	1.25‡	2.43	–	–
Average family satisfaction with usual sources (1 = very satisfied → 4 = very dissatisfied)	1.15	1.18	1.34‡	2.22
Least satisfaction reported with any usual source (1 = very satisfied → 4 = very dissatisfied)	1.31	1.35	1.59‡	2.66
Subscriber's satisfaction with usual sources (1 = very satisfied → 4 = very dissatisfied)	1.24	1.29	1.49‡	2.54
Appointment acquisition time—family average (days)	9.43*	6.98	11.22	12.35
Appointment acquisition time—highest reported by a family member (days)	11.93*	9.34	13.65	15.51
Travel time to appointments—family average (minutes)	18.34	17.01	20.28	21.66

Continued

APPENDIX: Continued

VARIABLE	GROUP BC	BC-UHC	GHC	GHC-UHC
Travel time to appointments—highest reported by a family member (minutes)	20.89	19.36	22.24	23.90
Waiting time in office—family average (minutes)	22.74	24.12	19.65‡	35.15
Waiting time in office—highest reported by a family member (minutes)	25.97	28.22	21.91‡	40.49
Financial Capability				
Gross family income (01 = lowest category → 12 = highest: $44,000 +)	7.05*	6.35	5.91	5.70
Per capita income (01 = lowest category → 12 = highest: $44,000 +)	3.76†	3.39	3.32	3.28
Subscriber's occupation (1 = pro/mgt; 2 = nonpro/mgt)	1.39*	1.46	1.39‡	1.59
Subscriber's education (years)	15.99*	15.51	15.79‡	14.79
Average education of subscriber and spouse (years)	15.67	15.36	15.63‡	14.69
Other health insurance coverage for subscriber July 1977-July 1978 (1 = yes, 0 = no)	0.32*	0.26	0.20	0.27
Number of other policies in family (controlled for eligible family members)				
July 1975-June 1976	0.48	0.41	0.33†	0.49
July 1976-June 1977	0.43	0.38	0.28*	0.39
July 1977-June 1978	0.41	0.35	0.25†	0.37
Sum of policies 3 years	1.32	1.14	0.86†	1.24
Sum of mean number of other policies in family July 1975-June 1978 while a state employee	0.90	0.75	0.51	0.69
Number of subscriber's other policies July 1975-June 1978 regardless of employment	1.12	0.95	0.76	1.07

Continued

APPENDIX: Continued

VARIABLE	*GROUP*			
	BC	*BC-UHC*	*GHC*	*GHC-UHC*
Experience with Plan				
Months of state employment July 1977–July 1978	11.69	11.69	11.54	11.27
Total months of state employment July 1975–July 1978	31.82*	32.95	30.66	28.83
Months of state BC coverage July 1977–July 1978	11.63	11.57	0.05	0.00
Months of state BC coverage July 1975–July 1978	30.09	30.65	1.36‡	4.56
Months of state GHC coverage July 1977–July 1978	0.02	0.00	11.48	11.15
Months of state GHC coverage July 1975–July 1978	0.49†	1.18	28.89‡	23.16
Months of BC coverage from any source, controlled for employment, July 1977–July 1978	11.69	11.67	0.65	1.02
Months of BC coverage from any source, controlled for employment, July 1975–July 1978	30.53	31.05	2.68‡	6.04
Months of GHC coverage from any source, controlled for employment, July 1977–July 1978	0.50	.29†	11.60*	11.23
Months of GHC coverage from any source July 1975–July 1978	1.50	1.70	29.15‡	23.60
Months of BC coverage from any source, not controlled for employment, July 1975–July 1978	31.26	31.79	3.29‡	7.41
Months of GHC coverage from any source, not controlled for employment, July 1975–July 1978	1.74	1.76	29.81‡	24.03
Report of problems with plan (0 = no, 1 = yes)	0.28‡	0.47	0.06	0.04
Report of problems with providers while covered by plan (0 = no, 1 = yes)	0.07	0.07	0.17‡	0.34
Out-of-pocket costs reported for January-June 1978	121.49	128.78	22.54‡	51.01

Continued

APPENDIX: Continued

VARIABLE	GROUP BC	BC-UHC	GHC	GHC-UHC
Costs as percent of income (Income = 1–12)	19.29	21.46	3.80*	9.57
Satisfaction with out-of-pocket costs (1 = satisfied → 3 = dissatisfied)	1.41*	1.80	1.16	1.23
Changed plans between July 1975–July 1978 (0 = no, 1 = yes)	0.06	0.10	0.10‡	0.31
Family's average utilization of all services for 6 months prior to switching (January 1978–June 1978)	167.35	134.07	142.90	84.03

*$p < .05$ (t or X^2).
†$p < .01$ (t or X^2).
‡$p < .001$ (t or X^2).

REFERENCES

1. Health Insurance Institute. The Adequacy of Private Health Insurance Coverage, 1980.
2. Moore, S. A., D. P. Martin, and W. C. Richardson. Does the primary care gatekeeper control the costs of health care: Lessons from the SAFECO experience. *New England Journal of Medicine* 309(22):1400, 1983.
3. Grazier, K. L. Factors Affecting Choice of Health Care Plans. Doctoral dissertation, University of California, Berkeley, 1980.
4. Richardson, W. C., et al. Consumer Choice and Cost Containment: An Evaluation of Safeco's United Healthcare Plan. Appendix VI.5. National Technical Information Service, PB82-264912, 1982.
5. Richardson, W. C., et al. Consumer Choice and Cost Containment: An Evaluation of Safeco's United Healthcare Plan. Volume I. National Technical Information Service PB82-264912, 1982.
6. Bice, T. W. Risk vulnerability and enrollment in a prepaid group practice. *Medical Care* 13(8):698–703, 1975.
7. Langner, T. S. A twenty-two item screening score of psychiatric symptoms indicating impairment. *Journal of Health and Human Behavior* 2(4):269–72, Winter 1962.
8. Berki, S. E., et al. Enrollment choices in different types of HMOs: A multivariate analysis. *Medical Care* 16(4):682–97, 1978.
9. Ashcraft, M. L. The Impact of Previous Medical Care Experiences on Enrollment in Prepaid Group Health Plans. Doctoral dissertation, University of Michigan, 1978.
10. Scitovsky, A. A., N. McCall, and L. Benham. Factors affecting the choice between two prepaid plans. *Medical Care* 16(4):660–81, 1978.

CHAPTER EIGHT

Ordinary Least-Squares Regression Analysis

A research problem is often suggested after a policy solution has already become accepted. The article by Elnicki and Schmitt offers an example of this situation, where it has been assumed by regulators that hospital and patient characteristics contribute to adverse patient events and hospitals thus have been required to determine what those characteristics were and to correct them. In this case, the authors attempted to prove a null hypothesis, that is, that the types of adverse incidents were not related to patient, hospital, or environmental characteristics. They explored the options of using logit and probit analysis because of the bivariate dependent variable, but settled on a linear model for the presentation of results when the results of a log-linear analysis were essentially the same.

The analysis involved the specification of very large models that included 23 patient and hospital environment variables and 36 interactions regressed on the adverse-incident scores aggregated across nursing units and the time periods for which data were available. The results produced significant relationships, but they were not consistent across the units. The potential for the reduction of the variables was not borne out in the data.

The authors were essentially exploring the data to look for recognizable patterns. They were working with a very large matrix of variables and were attempting to consider all of the variables simultaneously. They solved the problem of dealing with a very large number of variables by repeating their analysis for each of the ten nursing units and the three classes of adverse incidents. There are alternatives to this type of repeated specification and model solution, but their approach was to develop descriptive measures and selected characteristics rather than develop a solution to a specific hypothesis of causation.

The fact that the authors depended, in the end, on the more

simple, linear ordinary least-squares model points to the fundamental interrelationship between multivariate models. Unless there is a well-understood and strong nonlinear relationship between the dependent variable and one or more independent variables, the general linear model will produce results that are as valid and useful as a more correctly specified model with nonlinear variable construction or non-linear coefficients.

Contribution of Patient and Hospital Characteristics to Adverse Patient Incidents

Richard A. Elnicki and John P. Schmitt

The 1974 medical malpractice "crisis" brought about extensive legislation and insurance regulation in the United States. Hospitals in many states are now required to support risk management programs that include investigation and systematic analyses of adverse patient incidents. However, no research supports the hypothesis that systematic analysis of adverse patient incidents can identify contributory factors. In this study, a simple prediction model was used to estimate relationships between adverse incidents and selected patient and environmental characteristics in a large hospital. While some of the incident-characteristic relationships were significant, none of the estimated equations yielded results that could be logically translated into policy recommendations for the hospital. These results point to the need for further research. The benefits that positive research results would have for patients, hospitals, and the bill-paying public are obvious. Additional negative results would suggest that many legislative bodies and regulatory agencies were presumptuous in requiring hospitals to conduct analyses of incidents.

A major component of the growth of hospital costs in the last decade is the insurance that must be taken out for professional liability or hospital malpractice. Hospital's premiums increased more than 80 percent in 1969 and 1970; thereafter, annual increases were on the order of 10 to 20 percent, until a 64 percent increase occurred in 1976 [1]. The American Hospital Association reports that, in 1972, $200 million was spent by hospitals for liability insurance; that figure had risen to $1.2 billion in 1977. Such insurance was estimated to account for 2.5 percent or more of overall hospital costs [2]. It has been estimated that, if

---

Address communications and requests for reprints to Richard A. Elnicki, Professor of Decision and Information Sciences, College of Business Administration, University of Florida, Gainesville, FL 32611. John P. Schmitt is Assistant Professor of Health and Hospital Administration at the University of Florida.

the present trend continues, these costs will have increased tenfold by 1989 [3]. Such cost increases illustrate the situation popularly labeled the medical malpractice "crisis." It has been increasingly argued that the best solution to this crisis is the prevention of occurrences that are not, or may not be, "consistent with the routine care" of a particular patient in a health care facility [4].

Throughout the United States, legislation has been initiated to require hospitals to implement patient-incident prevention programs, including the investigation and analysis of the frequency and causes of general categories and specific types of adverse incidents [5-9]. Further, a number of national health care organizations have supported the use of analytical methods in incident prevention programs as a basis for loss prevention efforts [10-12]. However, we found no research in related literature to support the hypothesis that systematic analytical studies yield information about various classes of patient incidents and the factors that contribute to them.[1]

The large Florida hospital that participated in the study preferred to remain anonymous. This significantly reduced the specific data that could be included in this report of the results. Such data on location, demographics, occupancy, and case mix, for example, could have provided the reader with useful insights on the research results.

Hospital Risk Management Programs

Hospital risk management, or liability control, refers to a systematic, hospital-wide program designed to reduce preventable injuries and accidents and to minimize the severity of financial claims [13]. Few such programs existed before the 1974 medical malpractice crisis. As insurance companies began to withdraw from the professional liability market, hospitals throughout the country were left with the risk of financial loss arising from malpractice claims. As a result, hospital risk management programs were implemented by several concerned hospitals and medical centers. Many state legislatures, eager to remedy the crisis, required hospitals throughout their respective states to adopt similar measures [6-8].

Some state legislatures have explicitly stated that hospital risk management programs should contain certain components. For example, in 1976, Florida's legislature passed an act requiring all hospitals to implement risk management programs that include:

1. Investigation and analysis of the frequency and causes of general categories and specific types of adverse incidents causing injury to patients
2. Development of appropriate measures to minimize the risk of injuries and adverse incidents to patients through the cooperative efforts of all personnel
3. Analysis of patient grievances that relate to patient care and the quality of medical services
4. Development and implementation of an incident-reporting system based upon the duty of all health care providers and all agents and employees of the health care facility to report injuries and adverse incidents to the hospital risk manager [6].

Support for these features can be found in publications of a number of national health care organizations [10–12, 14].

As evidenced by the Florida legislation, there is a consensus that risk management programs should employ analytical methods to prevent patient injuries. One of the strongest endorsements of this approach appears in a recommendation made by the Secretary of Health, Education and Welfare's Commission on Medical Malpractice:

> The Commission RECOMMENDS the development of intensified medical injury prevention programs for every health care institution in the nation, such programs to be predicated on the following:
>
> 1. [I]nvestigation and analysis of the frequency and causes of the general categories and specific types of adverse incidents causing injury to patients
> 2. [D]evelopment of appropriate measures to minimize the risk of injuries and adverse incidents to patients through the cooperative efforts of all persons. [12]

The hypothesis underlying this recommendation is that quantitative, or analytic, studies of patient incidents will identify contributory factors which, when controlled, will prevent the occurrence of adverse patient incidents.

Our research was motivated by the possibility that incidents could be related probabilistically to patient and hospital environmental characteristics as suggested by [10–12]. This possibility is consistent with a risk management concept concerning liability: loss reduction is the reduction of hazards found in hospital situations and conditions and in patient actions and attitudes [13]. If such relationships could be established, and if incidents could be related probabilistically to patient health impairment, court cases, and settlements, then a method of systematic reduction of the latter was also possible. Hence, we focused on whether incidents could be related to patient and hospital environmental characteristics. If, say, staffing was related to incidents, the hospital could change staff. Similarly, if patients with a given personal characteristic were associated with more frequent adverse incidents, the hospital might be able to adjust resources or resource allocations accordingly. If incidents increased when there was a full moon because bright nights kept patients awake and walking in rooms and corridors, different window shades might lower the number of incidents by allowing patients to sleep. No literature was found to support or help direct the study of these kinds of questions.

The quantitative research we found in the literature was limited to listings and sorts by various characteristics included in actual incident reports [14–16]. Such data indicate what characteristics existed in settings in which adverse incidents occurred—they do not indicate whether the same characteristics existed in settings in which there were no incidents. Therefore, they do not indicate whether given characteristics are probabilistically related to incidents.

Research Hypothesis, Study Variables, and Sources of Data

The lack of systematic research on the relationship between incidents and various patient hospital environmental characteristics led us to develop a simple prediction model. The number of types of incidents per day on a nursing service was estimated given patient characteristics, hospital environmental characteristics, and their interactions on that service that day. Three types of incidents were estimated: falls, medication errors, and others. The null hypothesis is that the types of patient incidents are not a function of patient characteristics, hospital environment characteristics, or their interactions.

In testing the hypothesis, we assumed that ten nursing service units were appropriate observation units (see Table 1). For example, the importance of various numbers of a set of factors influencing incidents in a psychiatric unit was considered to be different in a surgical unit. In addition, the choice of nursing service provided a weak measure of case mix. Incidents occurring in other services such as the emergency room, clinics, and surgical suites are not included. A linear

Table 1: Nursing Units

Nursing Unit	*Percentage of All Beds*
Psychiatric	7
Pediatric	10
General Surgery	9
Surgical Specialties	13
Medical	12
Obstetrics and Gynecology	9
Ambulant	5
Adolescent	7
Surgical-Two	5
Medical-Two	3
Total*	80

*The hospital had over 10,000 emergency room visits and over 50,000 other outpatient visits during the study period, but incidents occurring in these areas are not included.

relationship was estimated for each of the three types of incidents for each of the ten nursing service units using ordinary least squares.

Appendix A discusses the considerations and limitations that led to the simple predictive model, the observation basis, and the use of ordinary least squares for estimation. The dependent variable is the number of patients who had an adverse incident during a given day in a given setting. We used frequency of incidents rather than actual claims because claims grow out of incidents and amount to less than 1 percent of reported incidents in the hospital. The independent variables include patient characteristics, hospital environment factors, and interactions in the settings. Patient days, a weighted census discussed further on, and other factors are included in the hospital environment variable set to reflect the total care setting. This eliminated the major shortcoming of earlier studies, which considered various incidents and sets of characteristics without considering the same sets of characteristics when no incidents occurred [14–16].

Classes of the dependent variable were established by dividing the hospital's incidents into the principal injury categories used by the National Association of Insurance Commissioners (NAIC) [17]. The three most common were accidental falls, adverse effects of drugs (medication errors), and miscellaneous (other). This distribution is consistent with the distribution of claims reported to the NAIC. Appendix B contains definitions of the three incident classes.

The system used by the hospital for reporting incidents had been in existence for three years. Incidents are reported by physicians, nurses, ancillary professionals, or other hospital personnel who witness injuries or errors. The type, location, date, and other features of the incident are recorded on either an "incident report" or a "medication variance report" form. The forms are forwarded to the hospital's risk manager, who reviews them and oversees any related investigations. The reports are sorted into one of the three incident categories described above and are filed in chronological order. Incidents suggesting hospital liability have a supplementary claim file set up to facilitate additional investigation and monitoring. Effort is underway to automate the filing system to enhance loss prevention efforts.

Our study used 432 reported incidents (see Table 2). Data were collected for each day in January, March, May, July, September, and November 1977. We selected alternate months to control for possible seasonal effects. Each day in each recorded month was treated as an observation unit, yielding a total of 184. The patient factors included physical, medical, financial, religious, and attitude characteristics of patients in locations where incidents were reported. Similarly, hospital factors included physical, work load, staffing, education, and environmental characteristics of locations where patients received routine daily care.

We developed specific factors on the basis of a review of related literature [18, 19] and interviews with key hospital personnel. The limited availability of daily measures for each of the ten nursing units restricted the investigation to an analysis of 23 patient-characteristic and hospital-environment variables. Since the study was exploratory, we added several environmental factors that were available from hospital records but that were not found in related literature or suggested by hospital variables. This gave us 36 interaction variables, bringing the total number of explanatory variables studied to 59. Table 3 contains definitions of the dependent and independent variables used in the study.[2]

RESULTS

None of the 30 estimated equations gave results from which logical policy recommendations could be made. The highest R^2, 0.489, was for medication errors on the surgical-two unit (Table 4). Although significant at conventional levels, the findings did little to explain why incidents occurred. More important, the significant beta coefficients in the estimate did not allow us to develop recommendations that might help the hospital reduce incidents. Table 5 shows the beta coefficients signif-

Table 2: Distribution of Incidents by Type

*Incident**	*Number*	*Percent*
Accidental falls	166	38
Medication errors	137	32
Other incidents	129	30
Total	432	100

*In the aggregate, there was a 0.0081 chance of a patient experiencing an incident on any given day of the study (incidents per patient day = 0.0081).

icant at the 0.01 level from all 30 estimated equations. Other tests indicated that multicollinearity among patient and environment variables was not a problem.

The estimate for MEDERROR surgical-two unit did not include any hospital environment factor significant at the 0.01 level. Two patient characteristics, CHRISTN and OTHERELIG, were significant at 0.01. Significant (0.01) interaction variables gave contradictory results. Medication errors on the unit were negatively related to greater numbers of patients and greater numbers of indigent patients (INDI*PATDAY). Conversely, medication errors on the unit were positively related to more nursing staff on duty and to greater numbers of self-paying patients (SELF*NURS) but negatively related to more indigent patients and more nursing staff on duty (INDI*NURS). A more general interaction variable for nursing staff and patient day, which was included in preliminary estimates, was not found to be significant in any equation.

Overall, there was no consistent pattern of significant variables across nursing units at the 0.01 level (or at the 0.05 level). Of the 30 estimates, 17 did not include any significant beta coefficients at the 0.01 level (Table 6). Six of the estimates did not include significant coefficients at the 0.05 level. Only 28 (1.6 percent) of the 1,770 estimated beta coefficients were significant at the 0.05 level. Using a simple difference between proportions test (assuming the 0.05 is not too close to 0), it follows that these aggregate results could easily have been found by drawing sample data from random numbers (t = -0.055).

At the 0.01 level, only two hospital environment factors were significant: RNLESSEX for FALLS in the obstetrics and gynecology unit and EXHOKEEP for MEDERROR in the medical unit. Variables for the interaction of hospital environment and patient characteristics entered estimates only 13 times, while FULLMOON entered estimates independently or through interaction with other variables

Table 3: Definition of Variables

Variable	*Definition*
	Dependent Variables
FALLS	Unintentional falls by patients
MEDERROR	Erroneous administration of drugs and intravenous solutions
OTHERROR	Other adverse incidents
	Independent Patient Variables
LESSCARE	Needing less than routine care
INTCAREPT	Needing above average or intensive care
LONGSTAYPT	On a nursing unit 12 days or longer
PEDPT	Age 15 and under
ELDER	Age 60 and over
MALE	Men
MARRIED	Married
JEWISH	Jewish
CHRISTN	Protestant or Roman Catholic
OTHERELIG	Other religious denominations
SELFPAY	Full and personal responsibility for hospital charges
INSURPT	Some form of third party coverage for hospital charges
INDIGENT	Unable to pay hospital charges
COMPLNT	Written or verbal complaints filed with the patient relations department about nursing care, housekeeping, or other patient services
	Independent Hospital Variables
WORKLOAD	Number of patients processed for discharge or transfer out of the nursing unit
PATDAY	Number of patients on the unit at the census-taking hour, weighted by three nursing care factors
NURSTAFF	Full-time nursing staff on duty, including RNs, LPNs, and NAs
RNSTAFF	Ratio of RNs to total nursing staff
MNTVISIT	Equipment repairs, preventive maintenance checks, and emergency repairs or replacements on the unit
EXHOKEEP	Housekeeping staff is twice the average number
INSERVED	In-service education program on the unit
RNLESSEX	RNs with less than one month's working experience in the hospital
FULLMOON	Occurrence of a full moon
	Interaction Variables
INT*WORK	INTCAREPT with WORKLOAD
INT*PATDAY	INTCAREPT with PATDAY
INT*NURS	INTCAREPT with NURSTAFF
INT*RN	INTCAREPT with RNSTAFF
INT*RNLESSEX	INTCAREPT with RNLESSEX

Continued

Table 3: Continued

Variable	*Definition*
INT*FULL	INTCAREPT with FULLMOON
LONG*WORK	LONGSTAYPT with WORKLOAD
LONG*PATDAY	LONGSTAYPT with PATDAY
LONG*NURS	LONGSTAYPT with NURSTAFF
LONG*RN	LONGSTAYPT with RNSTAFF
LONG*RNLESSEX	LONGSTAYPT with RNLESSEX
LONG*FULL	LONGSTAYPT with FULLMOON
JEW*WORK	JEWISH with WORKLOAD
JEW*PATDAY	JEWISH with PATDAY
JEW*NURS	JEWISH with NURSTAFF
JEW*RN	JEWISH with RNSTAFF
JEW*RNLESSEX	JEWISH with RNLESSEX
JEW*FULL	JEWISH with FULLMOON
SELF*WORK	SELFPAY with WORKLOAD
SELF*PATDAY	SELFPAY with PATDAY
SELF*NURS	SELFPAY with NURSTAFF
SELF*RN	SELFPAY with RNSTAFF
SELF*RNLESSEX	SELFPAY with RNLESSEX
SELF*FULL	SELFPAY with FULLMOON
INDI*WORK	INDIGENT with WORKLOAD
INDI*PATDAY	INDIGENT with PATDAY
INDI*NURS	INDIGENT with NURSTAFF
INDI*RN	INDIGENT with RNSTAFF
INDI*RNLESSEX	INDIGENT with RNLESSEX
INDI*FULL	INDIGENT with FULLMOON
COMP*WORK	COMPLNT with WORKLOAD
COMP*PATDAY	COMPLNT with PATDAY
COMP*NURS	COMPLNT with NURSTAFF
COMP*RN	COMPLNT with RNSTAFF
COMP*RNLESSEX	COMPLNT with RSLESSEX
COMP*FULL	COMPLNT with FULLMOON

seven times at the 0.01 level. There was no difference in the occurrence of significant variables by type at the 0.05 level and higher. Using 30 equations, we estimated 1,080 beta coefficients for interaction variables, one fewer than the 55 that were significant at the 0.05 level or higher. Similarly, 5 percent of the variable beta coefficients estimated is 34; 33 were significant at the 5 percent level or higher. Hence, the results do not suggest the types of variables that should be used in future research.

Estimates were also made without using nursing unit partitions, thus expanding the replication of cases. Linear and log-linear estimates were made by pooling the dependent and independent variables. The results are shown in Table 7. While all the estimates were significant at

Table 4: MEDERROR Regression Data for the Surgical-Two Unit

Variable[†]	*Coefficient*	*Standard Error*	*F-Value*[‡]
Patient			
LESSCARE	-0.000	0.008	0.00
INTCAREPT	-0.012	0.009	1.81
LONGSTAYPT	0.080	0.075	1.13
PEDPT	0.000	0.007	0.00
ELDER	0.005	0.003	2.57
MALE	0.006	0.003	3.09
MARRIED	0.003	0.005	0.53
JEWISH	0.073	0.075	0.93
CHRISTN	-0.015	0.005	10.74[§]
OTHERELIG	-0.021	0.007	9.61[§]
SELFPAY	0.022	0.057	0.15
INSURPT	0.010	0.004	6.62[‖]
INDIGENT	-0.002	0.038	0.00
COMPLNT	0.000	0.000	0.00
Hospital			
WORKLOAD	-0.006	0.008	0.53
PATDAY	0.006	0.004	3.28
NURSTAFF	0.006	0.008	0.37
RNSTAFF	0.134	0.220	0.37
MNTVISIT	0.001	0.010	0.01
EXHOKEEP	0.011	0.017	0.37
INSERVED	0.005	0.034	0.02
RNLESSEX	-0.057	0.095	0.36
FULLMOON	0.141	0.261	0.29
Interaction			
INT*WORK	0.001	0.001	0.85
INT*PATDAY	0.000	0.000	1.81
INT*NURS	0.000	0.000	0.09
INT*RN	-0.018	0.014	1.57
INT*RNLESSEX	0.001	0.006	0.02
INT*FULL	-0.021	0.038	0.29
LONG*WORK	-0.000	0.003	0.00
LONG*PATDAY	-0.000	0.001	0.10
LONG*NURS	-0.003	0.004	0.63
LONG*RN	-0.090	0.105	0.74
LONG*RNLESSEX	0.040	0.066	0.37
LONG*FULL	0.016	0.054	0.09
JEW*WORK	-0.007	0.005	1.92
JEW*PATDAY	0.001	0.002	0.15

Continued

Table 4: Continued

Variable†	*Coefficient*	*Standard Error*	F-*Value*‡
JEW*NURS	-0.002	0.004	0.31
JEW*RN	-0.089	0.149	0.36
JEW*RNLESSEX	-0.089	0.098	0.84
JEW*FULL	0.025	0.120	0.04
SELF*WORK	-0.002	0.003	0.45
SELF*PATDAY	-0.004	0.000	24.63§
SELF*NURS	0.010	0.003	9.16§
SELF*RN	0.015	0.081	0.03
SELF*RNLESSEX	0.054	0.064	0.70
SELF*FULL	0.113	0.203	0.31
INDI*WORK	0.004	0.002	5.34‖
INDI*PATDAY	0.002	0.001	12.08§
INDI*NURS	-0.007	0.002	10.60§
INDI*RN	0.021	0.056	0.14
INDI*RNLESSEX	0.009	0.015	0.33
INDI*FULL	-0.006	0.028	0.05
COMP*WORK	0.000	0.000	0.00
COMP*PATDAY	0.000	0.000	0.00
COMP*NURS	0.000	0.000	0.00
COMP*RN	0.000	0.000	0.00
COMP*RNLESSEX	0.000	0.000	0.00
COMP*FULL	0.000	0.000	0.00

†Variable definitions are given in Table 3.
‡F (52, 113) = 2.08. Theoretical F (60, 120) = 1.47 @ .01; 1.32 @ 0.05. R^2 = 0.489.
§Significant at the 0.01 level.
‖Significant at the 0.05 level.

the 0.01 level (because of the size of n), they explain little; multicollinearity among patient and environment variables was a problem. Further, the R^2 values were all substantially lower than those found when nursing units were divided into categories (see Table 6). This finding tentatively suggests that nursing units may be of value as design partitions in future studies.

Conclusions and Implications

The results clearly imply that adverse patient incidents cannot be predicted by observing the patient-characteristic and hospital-environment factors used in this study. In no case did the results suggest policies or practices that hospital management might find useful in

Table 5: Variables from 30 Estimates (Significant at 0.01 Level)

Dependent Variable	*Nursing Unit*	*Independent Variable*	*Level of Significance*	
Accidental falls	Psychiatric	INTCAREPT	0.003	+
	Pediatric	FULLMOON	0.001	+
		INDI*FULL	0.001	-
		JEW*FULL	0.004	-
	Obstetrics and Gynecology	RNLESSEX	0.001	+
		INT*RNLESSEX	0.001	-
	Adolescent	CHRISTN	0.004	+
Medication errors	Pediatric	SELF*NURS	0.003	-
	General Surgery	JEW*WORK	0.010	+
	Medical	EXHOKEEP	0.001	+
		LONG*WORK	0.006	+
	Ambulant	INT*RNLESSEX	0.001	+
		INT*FULL	0.004	-
		INDI*RNLESSEX	0.007	-
	Adolescent	INDI*WORK	0.003	-
	Surgical-Two	CHRISTN	0.001	-
		OTHERELIG	0.002	-
		SELF*PATDAY	0.001	-
		INDI*PATDAY	0.001	+
		INDI*NURS	0.001	-
		SELF*NURS	0.003	+
Other incidents	Pediatric	JEW*RNLESSEX	0.003	+
		INDI*RNLESSEX	0.007	+
		JEW*FULL	0.010	-
		INDI*FULL	0.010	-
	Surgical-Two	LONG*RNLESSEX	0.003	-
	Medical-Two	MALE	0.001	+
		INDI*FULL	0.001	-

reducing the number of incidents. However, the results do suggest that the authors of related literature and legislation may have been presumptuous in assuming that patient injuries could be prevented by requiring hospitals to study the frequency and characteristics of incidents. Our study only maintained the null hypothesis for one hospital's experience, and we were constrained in our use of data. No research has demonstrated that the costly studies required of hospitals are effective.

One implication of the study's statistical results is that each incident may have a unique set of contributing factors, which would preclude the use of factor effects in making reliable predictions of similar incidents. This is not to say that incident, patient, and hospital environment data should not be recorded and stored for analysis: a major

Table 6: Summary Measures of Equation 7

*Type of Incident**	*Nursing Unit*	R^2	*F(52, 113)*†	*Significant Variables*‡ (at 0.05)	*Significant Variables*‡ (at 0.01)
Accidental falls	Psychiatric	0.243	0.70	2	1
	Pediatric	0.352	1.18	1	3
	General Surgery	0.190	0.48	0	0
	Surgical Specialties	0.249	0.72	0	0
	Medical	0.267	0.77	1	0
	Obstetrics and Gynecology	0.394	1.39	1	2
	Ambulant	0.230	0.62	0	0
	Adolescent	0.331	1.16	4	1
	Surgical-Two	0.272	0.81	0	0
	Medical-Two	0.323	0.17	5	0
Medication errors	Psychiatric	0.138	0.35	0	0
	Pediatric	0.370	1.28	5	1
	General Surgery	0.348	1.09	1	1
	Surgical Specialties	0.303	0.94	1	0
	Medical	0.391	1.36	3	2
	Obstetrics and Gynecology	0.274	0.80	3	0
	Ambulant	0.408	1.44	1	3
	Adolescent	0.372	1.38	4	1
	Surgical-Two	0.489	2.08	2	6
	Medical-Two	0.317	1.04	3	0
Other incidents	Psychiatric	0.357	1.21	2	0
	Pediatric	0.329	1.06	5	4
	General Surgery	0.257	0.70	2	0
	Surgical Specialties	0.331	1.07	2	0
	Medical	0.251	0.71	2	0
	Obstetrics and Gynecology	0.222	0.61	2	0
	Ambulant	0.199	0.52	1	0
	Adolescent	0.172	0.49	0	0
	Surgical-Two	0.278	0.84	4	1
	Medical-Two	0.457	1.88	3	2

*The types of incidents are defined in Appendix B.
†Theoretical $F(60, 120) = 1.47$ @ 0.01; 1.32 @ 0.05.
‡Total variables significant at the 0.05 level or better, 88; at the 0.01 level or better, 28.

limitation of this and other related research has been the unavailability of such data [16, 20–22]. Rather, injury prevention programs should focus on the details of each incident as it occurs. Investigative findings may lead to specific corrective action.

As more complete data on patient injuries become available, hos-

Table 7: Estimates of Incidents Pooled over Nursing Stations

Dependent Variable	*Estimation Form*	R^2	$F(57, 1615)$*
Accidental falls	Linear	0.056	1.67
	Log-linear	0.054	1.63
Medication errors	Linear	0.079	2.43
	Log-linear	0.065	1.99
Other incidents	Linear	0.054	1.62
	Log-linear	0.068	2.09

*Theoretical $F(60, \infty) = 1.47$ at 0.01.

pitals may be able to develop prevention policies using empirical studies [23]. However, legislators and national health care spokesmen must recognize that it is erroneous to assume that health care organizations that are not recording sufficient data can conduct more meaningful analytic studies. Moreover, governmental bodies should support research efforts, which could lead to greater cost effectiveness in hospitals. They should not aggravate an already critical situation by imposing costly requirements that have no basis in theory or practice.

The results also suggest some directions for future research. Categorizing patients by the type of nursing care they require, for example, appears preferable to the pooling of all patients. Our design, which encompassed daily observations of incidents, patient characteristics, and hospital environment factors for a single hospital, was not useful. A nursing shift as an observation unit was considered early in this research, but limitations on our data precluded its use. Perhaps a design that includes data collection over a planned period would eliminate many of the limitations imposed on this study by available data.

In this study, patients' incident and related data for each day at a nursing station were aggregated for observations. A logical alternative would be to measure incident and related data for each patient day at a nursing station or for each patient at each shift at a nursing station (per Equation 2 in Appendix B). The incident measure would be 1 for an incident and 0 for no incident. The relationship between the (0,1) dependent variables and independent variables could be estimated with a logit procedure. The resulting beta weights would give incident probabilities related to the explanatory variables.

It should be noted that this study was a first step in the systematic analysis of patient incidents. The results are not sufficient to allow a conclusion on whether or not such studies can provide an empirical basis for reducing adverse patient incidents in hospitals. This attempt at formal incorporation of hospital practices, professional opinions, and legislative requirements in a simple predictive model for one hospital proved unsuccessful. Similar results could be found by sampling from random numbers. However, this initial research effort prompts a number of questions. Is the model erroneously specified? Are preventive ideas in the literature and legislation wrong? Are incidents in hospitals correctly described as a random process? Researched answers to these questions could help in the formulation of reasoned public policy for countering the nation's malpractice crisis.

APPENDIX A

MODEL DEVELOPMENT AND ESTIMATION METHODOLOGY

We attempt to answer a question about risk management that has apparently been assumed as validated by various legislative bodies throughout the country. Can incidents be predicted for given patient (P) and hospital environment (E) characteristics? The development of the predictive model used in this study to address the question included the following considerations. The literature suggests that incidents (Y) are a function of P, E, and/or their interaction (PE):

$$Y = f(P, E, PE) \quad (1)$$

For example, an alert ambulatory patient could fall while walking in an area with no hazards, $Y = f(P)$. An alert patient could fall after being given the wrong medication, $Y = f(E)$. A sedated patient, otherwise alert, could fall from a bed because the attendant moving him slipped on a wet floor, $Y = f(PE)$. We record the actual incident experienced by the patient and place it in one of three categories: accidental falls, medication errors, and other incidents.

In a given time frame, a patient with a set of measurable characteristics in a hospital location with a set of measurable characteristics either does or does not experience an incident. If no incident occurs, Y is zero for that patient. If an incident does take place, the question arises, How should Y be measured? Marginal impairment of patient health and marginal cost to the hospital were ruled out as possibilities because of quantification problems in making direct estimates for all patients experiencing incidents. If the only patients considered were those who experienced incidents requiring negotiated or court settlements, the number of nonzero dependent variables would be too small for any significant statistical results. Hence, the available information on a patient's incident was used, the condition 1 indicating that an incident took place. This is a gross measure, one dictated by the realities of measurement limitations.

Thus the basic model construct was established. In a given time frame for n patients with a set P and a set E, there exists a matrix:

Patient	Y	P	E	
1	0	$p_{1,1}, p_{1,2}, \ldots, p_{1,m}$	$e_{1,1}, e_{1,2}, \ldots, e_{1,k}$	
2	0	$p_{2,1}, p_{2,2}, \ldots, p_{2,m}$	$e_{2,1}, e_{2,2}, \ldots, e_{2,k}$	
3	1	$p_{3,1}, p_{3,2}, \ldots, p_{3,m}$	$e_{3,1}, e_{3,2}, \ldots, e_{3,k}$	(2)
	. . .			
n	0	$p_{n,1}, p_{n,2}, \ldots, p_{n,m}$	$e_{n,1}, e_{n,2}, \ldots, e_{n,k}$	

One objective of the research was to determine whether any systematic relationships could be found. Such relationships suggest that the hospital management either modify controllable E characteristics or plan procedures that anticipate given E and P characteristics, when possible, so the number of incidents could be reduced. The data construct in Equation 2 could be analyzed using logit procedures, but practical realities constrained the research. Data did not exist to build the construct in Equation 2. Enough hospital reports did exist to build the following vector for n patients in each nursing unit for each day for each type of incident:

$$\sum_n Y \quad \sum_n p_1 \quad \sum_n p_2 \quad \ldots \quad \sum_n p_m \quad \sum_n e_1 \quad \sum_n e_2 \quad \ldots \quad \sum_n e_k \tag{3}$$

We initially thought the aggregations in Equation 3 could be done by nursing shift, instead of by day. However, data by shift were not available for many variables.

Equation 3, a column-by-column summation of Equation 2, can be restated in the form used in Equation 1, where $X = \Sigma Y$. X is the number of incidents on a nursing service for a day for each of the three types of incidents considered in the study.

$$X = f(P, E, PE) \tag{4}$$

The relationship in Equation 4 in the context of the study observation base is

$$X_t = f(p_{i,t}, e_{i,t}, pe_{i,t}) \tag{5}$$

where X_t is the number of incidents in each injury classification in the t th time period (24 hours), $e_{i,t}$ is the ith environment factor of a nursing service in the t th time period, and $p_{i,t}$ is the ith characteristic of patients in a nursing station in the t th time period; $pe_{i,t}$ are interaction terms.

A set of 23 patient and environment factors was considered, $e'_{i,t}$ and $p'_{i,t}$, as a subset of all possible factors. Hence, the excluded factors, $e''_{i,t}$ and $p''_{i,t}$, are assumed as given, with randomly distributed effects. Therefore, the relationship estimated for each nursing station and type of incident is

$$X_t = f(e'_{i,t}, p'_{i,t}, pe'_{i,t} \mid e''_{i,t}, p''_{i,t}) \tag{6}$$

A linear relationship was estimated for each nursing station

$$X_t = B_o + B_i e'_{i,t} + B_j p'_{j,t} + B_k pe'_{k,t} + v_t \tag{7}$$

using ordinary least squares, assuming the error term is normally distributed with a mean equal to 0 and a variance of σ_t^2, $[v_t \sim N(0, \sigma_t^2)]$. This estimation method is supported by conclusions in [10, 12, 24].

The estimation form was motivated by the nature of the variables available for study. Most of the included variables were continuous (cardinal) measures of patient and environment characteristics. Hence, the linear form was first used, since the variable coefficients permitted marginal measures of contributions by the various characteristics to incidents. The results of the linear analyses led to the association measures given by Spearman rank correlation coefficients; they did not differ in substance from the results reported in this article.

Other estimation forms were considered. As noted above, data limitations precluded the use of logit. Another alternative was to divide the dependent variable (the number of incidents) by patient days (midnight census), exclude patient days from the independent variables (to avoid specification errors), and use probit for the estimations. This choice was not aided by theory, and the lack of multicollinearity problems led to the presentation of ordinary least-squares results.

APPENDIX B

DEFINITIONS OF INCIDENT CLASSES

Accidental Falls (FALLS). An accidental fall was defined as an unintentional fall by a patient. Falls of visitors and staff members were not used in the study. The following types of recorded falls were included in this category:

Falls—different levels
  From bed
    Rails up

Rails down
Rail position not indicated
From chair, wheelchair, stool
From stretcher
From table
Not otherwise classified
Falls—same level
Patient room
Patient bathroom
Corridor
Waiting area
Not otherwise classified
Falls—transportation
Falls—equipment malfunction.

Medication Errors (MEDERROR). A medication error was defined as an erroneous administration of either drugs or intravenous solutions. The following types of reported incidents were included in this category:

Drug variances
Wrong patient
Wrong drug
Wrong dosage
Wrong route
Wrong time
In wrong site
Out-of-date drug
Out-of-date order
Adverse drug response
Medication self-administered
Medication not given
Discontinued medication given
Communication
Drugs unavailable
Pharmacy error
Drug incompatibility
Defective equipment
Not otherwise classified
Transfusion-intravenous solution
Wrong dosage
Wrong rate

- Wrong time
- Without permit
- Equipment malfunction
- Not otherwise classified

Diagnostic procedures

- Wrong time
- Wrong patient
- Wrong body part
- Wrong procedure
- Without permit
- Incomplete permit
- Equipment malfunction
- Not otherwise classified

Miscellaneous

- Temperature extremes
- Struck by
- Struck against
- Caught in, on, between (pinch points)
- Smoking
- Intentional self-harm
- Assault or battery
- Animal or insect bite
- Human bite
- Patient behavior
- Procedure variance
- Equipment failure.

Notes

1. The literature review included the following insurance journals and trade publications from January 1975 to January 1980: *Journal of Risk and Insurance, Bests' Review, Risk Management, Insurance Law Journal, Journal of American Insurance, Rough Notes, National Underwriter, Weekly Underwriter,* and *Insurance Salesman*. It also included the following health care journals: *Inquiry, Health Services Research*, and *Hospitals, Journal of the American Hospital Association*.
2. A table containing the means and standard deviations of the variables (with 1,240 entries) is available from the authors.

REFERENCES

1. Munch, P. *Causes of the Medical Malpractice Insurance "Crisis": Risks and Regulations*. Santa Monica, CA: The RAND Corporation, 1976.
2. Vanderpool, W. Case notes on cost containment and malpractice insurance. *Appalachian Business Review* 6(3):38, 1979.
3. Rubsamen, D. S. Medical malpractice. *Scientific American* 235(2):18, 1976.
4. Florida Department of Insurance. *Rules of the Department of Insurance Chapter 4-40 Medical Incident Patient Compensation Program*. Tallahassee, FL: Department of Insurance, 1976.
5. National Association of Insurance Commissioners. *NAIC Malpractice Claims* 2(3):1976.
6. State of Florida. *An Act Relating to Medical Malpractice and Medical Liability Insurance Amending s627.352(5)*. Florida Statutes Sec. #395.18, c. 76-260, no. 586, 1976.
7. State of Michigan. *Plan of Operation, Review, Approval, Amendment, Reports*. Michigan Statutes, Sec. 500.2507, P.A. 1975, No. 43, 1975.
8. State of Pennsylvania. *Chapter 5A—Health Care Services Malpractice*. Pennsylvania Statutes, Sec. 810, P.L. 390, No. 111, 1975.
9. Thistle, M. G. A look at the causes and possible solutions. *Risk Management* 24(7):7, 1977.
10. Federation of American Hospitals. Hospitals cautioned to identify areas of problems before incident occurs. *Review* 10(1):37, 1977.
11. Maryland Hospital Education Institute. *Controlling Hospital Liability: A Systems Approach*. Chicago, IL: American Hospital Association, 1976, p. 1.
12. U.S. Department of Health, Education and Welfare. *Report of the Secretary's Commission on Medical Malpractice*. Washington, DC: Government Printing Office, 1973.
13. Mehr, R., and B. A. Hedges. *Risk Management Concepts and Applications*. Homewood, IL: Richard D. Irwin, 1974, p. 99.
14. Ashby, J. L., and S. B. Pearson. *Study of Hospital Injury Prevention Programs*. Rockville, MD: Applied Management Sciences, 1976.
15. Federation of American Hospitals. FAH manual outlines control programs on risk management for hospital use. *Review* 10(1):13, 1977.
16. Korsak, A. WESTAT 1976 study focuses on closed claims in hospital settings. *Hospitals, Journal of the American Hospital Association* 53(6):48, 1979.
17. National Association of Insurance Commissioners. *NAIC Malpractice Claims* 1(1):1975.
18. Doherty, E. G., and C. O. Haven. Medical malpractice and negligence—Sociodemographic characteristics of claimants and nonclaimants. *Journal of the American Medical Association* 238(15):1656, 1977.
19. Peterson, J. L. *Department of Health, Education, and Welfare's Report of the Secretary's Commission on Medical Malpractice Appendix*. Washington, DC: Government Printing Office, 1973, pp. 658–91.
20. Federation of American Hospitals. Research called key to minimizing damage suits filed against hospitals. *Review* 10(1):33, 1977.

21. Mikolaj, P. J. Hospital association determines nature of closed claims in state. *Hospitals, Journal of the American Hospital Association* 52(6):53, 1978.
22. Rudov, M. H., T. I. Myers, and A. Mirabella. *Department of Health, Education, and Welfare's Report of the Secretary's Commission on Medical Malpractice Appendix*. Washington, DC: Government Printing Office, 1973, pp. 1–25.
23. Korsak, A. Risk management: Idea and effort widely supported, but appropriate methods debated. *Hospitals, Journal of the American Hospital Association* 53(7):175, 1979.
24. Federation of American Hospitals. Reviewers are high in praise of FAH for its publication of risk manual. *Review* 10(3):36, 1977.

CHAPTER NINE

Regression Model Building: Recursive and Nonrecursive Models

The interrelationship of the health and behavioral characteristics of patients presents a daunting challenge to the analyst. Health status and patient health-related behavior or choice may be a cause or an effect of utilization, or both. Likewise, one component of health behavior may lead to another or may itself be influenced. This fundamental problem can arise in many contexts, affecting many specific instances where health status, utilization, and health care behavior are analyzed. The article by Kuder and Levitz explores the relationship between use of services and whether or not the patient has a usual source of care. The authors posit three models of relationships and seek to determine which is most explanatory.

The authors describe two unidirectional models relating usual source of care to utilization measured in visits. These models are analyzed using ordinary least-squares regression. The third model assumes a two-directional relationship between the variables and requires a two-stage equation approach that includes an intermediate predictor or instrument based on the other variables in the final model. The two-stage regression approach accounts for feedback among variables and is a common method to reduce bias in regression models with complex causal paths. In this instance, rather than using the same technique for all three models, the authors chose to reduce bias further in their estimates by estimating the instrument for the third model using the probit maximum-likelihood technique.

The fact that the three models produce different results testifies to the presence of interactive or feedback effects of variables in complex systems of causation. As the authors point out, the dimensions of the observed effects can lead to diverging conclusions concerning the impact and effectiveness of programs and projects. The model that takes into account mutual causation, however, more closely reflects the reality of the relationship.

Visits to the Physician: An Evaluation of the Usual-Source Effect

John M. Kuder and Gary S. Levitz

Having a regular or usual source for medical care has frequently been found to be an important correlate of ambulatory visits to the physician. However, it remains unclear whether having a usual source is a determinant of visits, a consequence of visits, or both. This article addresses the question, how do these alternative theoretical relationships affect estimates of the relative impact of having a usual source on illness-related visits? The empirical results of a household interview survey generally support the significance of a usual-source variable as a determinant of illness-related visits, but they indicate that use of a single equation-estimation technique may overestimate the magnitude of this effect.

INTRODUCTION

Researchers investigating the utilization of physician services generally assume (often implicitly) either (1) that people who do not have a usual or regular source of medical care face an additional barrier to access compared to individuals with a usual source and, therefore, that they are likely to make fewer visits to the physician; or (2) that having or not

---

The research reported here is based on a project supported by the Veterans Administration Health Services Research and Development Field Program, Ann Arbor, Michigan.

At the time the research was completed, both authors were assistant professors in the Graduate Program in Hospital and Health Administration, The University of Iowa. John Kuder, Ph.D. is currently Director, Center for Applied Research at Henry Ford Hospital in Detroit; and Gary Levitz, Ph.D. is Assistant Director for Special Projects, The University of Iowa Hospitals and Clinics, Iowa City, IA, and Adjunct Associate Professor, The Graduate Program in Hospital and Health Administration, The University of Iowa. Address communications and requests for reprints to John M. Kuder, Director, Center for Applied Research, Henry Ford Hospital, 2799 West Grand Boulevard, Detroit, MI 48202.

having a usual source of care is a consequence of utilization and therefore does not directly affect the number of visits made to a physician. We examine three alternative models of the usual source-utilization relationship to determine if they yield different results and thus yield different policy implications. The analysis presented is insufficient to determine which of the models best reflects the true causal relationship; however, the comparison of the models and the interpretation of coefficients across each model is designed to indicate the likely differences and potential biases that can occur when employing any one of the models in deference to the others. The clarification of this issue is important for our understanding of the impact that having a usual source has on medical service use. It is also relevant to the growing body of literature which indicates that having or not having a usual source is an important determinant of consumer choices among alternative delivery systems—and of the subsequent utilization of services once that choice is made [1, 2].

BACKGROUND

Studies of health services utilization have found an association between individuals and families who report an established relationship with a regular source of medical care and their utilization of medical care services [3–7]. Having a regular or usual source of care has frequently been identified as a facilitator of access and as an indicator that the individual is not alienated from the health delivery system [8–10]. For example, Luft, Hershey, and Morrell found in their study of physician utilization in a rural California sample that individuals reporting no usual source received far fewer physician services than individuals reporting a usual source of care [11]. Adjusting the data for differences in health status, age, sex, and insurance coverage, Luft et al. found individuals without a usual source to have had one-third fewer physician visits and to be less than half as likely to have had a checkup during the year prior to the interview when compared with individuals reporting a usual source. Lave et al., using a large sample of individuals in East Palo Alto, California, found that 50 percent of adults with a usual source made a preventive visit during the year before the interview while only 28 percent of adults without a usual source made such a visit [12].

A recent report of data from the National Health Care Expenditures Study estimates that about 14.2 percent of the U.S. population was without a usual source of care in 1977, up from the 1970 figure of 11 percent [13]. This study also estimated that about 4 million of those people were without a usual source of medical care because their usual source was no longer available. The number of visits to a physician was found to be much lower for those individuals without a usual source. Among individuals 65 years of age and older reporting no usual source because their usual source was no longer available, the annual mean number of physician visits was 2.4, while for those 65 and over with a usual source, the annual mean number of visits was 6.5.

Even though the evidence strongly suggests a significant usual-source effect, conclusions drawn from recent studies are problematic and have been criticized because of the use of an explicit one-way causation paradigm. The general form of these one-way models is exhibited as Model I in Figure 1. Critics have focused specifically on the point that the often-assumed relationship from usual source to use is a misspecified model. Sloan and Bentkover point out that, although several studies have related usual source to ambulatory care use, "such links are somewhat suspect since it is difficult to assume a one-way causation from usual source to use. Heavy users are more likely, holding other factors constant, to obtain a regular source." [14] As a result, having a usual source is generally regarded as a correlate of visits, but it is unknown to what extent it is a determinant of use, a consequence of use, or both. Model II in Figure 1 presents the general form of a model where usual source is only a consequence of use, and Model III presents a model where usual source is both a determinant and a consequence of use. The resolution of this point has significant implications for the conclusions of previous studies utilizing one-way models.

Analytic Framework

The analysis employs a model that is limited to illness-related ambulatory care utilization. Following the Andersen and Aday framework, our model of physician visit demand postulates three categories of explanatory factors: (1) health status/need factors; (2) predisposing factors which reflect social correlates of health-related behavior and the perceived efficacy of the health production process; and (3) enabling factors, including insurance, income, and time factors [15, 16]. The analytic procedures we employed were designed to estimate and compare three models. The models are distinguished by their alternative

Figure 1: Alternative Model Specifications

	Model	Equation(s)	*Variable Relationships Without Error Terms*
I	Usual source as a determinant of visits	(1) $v = f(x,y,US)$	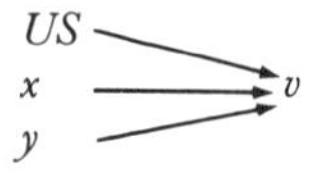
II	Usual source as a consequence of visits	(2) $v = f(x,y)$	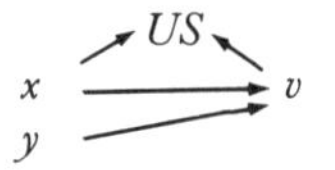
III	Usual source as *both* a determinant and consequence of visits	(3a) $v = f(x,y,US)$ (3b) $US = g(x,z,v)$	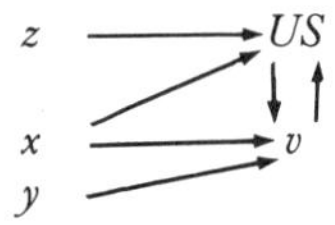

Where: v = illness-related visits to the physician.
US = usual source of medical care.
x,y,z = vectors of need, predisposing, and enabling variables.
f,g = functional operations.

specifications of the relationship between utilization and a variable measuring usual source of care (see Figure 1).

One model (Model I) is based on the assumption that the relationship is one-directional—that having a usual source increases utilization. In this model, usual source is included in a multivariate analysis as an independent explanatory variable. The number of illness-related visits that an individual makes is a function of whether an individual has a usual source of care and other health status/need, predisposing, and enabling variables.

The second model (Model II) is based on the assumption that the relationship is one-directional, but opposite in direction to that assumed in Model I. Therefore, in Model II the usual source variable is not included as a determinant of utilization (since it is a consequence, not a cause). Model II has not had advocates in the literature; however, whenever usual source is omitted from utilization models due to insufficient data or other reasons, this model is the result [17, 18].

The final model (Model III) is based on the assumption that a two-directional relationship exists between usual source and utilization, i.e., that visiting the physician increases the likelihood of having a usual source but that having a usual source also enhances access to a physician and thus increases use. In this model, as in Model I, the number of visits that an individual makes is a function of whether that individual has a usual source of care, and other health status/need, predisposing, and enabling variables. However, in Model III we postulate, in addition, that whether or not the individual has a usual source of care is a function of the number of illness-related visits made, certain health status/need, predisposing, and accessibility variables, plus additional exogenous variables. A more comprehensive development of these alternative models is provided elsewhere [19].

The analysis of these three models employed cross-sectional survey data. As a result, the data are insufficient to determine which model represents the true causal relationship between visits and usual source. The exact nature of the causal relationships might be determined more appropriately in an analysis which somehow establishes the chronological order of events between visits and the establishment of a usual source of care (e.g., a longitudinal panel study). The data employed here do not permit such an analysis.

If a one-directional relationship is estimated when the causal relationship is actually two-directional, regression coefficients of the independent variables will be biased. This potential coefficient bias results from a correlation between the error terms of the explanatory function and the independent variables [20]. In this case, an increase in visits, due to some unknown factor, may be accompanied by an increase in individuals identifying a usual source (via Equation 3(b) in Figure 1). Likewise an increase in the proportion of individuals with a usual source will increase the number of visits in Equation 3(a). Thus, when estimating the influence of usual source on visits using only Equation 3(a), the error terms in the visit function and the usual-source variable are positively correlated. The ordinary least-squares regression technique attributes both of these increases in visits (that due to the unknown factor and that due to increases in the proportion of individuals with a usual source) to the usual-source variable. This implies that if only Equation 3(a) is estimated, and the true model is represented by the two-equation system, Equations 3(a) and 3(b), the estimate of the usual source coefficient will be biased upward. Therefore, in order to obtain unbiased estimates of equation parameters in Model III, the use of a statistical technique for estimating simultaneous equations is required. When appropriately identified, such approaches yield unbiased and consistent estimates of the structural parameters (e.g., the coefficient estimates for the explanatory variables in Model III) [20].

THE DATA AND SAMPLING PROCEDURES

The data are from a household interview survey of residents of Washtenaw County, Michigan. Interviews were conducted to determine health services use, health attitudes, health beliefs, and health behavior. The recall period of the survey was 6 months. Households that were occupied by persons who were residing in the county primarily for the purpose of attending a college or university were not eligible households for purposes of the interview and thus were excluded. The sample was obtained using a multistage sampling technique. An objective selection of a single primary adult respondent (defined as over 17 years of age or married) was made from each household. In this manner, 851 primary adult interviews were completed (77.2 percent response rate). With the further exclusion of women who were pregnant during the recall period, the sample used became 820 adults.

Washtenaw County has a diverse population and economy. The economy includes heavy and light industry, agriculture, and two state universities. This diversity is represented in the sample (see Table 1). On average, the sample is fairly well educated, with over half having at least some college education. The most distinguishing feature of the sample is the completeness of reported insurance coverage. Ninety-three percent reported at least some health insurance, and 69 percent reported at least some coverage for ambulatory care. In addition, there are some substantial differences between individuals reporting a usual source and those without a usual source (see Table 2). Respondents with a usual source reported substantially more illness-related visits to the physician, had more disability days, were slightly older and, on average, had somewhat better health insurance coverage than those without a usual source. Therefore, in order to identify a usual-source effect, we must make a careful attempt to disentangle how much of the increased number of visits is due to having a usual source—independent of the influence of all other factors.

DEFINITION AND MEASUREMENT OF VARIABLES

Table 3 displays the independent variables, their measurement, and their expected impact on the number of illness visits, and Table 4 displays the zero-order correlation matrix of these variables. The explanatory variables and their measurement are common to most

Table 1: Descriptive Statistics for Exogenous Variables

Variable	*Mean*	*Standard Deviation*
No need	2.40	0.66
Chronic	0.64	0.79
Injury	0.17	0.38
Hosp	0.07	0.25
Dis days	4.46	11.73
Age	41.02	16.68
Age^2	1,960.70	1,580.50
Sex	0.55	0.50
Educ	0.55	0.50
Income	7,859.20	5,781.50
Ins A	0.40	0.49
Ins B	0.29	0.46
Ins C	0.24	0.43
Time	48.11	29.62
Appt	2.28	1.11

Table 2: Description of Usual Source Strata by Selected Variables

	Individuals Without Usual Source		*Individuals with Usual Source*	
Variable	*Mean*	*Std. Dev.*	*Mean*	*Std. Dev.*
Illness visits	.23	.68	.77	1.25
Dis days	2.33	7.81	5.00	12.49
No need	2.61	0.56	2.34	0.67
Chronic	0.46	0.71	0.68	0.79
Age	35.85	15.12	42.35	16.82
Income	7,769.40	6,120.90	7,882.30	5,695.50
Ins A	0.33	0.47	0.42	0.49
Ins B	0.35	0.48	0.27	0.45
Ins C	0.20	0.41	0.25	0.43
N =	168		652	

studies of ambulatory care utilization and were chosen because of their demonstrated significance, reliability, and validity. Other often used variables (race, marital status, and employment status) were omitted, because earlier regression estimations found them to be statistically and substantively insignificant as explanatory variables in all models.

The dependent variable, illness visits, is measured by the number of reported illness-related visits to a physician during the recall period

Table 3: Exogenous Variables in Utilization Equation 1

Variable Number	*Name*	*Description*	*Expected Effect on Log Visits*	*Measures*
1	No need	Perceived need for health care compared to persons same age	–	1 = More need for care 2 = About the same 3 = Less
2	Chronic	Number of chronic conditions reported	+	0 = Zero 1 = One 2 = Two or more
3	Injury	Did an injury occur during recall period?	+	0 = No injury 1 = Yes, injury or injuries occurred
4	Hosp	Did a hospitalization occur during recall period?	+	0 = No hospitalization 1 = Yes, at least one episode of hospitalization
5	Dis days	Number of bed-days and/or number of restricted-activity days	+	Number reported during recall period
6	Age	Age of respondent	+	Age reported
7	Age squared	Age^2	–	(Age × age)
8	Sex	Sex of respondent	+	0 = Male 1 = Female
9	Educ	Did respondent attend college?	–	0 = No college 1 = Yes, at least some college attended
10	Income	Income per family member	+	Reported annual family income divided by the number of family members

11	Ins A	Insurance coverage of ambulatory visits to physician, with no deductible	+	0 = No, does not have this type coverage 1 = Yes, does have this type coverage
12	Ins B	Insurance coverage of ambulatory visits but with a deductible	+	0 = No, does not have this type coverage 1 = Yes, does have this type coverage
13	Ins C	Insurance coverage of hospitalization only	+	0 = No, does not have this type coverage 1 = Yes, does have this type coverage
14	Time	Usual travel time to usual source plus expected office wait	-	Combined time in minutes
15	Appt	Usual time between making of appointment and seeing the provider	-	Time in usual days of wait
16	US	Reporting of usual source of care	+	0 = No 1 = Yes
17	PUS	Probit equation prediction of whether individual has usual source of care or not	+	Predicted probability of having a usual source of care based upon probit-equation (maximum likelihood) estimation

Table 4: Zero Order Correlations Between Explanatory Variables

	1	*2*	*3*	*4*	*5*	*6*	*7*
1. No need	1.000						
2. Chronic	-.2589	1.000					
3. Injury	.0501	.0483	1.000				
4. Hosp	-.1301	.2245	-.0491	1.000			
5. Dis days	-.2321	.3260	.0373	.3460	1.000		
6. Age	.0418	.3071	-.1123	-.1466	.1417	1.000	
7. Age squared	.0318	.3080	-.1072	.1452	.1333	.9848	1.000
8. Sex	-.0696	.0236	-.0624	.0236	.0425	.0853	.0937
9. Educ	.0658	-.1047	.0188	-.0998	-.0524	-.1665	-.1727
10. Income	.1202	-.0458	-.0186	-.0152	-.0579	.1101	.0820
11. Ins A	-.0175	-.0186	-.0073	.0832	.0613	.0844	.0687
12. Ins B	.0409	-.0324	-.0323	-.0599	-.0455	.0064	.0165
13. Ins C	-.0480	.0514	-.0210	-.0175	-.0382	-.0167	-.0205
14. Time	-.0611	.0815	-.0129	.0837	.0666	.0095	.0081
15. Appt	.0144	.0048	-.0381	-.0246	-.0070	.0616	.0496
16. US	-.3155	.2669	-.0221	.1342	.2538	.3126	.2875

transformed into natural logarithms. Illness visits are differentiated from well or preventive visits by (1) deleting from the total visits reported the number of "checkup" visits made, and (2) by analyzing further the conditions listed as the "reason for the visit." When chronic, acute, and/or symptomatic conditions were listed, visits were designated as illness related.

The usual source of care variable required two formulations, one for Model I (usual source, US) and one for Model III (predicted usual source, PUS). The reported usual source variable (US) was based on the respondent's answer to two questions in the survey: (1) Is there a *usual* place or doctor that you go to when you are sick or want advice about your health? and (2) During the time you have lived in Washtenaw County, is there a place or person you have gone to for health care three or more times in the last 5 years? If a "yes" answer was given to *either* of the questions, the respondent was coded as having a usual source of care. The creation of PUS is described below.

EQUATION SPECIFICATIONS AND METHODS

The equation specification of Model I can be summarized in equation form as:

Table 4: Continued

8	*9*	*10*	*11*	*12*	*13*	*14*	*15*	*16*
1.000								
-.0971	1.000							
-.0953	.2615	1.000						
-.0170	-.0963	.0539	1.000					
-.0263	.1670	.0568	-.5199	1.000				
.0809	-.0533	-.0292	-.4514	-.3593	1.000			
.0644	-.1186	-.0748	.0511	-.0874	.0022	1.000		
.1499	.1163	.1337	.0398	-.0414	.0419	-.0038	1.000	
.2070	-.1628	.0120	.0838	-.0383	-.0094	.0687	.0760	1.000

$$\begin{aligned}\text{Log Visits} = f(&\text{No need, Chronic, Injury,}\\ &\text{Hosp, Dis days, Age, Age}^2\text{, Sex,}\\ &\text{Educ, Income, Ins A, Ins B,}\\ &\text{Ins C, Time, Appt, US).}\end{aligned} \qquad (4)$$

The equation specification of Model II is identical to Equation 4, except that US has been omitted as an independent variable.

Models I and II were estimated using single-equation, ordinary least-squares regression techniques. Whereas least-squares assumptions are not formally met because of the measurement and distribution of the dependent variable used, alternative maximum likelihood estimates have been found to provide quite similar results at a much higher cost than the least-squares results reported here. These results are in line with work reported elsewhere [21].

In order to estimate Model III, a statistical procedure designed for multi-equation, two-directional causation models was employed so that the biases, discussed earlier, could be removed from parameter estimates. The method used is similar to a two-stage least-squares method, but here, instead of estimating the instrument to replace the reported usual-source variable (US) via least-squares regression, it was estimated by a probit/maximum likelihood technique. The resulting probability values of the usual-source variable (PUS) were then used as an instrumental variable replacing the reported usual-source variable (US). For any given sample observation, PUS is the probability that the individual has a usual source of care. According to Heckman, the use of a probit estimate of a dichotomous variable yields estimates superior on a consistency basis to those generated by the use of a least-squares predicted instrument [22].

The use of this two-stage approach required estimation of an equation to generate the predicted usual-source variable (PUS). The equation used incorporated nine independent variables from the visit equation and two additional exogenous variables found to be significant correlates of US but not significant correlates of visits. The two exogenous variables were the respondent's estimate of the usual frequency of well visits to the physician for checkups, and a variable indicating if the respondent had recently moved into the county. Because the purpose was to generate a measure of the likelihood of having a usual source that is not determined by the number of illness visits actually made, the illness-visit variable was necessarily excluded from this equation. The full specification of this equation and the results of the estimation are available from the authors. The resulting equation system representing Model III met the statistical requirements (rank and order conditions) for using the two-stage estimation technique [20]. The resulting illness-visit equation representing Model III is:

$$\begin{aligned}\text{Log Visits} = f(&\text{No need, Chronic, Injury, Hosp,}\\ &\text{Dis days, Age, Age}^2\text{, Sex, Educ,}\\ &\text{Income, Ins A, Ins B, Ins C, Time,}\\ &\text{Appt, PUS}).\end{aligned} \tag{5}$$

RESULTS

The choice of which model to use and how to compare them depends upon the purpose for which the results are to be used. Often for descriptive purposes the researcher wishes to explain as much variation as possible with the fewest explanatory variables. In this case, the model with the maximum adjusted multiple correlation coefficient ($\bar{R}^2$) is often preferred. When accurate prediction or forecasting of the value of the dependent variable is the primary goal, researchers generally prefer the model with the minimum mean-square error and/or the minimum residual mean-square [23]. Frequently, in policy analysis, researchers are called upon to estimate the magnitude of the independent effect of changes in the size of a single explanatory variable on the dependent variable. In this case, the analyst would like to minimize the bias and the standard error of the estimated regression coefficients.

The results are reported so that any of these comparisons can be made. However, the discussion emphasizes the comparison of how the estimated effect of each of the explanatory variables changes across the three models. We begin by reporting the results obtained by estimating Model III and then proceed to a comparison of these results with estimates of Models I and II.

MODEL III

The results of the regression procedures used to estimate the log illness-visit equation (Equation 5) are summarized in Table 5. The results in the right-hand columns of the table were obtained when the full sample of 820 individuals and the predicted usual-source variable PUS were used in the estimation procedure. The model explained approximately 30 percent of the variance in the dependent variable ($\bar{R}^2 = 0.3006$).

As expected, the health status/need variables were found to be important predictors of the number of illness visits made to a physician. Each of these health status/need variables (*No need, Chronic, Injury, Hosp,* and *Dis days*) was found to have a coefficient with the sign as predicted. Only *Injury* was not found to be statistically significant.

Once the several dimensions of health status/need were controlled, the demographic variables measuring age (*Age* and *Age*^{2}) and education (*Educ*) were found not to be statistically significant. *Sex* was found to be a significant predictor of the number of illness visits: being female was found to be associated with having more illness visits to a physician.

The coefficient of *Income* was found to have the expected positive sign and was statistically significant. However, the size of the estimated coefficient indicates that once other variables in the model were held constant, even very large differences in family per capita incomes were associated with only small differences in the number of illness visits.

Each of the insurance variables (*Ins A, Ins B,* and *Ins C*) was found to have statistically significant coefficients, and all had the expected positive sign. As anticipated, individuals who reported having health insurance coverage (in any of the three categories) were found to have increased illness visits as opposed to individuals who reported having no health insurance coverage.

Combined expected travel and waiting room times (*Time*) do not seem to act as a barrier to visits in this sample. However, appointment delay (*Appt*) was found to be statistically significant, with the expected negative sign. This result implies that the expected long delays between making an appointment and the date of the actual appointment are associated with reduced use of the physician.

The usual-source variable, PUS (the predicted probability of having a usual source of care), was found to be statistically significant, and its coefficient had the expected positive sign. As anticipated, the greater the projected probability of a usual source of care for an individual, the greater the number of illness-related visits to the physician, *ceteris paribus*.

COMPARISON OF MODEL III WITH MODELS I AND II

Table 5 also presents parameter estimates for Models I and II. Comparing the coefficient estimates of the usual-source variables for Models I and III, we find that the size of the coefficient changed as did the standard error of the coefficient. The size of the *beta* coefficient for the reported usual source (US) was approximately four times as large as the coefficient reported for the predicted usual source (PUS). The effect of having a usual source of care on illness-related utilization of the physician is substantially different for the alternative models. Employing estimates from Model III, an approximate 5 percent increase in utilization is associated with having a usual source. In contrast, the estimates from Model I indicate that a 21 percent increase in utilization is associated with having a usual source. The formula for calculation of the percentage effect of a dummy variable in a log-linear model is given by Halvorsen and Palmquist [24]. The standard error for the reported usual source in Model I is 0.0585 but was lower for the predicted usual source in Model III (0.0235). Thus, the choice of theoretical model is important for evaluating the importance of having a usual source. If Model I is chosen, having a usual source increases the number of illness visits. If Model II is chosen, the analyst is, by definition, excluding any possible impact of usual source on illness visits. Finally, if Model III is chosen, usual source does significantly influence the number of illness visits made, but the effect is much smaller than that estimated using Model I.

Except for the usual-source variable, the remaining features of the three models are relatively similar. The health status/need variables have a somewhat smaller impact on visits in Model III, but the difference is small. Also, *Sex* was found to have a slightly stronger impact on visits in Model I. The adjusted R^2 and the residual mean-square for the

Table 5: Multiple Regression Results for Three Models of Illness Visit Demand (Dependent Variable: Log Illness-Related Visits to the Physician, N = 820 Adults)

	Model I (US)		*Model II (US Omitted)*		*Model III*	
Independent Variable	*Coefficient* (*t-ratio*)	Beta (*Normalized*) *Coefficient*	*Coefficient* (*t-ratio*)	Beta (*Normalized*) *Coefficient*	*Coefficient* (*t-ratio*)	Beta (*Normalized*) *Coefficient*
Constant	.216 (1.04)		.336* (1.63)		.288 (1.39)	
No need	-.197‡ (-5.25)	-.167	-.215‡ (-5.77)	-.18	-.191‡ (-4.89)	-.162
Chronic	.179‡ (5.41)	.181	.182‡ (5.45)	.183	.177‡ (5.30)	.179
Injury	.098* (1.61)	.048	.102* (1.66)	.049	.099* (1.61)	.048
Hosp	.692‡ (7.17)	.228	.691‡ (7.12)	.226	.693‡ (7.15)	.277
Dis days	.013‡ (6.01)	.196	.103‡ (6.04)	.196	.013‡ (5.79)	.190
Age	.009 (1.07)	.193	.011 (1.38)	.237	.008 (0.95)	.168
Age squared	-.0001* (-1.46)	-.203	-.00014* (-1.69)	-.203	-.0001* (1.37)	-.239
Sex	.166‡ (3.50)	.127	.186‡ (3.93)	.188	.168‡ (3.50)	.108
Educ	-.059 (-1.19)	-.04	-.064 (-1.28)	-.041	-.064 (-1.29)	-.042
Income	.00001‡ (2.55)	.074	.00001‡ (2.58)	.089	.00001‡ (2.55)	.081
Appt	-.056‡ (-2.68)	-.080	-.056‡ (-2.63)	-.079	-.059‡ (-2.77)	-.084
Time	.001 (1.35)	.038	.0008 (1.13)	.031	.0009 (1.11)	.033
Ins A	.200† (2.14)	.126	.215† (2.28)	.135	.215† (2.29)	.135
Ins B	.207† (2.17)	.121	.210† (2.19)	.122	.211† (2.21)	.124
Ins C	.190† (1.95)	.103	.202† (2.05)	.111	.207† (2.11)	.114
US	.193‡ (3.30)	.100	– –	–	– –	–
PUS	– –	–	– –	–	.047† (2.02)	.025
F-statistic	23.62		24.17		22.99	
R^2	.3200		.3107		.3142	
Adjusted R^2	.3064		.2979		.3006	
Residual mean-square	.4181		.4233		.4217	

Statistical significance levels:
* = .10.
† = .05.
‡ = .01.

three models were found to be quite similar. Models I and III, which include a usual-source variable, explain slightly more of the variance in visits and yield somewhat more precise estimates of the number of visits—but, again, these differences are very small.

CONCLUSIONS

All three models yield similar results if our purpose is general prediction or description. However, if our goal is to estimate accurately the impact of a policy program or a demographic trend which changes the proportion of individuals with a usual source of care, then the three models yield different results. The impact of usual source on visits appears to be much lower when the two-directional model is employed as compared to use of an alternative one-directional model including usual source (Model I). The evidence is clear that individuals who report having a usual source of care more frequently visit the physician for illness-related reasons, even when other access and health/need factors are statistically held constant. For this sample, the reporting of a usual source of care appears to be a more important determinant of illness-related physician use than either family per capita income or the expected travel and waiting time associated with a provider. The results provide further evidence that the absence of linkages with a regular source of care is a significant barrier to ambulatory visits to the physician and that population heterogeneity regarding such linkages is associated with variations in ambulatory care utilization. If public policy is to emphasize the equitable distribution of medical care, emphasis should be placed on establishing programs which encourage specific entry points to the medical care system to serve as regular sources of advice, treatment, and referrals.

A more thorough understanding of the usual-source effect is also important for our understanding of self-selection biases that potentially can occur during enrollment in alternative delivery systems. Differences between HMO and fee-for-service utilization experiences are not only a function of the financing and organizational characteristics of these alternatives; they also are related to differences in the characteristics of their enrollees. Since the provider-patient relationship is an important factor which distinguishes groups which enroll in different plans, this factor may in part explain differences in plan performance and may be important even after health status and other enrollee characteristics are taken into account.

Other questions raised by the results of this study are important to our current understanding of the impact of a usual source on physician utilization. The results of this study call attention to the need to study the factors which influence an individual's identification with a regular source of care and the barriers to establishing those relationships. For example, we do not know the importance of the interrelationships between provider characteristics and individual characteristics in the processes of establishing a usual source and visiting the physician.

ACKNOWLEDGMENTS

The authors would like to express their gratitude to the University of Michigan Health Services Research Center for providing access to the data. We also thank S. E. Berki, Avedis Donabedian, John R. C. Wheeler, and Daniel L. Rubinfeld for their advice during the completion of this research.

REFERENCES

1. Berki, S. E., and M. Ashcraft. HMO enrollment: Who joins what and why: A review of the literature. *Milbank Memorial Fund Quarterly* 58(4):588, Fall 1980.
2. Luft, H. S. Assessing the evidence on HMO performance. *Milbank Memorial Fund Quarterly* 58(4):501, Fall 1980.
3. Berki, S. E., and M. Ashcraft. On the analysis of ambulatory utilization. *Medical Care* 17(12):1163, December 1979.
4. Hershey, J. C., H. S. Luft, and J. M. Gianaris. Making sense out of utilization data. *Medical Care* 13(10):838, October 1975.
5. Kennedy, V. C. Rural access to a regular source of medical care. *Journal of Community Health* 4(3):199, Spring 1979.
6. Aday, L. A., and R. L. Eichorn. *The Utilization of Health Services: Indices and Correlates—A Research Bibliography.* DHEW Publication No. (HSM) 73-3003. Washington, DC: U. S. Government Printing Office, 1972.
7. Aday, L. A. Economic and noneconomic barriers to the use of needed medical services. *Medical Care* 13(6):447, June 1975.
8. Solon, J. A., C. G. Sheps, and S. S. Lee. Delineating patterns of medical care. *American Journal of Public Health* 50(12):1113, December 1960.
9. Aday, L. A., and R. Andersen. *Development of Indices of Access to Medical Care.* Ann Arbor, MI: Health Administration Press, 1975.
10. Andersen, R., et al. Exploring dimensions of access to medical care. *Health Services Research* 18(1):49, Spring 1983.
11. Luft, H. S., J. C. Hershey, and J. Morrell. Factors affecting the use of physician services in a rural community. *American Journal of Public Health* 66(9):865, September 1976.

12. Lave, J. R., et al. Characteristics of individuals who identify a regular source of medical care. *American Journal of Public Health* 69(3):261, March 1979.
13. Kasper, J., and G. Barrish. *Usual Sources of Medical Care and Their Characteristics*. DHHS Publication No. (PHS) 82-3324. Washington, DC: U.S. Government Printing Office, 1982.
14. Sloan, F., and J. Bentkover. *Access to Ambulatory Care and the U.S. Economy*. Lexington, MA: Lexington Books, 1979.
15. Aday, L. A., and R. Andersen. A framework for the study of access to medical care. *Health Services Research* 9(2):208, 1974.
16. Anderson, J. G. Health services utilization: Framework and review. *Health Services Research* 8(2):184, 1973.
17. Phelps, C. E. Effects of Insurance on Demand for Medical Care. In R. Anderson, J. Kravits, and O. Anderson (eds.). *Equity in Health Services*. Cambridge, MA: Ballinger, 1976.
18. Newhouse, J. P., and C. E. Phelps. New Estimates of Price and Income Elasticities of Medical Care Services. In R. N. Rosset (ed.). *The Role of Health Insurance in the Health Services Sector*. New York: Neale Watson, 1976.
19. Kuder, J. M. *Prices and the Distribution of Ambulatory Medical Visits*. Doctoral Dissertation. Ann Arbor: The University of Michigan, 1982.
20. Koutsoyiannis, A. *Theory of Econometrics*. New York: Barnes and Noble, 1973.
21. Kobashigawa, B., and S. E. Berki. Alternative regression approaches to the analysis of medical care survey data. *Medical Care* 15(5):396, May 1977.
22. Heckman, J. J. Simultaneous Equation Models with Continuous and Discrete Endogenous Variables and Structural Shifts. In S. Goldfield and R. Quandt (eds.). *Studies in Nonlinear Estimation*. Cambridge, MA: Ballinger, 1976.
23. Chatterjee, J., and B. Price. *Regression Analysis by Example*. New York: John Wiley and Sons, 1977.
24. Halvorsen, R., and R. Palmquist. The interpretation of dummy variables in semi-logarithmic equations. *American Economic Review* 70(3):474, June 1980.

CHAPTER TEN

Probit Economic Models

The observation is often made in health services research that there are fundamental differences in the way economists see problems versus the way sociologists or epidemiologists or political scientists view them. This perception is often exacerbated by the tendency of economists to choose one particular set of analytical methods to work with, while researchers trained in other disciplines attack similar problems with different conceptualizations and analytical tools. The article by Cromwell and Mitchell is a classic example of how the operation and performance of a particular class of organizations are examined from the economic point of view. Although the authors are focusing on a "demand" conceptualization interpreted in the light of competition, pricing mechanisms, profit maximization, and the effect of marginal decision on the part of the firm, their general approach is similar to the other investigations included in this volume in that they posit a model of behavior and test that model with a statistical technique that best suits the data used to answer the fundamental research question: What are large Medicaid practices like?

Economists have pioneered the use of probability-based regression techniques that accommodate dependent variables not normally distributed, or restricted in some way. In this case, the technique of choice is the probit model. It remains a linear, additive model of behavior and is derived, essentially, from the general linear modeling technique upon which least-squares regression is drawn.

Another characteristic of analyses that follow the econometrician's lead is the extensive development of the variables that are entered into the model. This article provides an excellent example of the depth to which each independent variable and the dependent variable should be described in a research article where space may be of concern.

The economic model presented here has important implications for policy and those implications do not fit exclusively into economic categories. Regulatory options are involved, but behavioral and organizational alternatives are offered as well.

An Economic Model of Large Medicaid Practices

Jerry Cromwell and Janet B. Mitchell

Public attention given to Medicaid "mills" prompted this more general investigation of the origins of large Medicaid practices. A dual market demand model is proposed showing how Medicaid competes with private insurers for scarce physician time. Various program parameters—fee schedules, coverage, collection costs—are analyzed along with physician preferences, specialties, and other supply-side characteristics. Maximum likelihood techniques are used to test the model. The principal finding is that in raising Medicaid fees, as many physicians opt into the program as expand their Medicaid caseloads to exceptional levels, leaving the maldistribution of patients unaffected while notably improving access. Still, the fact that Medicaid fees are lower than those of private insurers does lead to reduced access to more qualified practitioners. Where anti-Medicaid sentiment is stronger, access is also reduced and large Medicaid practices more likely to flourish.

One of the major goals of the Medicaid program was to integrate the poor into mainstream medicine. To this end, an insurance scheme was devised that allowed Medicaid eligibles the discretion to choose among hospitals, physicians, and other providers. Provider participation—particularly among physicians—was strictly voluntary so long as they were willing to accept the Medicaid-allowed charge as payment in full.

Whether the program has been a success, therefore, depends in no small way on how physicians have responded to the fee schedules and to the accompanying rules and regulations regarding payment. Distressing in this regard is the anecdotal evidence of serious fraud and abuse of the system by physicians, especially in practices concentrating

---

This article was funded by the Health Care Financing Administration, Office of Research, Demonstrations, and Statistics under Contract No. 500-78-0051.

Jerry Cromwell, Ph.D. is President of Health Economics Research Inc., 75 Second Avenue, Suite 100, Needham, MA 02194. Janet B. Mitchell, Ph.D. is Vice-president of Health Economics Research Inc. Address communications and requests for reprints to Dr. Cromwell at the above address.

on the Medicaid population [1]. While large Medicaid practices (LMPs) are not necessarily "mills," the maldistribution of Medicaid patients is a legitimate concern. If the majority of the poor are being relegated to a few physicians, both their access to office-based care and the quality of care they receive may be jeopardized. For example, several studies have shown that physicians with large Medicaid caseloads are older, in general practice, lacking in hospital affiliation, and trained abroad [2–6].

Because LMP physicians generally are less credentialled, serious consideration must be given to changes in program policy that might exacerbate the distribution problem even further. Several studies have already shown that physicians are more likely to participate in Medicaid when fees are higher [7–11], but that participants also expand their Medicaid caseloads when enticed by higher fees, leaving unclear the ultimate impact of fees on maldistribution. Sloan, Mitchell, and Cromwell [12], for example, found positive, statistically significant effects of Medicaid fees on physician participation, defined either as a dichotomous decision to accept Medicaid patients or to expand on existing Medicaid caseloads. Policymakers have voiced concern over raising fees for fear that Medicaid mills will reap most of the benefit [13]. Whether these fears are well founded or not remains an empirical question to be addressed in this article.

Also of concern is program scope and patient maldistribution. In states with large numbers of Medicaid eligibles relative to office-based physicians, will the maldistribution problem be more acute, or will more physicians choose to participate and keep LMP growth within bounds?

Answers to these and other questions require a theory of physician participation in Medicaid that simultaneously deals with non-, small, and large participants. It is not enough to consider solely the decision to participate; the physician's decision to expand his Medicaid practice also requires study. The next section examines an economic theory of the size distribution of Medicaid practices, taking into consideration: (1) competition from private markets and other physicians, (2) eligibility limits, (3) discrimination, and (4) factors affecting physician supply. This is followed by a brief discussion of data sources. An empirical test of the model is then made, focusing not on the participation decision per se (which has been investigated elsewhere), but rather on the probability of observing a large Medicaid practice among participants. The last section discusses the findings from both a behavioral and a policy perspective.

THEORY

The origins of large Medicaid practices can be considered in terms of a two-market demand model.[1] In one market, the physician sets prices, demand is downward sloping, and additional visits are demanded only at lower prices. In the second market, fees are predetermined and the physician serving this market can provide as much as he chooses, within limits, at a fixed price. While several insurers have fixed payment schedules, we consider only the fixed-payment Medicaid program here.

Assuming profit maximization (to be relaxed momentarily) for each visit level, the physician moves down along his marginal revenue curve, AB, in Figure 1, until marginal revenue falls below the fixed Medicaid fee, f_m.[2] The physician then begins to participate in the Medicaid program until the pool of Medicaid patients is exhausted.[3] Demand segment, BC, corresponds to the potential pool of Medicaid patients upon which each physician may draw. The introduction of Medicaid effectively segments marginal revenue into two parts—one above, one below—the Medicaid fee, f_m. Marginal patients in the upper segment, AB, are willing and able to pay higher fees than f_m, while in segment CD, they will only pay less than f_m.

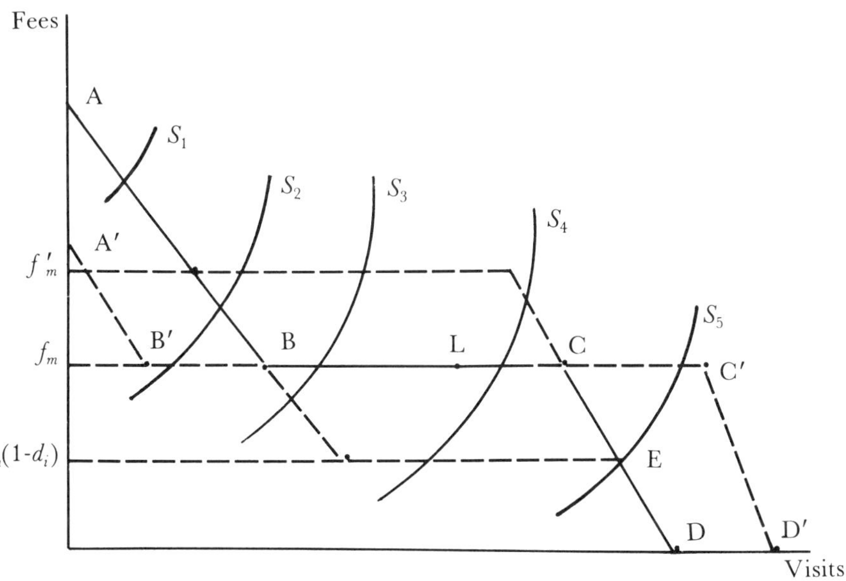

Figure 1: Medicaid Participation Model

If a physician's supply curve is S_3 he can be said to be operating a small Medicaid practice (SMP), as the majority of his visits are with private patients. (A more precise definition of an SMP will be given later.) If physician supply is farther to the right, say S_4, then this practice can be considered an LMP, as a majority of patient visits are devoted to Medicaid patients. If supply is far to the left, say S_1, then the physician is not accepting any Medicaid patients.

Thus, the physician's decision to participate in Medicaid, as well as the level of his participation, depends on supply and private-plus-Medicaid demand. Private physician demand can be considered a function of patient health status, income, and insurance, plus the physician's credentials and his/her competition. Considerable empirical research has documented the effects of health status, income, and insurance on private demand [14,15]. Patients should also be willing to pay higher fees to see better-trained specialists [10,12]. Holding these factors constant, private demand per physician should be lower in physician-rich areas because of competition, with limited numbers of patients spread among a larger number of physicians.[4] Factors limiting private demand shift marginal revenue inward (see $A'B'$, in Figure 1), increasing the Medicaid participation rate for a given physician, *ceteris paribus*. Reduced demand also draws into the program marginal non-participants (represented by supply S_2).

MEDICAID COVERAGE AND GENEROSITY

Medicaid coverage and generosity of payment definitely affects the level and nature of physician participation. Consider first an increase in Medicaid fees from f_m to f'_m without a change in program eligibility. If physician supply is S_2, an increase in fees to f'_m will draw the physician into the Medicaid market as an SMP. If supply is S_3, the effect of a Medicaid fee increase may be to turn an SMP into an LMP. Note that while total visits have increased with higher Medicaid fees, private visits have generally decreased, implying some substitution at the margin of poorer Medicaid for wealthier (or previously better insured) patients. Physicians with supply S_1 and S_5 are unaffected by the fee increase—the former still not seeing any Medicaid patients and the latter seeing all who ask for an appointment.

The net effect of Medicaid fees on the probability distribution of SMPs and LMPs in an area is generally ambiguous. Higher Medicaid fees do not necessarily foster LMPs (at least as a percentage of participants) if significant numbers of new physicians (like S_2) enter the Medicaid market as SMPs.

An increase in program eligibility or scope of benefits should have different effects. Increasing the Medicaid-eligible pool per physician has the effect of "lengthening" the Medicaid line from BC to BC′. This should have no effect on nonparticipating physicians: Medicaid fees have not increased, so marginal revenues from private patients still exceed the Medicaid fee.[5] Nor does it have any effect on participating practices that have not exhausted their potential pool of eligibles, again for the same reasons. Some practices, however, may be seeing all of the Medicaid patients who apply and some non-Medicaid poor in addition, e.g., S_5. An extension of Medicaid coverage will have a positive effect on participation (as well as on total visits) as these physicians substitute better-paying Medicaid for poorer-paying private patients. If Medicaid-extended coverage is for the poor who are already part of the physician's caseload—say, CE—then no substantial improvement in access will obtain (unless S_5 is quite elastic)—only a reduced out-of-pocket burden for the new eligibles. If coverage is extended to patients in segment ED, however, then the near-poor comprising CE will suffer as a result of expanded Medicaid coverage to the very poor.

A practice characterized by S_5 highlights an interesting point. A physician may be seeing all of the Medicaid patients that apply, but because the eligible population is so limited (at least before the program expanded), his practice may still be an SMP. Furthermore, the length of the horizontal line, which is based on the Medicaid population, is clearly related to private demand factors such as income. For this reason, we would expect both participation rates and the number of LMPs to be higher in poorer neighborhoods, inner cities, and rural areas. This may be offset, on the other hand, by a shortage of physicians in these areas, which would shift out *pro rata* private demand and reduce Medicaid participation. Thus, we have the rather surprising conclusion that, depending on the geographical match between physicians and patients, the number of *both* nonparticipants and LMPs in a low-income, high-Medicaid area may be higher than elsewhere if physicians are particularly scarce—as they generally are in these areas. Physicians, knowing the inner-city poor have access to outpatient facilities, also may restrict their practices to non-Medicaid patients.

Summarizing on the demand side, theory predicts that any factor raising (lowering) private demand per physician (e.g., patient income, insurance, health status; physician credentials and specialization; the physician-population ratio) should decrease (increase) the probability of participation as an SMP and of the participating practice expanding to an LMP, *ceteris paribus*. Similar predictions obtain for an increase in Medicaid fees. Whether higher Medicaid fees would exacerbate the distribution of patients between SMPs and LMPs becomes strictly an empirical question. Extensions in program eligibility, by contrast, should have definite effects on the size distribution of Medicaid practices, essentially skewing the distribution toward more LMPs.

DISCRIMINATION

The analysis so far has implicitly assumed that physicians do not discriminate among patients on factors other than ability to pay. Some physicians, however, may have a distaste for Medicaid patients or for the program as a whole. Some of their reasons may be objective (e.g., fee schedules too low, long payment delays, too much red tape, few Medicaid eligibles), others more personal. In a 1976 physician survey, nearly 40 percent of nonparticipants cited an "opposition to government in medicine" as a very important reason for not participating in the Medicaid program. Twenty-five percent also cited a "dislike for the kinds of patients enrolled" as a reason for not participating [7, p. 122]. Subjective responses like these suggest strongly that physicians discriminate against Medicaid patients for reasons other than economic.

Faced with a stated Medicaid fee, f_m, some physicians act as if f_m $(1 - d_i)$is the *net* fee, where d_i reflects the strength of the ith physician's discrimination coefficient in line with Becker [20].[6] This has the effect of lowering the flat Medicaid portion by an amount, $f_m d_i$, which clearly will vary by individual physician, unlike f_m, which all physicians receive as a nominal payment.[7] The effect of discrimination will be to lower participation and physician gross revenues—but not always. For example, it is immaterial whether the physician with supply S_1 discriminates or not, for he would not participate in Medicaid in any event. For physicians with supply S_3 or S_4, however, discrimination does make a difference. The "potential" SMP physician with supply S_3, if he has a positive discrimination coefficient, d_i, will not participate in Medicaid, even though he should on objective financial grounds. The "potential" LMP physician with supply S_4, will only be an SMP, choosing instead to move farther down his private demand curve before (begrudgingly) entering the program.

Discrimination in this context costs the physician because he chooses to see poorer-paying private patients at the margin rather than better-paying Medicaid patients. Economic losses to physicians naturally increase with d_i.[8] In the extreme where $d_i > 1$, the physician limits himself strictly to non-Medicaid patients whatever his objective supply. For these physicians the economic loss may be a high price to pay for refusing to accept Medicaid patients, particularly if private demand is limited. This does not necessarily mean that the physician is not seeing poor patients—on the contrary, he may be seeing many of the poor. He simply is not receiving directly from them as much as he could be if he had chosen to accept them as Medicaid patients.

The size distribution of Medicaid practices will vary depending on the mean and variation in d_i. Holding other factors like private demand and the distribution of practices constant, an inverse correlation between discriminatory preferences and supply (i.e., smaller suppliers with a greater distaste for the Medicaid program) should result in greater inequalities in Medicaid practice size. In this case, there should be more nonparticipants and fewer SMPs, leaving the bulk of the Medicaid population to be served by a few LMPs. Like Medicaid fees, a greater average level of discrimination in an area has an ambiguous effect on SMP/LMP inequalities. A positive correlation between discriminatory preferences and private demand will encourage LMPs, because discriminators tend to enjoy more lucrative private practices, leaving the nondiscriminators—who lack wealthy private patients—to treat the Medicaid population.

VARIATIONS IN PHYSICIAN SUPPLY

The ultimate impact of any shift in private or Medicaid demand on Medicaid participation rates in an area will depend on the locus and distribution of physician supply. Nationwide, Medicaid patients constitute 10–15 percent of all private physician caseloads [3]. If Medicaid patients and physicians were distributed equally across the general population, then participation rates would approximate 10–15 percent in any community. Because neither Medicaid recipients nor physicians are very equally distributed, however, it is possible for nearly all physicians in an area to be operating LMPs if few non-Medicaid patients exist. They do not have to be; need may simply be going unmet as particular physicians choose to see a limited number of patients *in toto*.

If the distribution of supply curves is uniformly distributed along the entire "visits" axis, as shown (roughly) in Figure 1, then a complete mix of nonparticipants, SMPs, and LMPs obtains. Shifts in demand will alter the mix, with increases in private demand (or reductions in Medicaid fees) resulting in more nonparticipants, fewer LMPs, and more or fewer SMPs, depending upon the distribution of practices around the "drop-out" kink (B) and some designated point L, the point where an SMP becomes an LMP.[9] If practices are more closely bunched around B than L, then increases in private demand or Medicaid fee reductions should reduce the relative number of SMPs to LMPs and exacerbate inequalities in the distribution of Medicaid patients across physicians.

The locus and distribution of area supply will depend on the mean of, and the variance in, the characteristics that underlie individual physician supply: (1) input prices, (2) productivity, (3) physician preferences for income and leisure, and (4) practice style. In areas where auxiliary wages are high, or where average productivity is low, total physician supply will be lower because physicians are financially limited in the visits they can provide profitably for a given fee. Specialists, for example, see fewer patients per hour. Therefore, in specialist-dominated areas, we would expect more limited supply and lower participation rates, *ceteris paribus*. If physicians in an area also have a higher average preference for leisure (e.g., older, semiretired physicians in Florida or Arizona), supply will be less than in areas where work (or income) preferences are stronger. Finally, in areas served by physicians whose practice style includes a significant number of high-quality inputs, amenities, and the like, supply will also be less as fees will cover only a limited number of more costly visits before marginal costs exceed marginal revenues.

Variations in physician supply are a function of variations in the same four categories. Presumably, all practices in an area face the same non-physician input prices, although certain exceptions may exist (e.g., black physicians may have to pay higher wages to attract white registered nurses in urban ghettos); thus, within-area variations in factor prices should not be a major contributor to supply differences or to the number of LMPs, although they may explain more of the *inter-area* variation.

Variations in physician productivity are considerable, however, as Reinhardt [24] has shown. Much of this variation tends to be specialty specific.[10] Any remaining output variation depends largely on the physician's managerial capacities and inclinations.

Physicians also vary considerably in the imputed wage they apply to their own efforts or, alternatively, their preferences for leisure. In addition to random variations in income-leisure preferences, physicians with significant nonpractice income or who are elderly—or female physicians who have children to raise—should have a greater disutility for work, *ceteris paribus* [12,25,26].

Finally, the most important variation from a policy perspective is physicians' choice of practice style, which is partly due to training and specialty choice, partly due to a desire to increase income. Variations in practice style include the time physicians spend with patients, the ancillaries they order, the quantity and quality of labor inputs used, the size of waiting rooms, and the like.

Consider first the use of ancillaries. Because these services are usually billed separately, it is appropriate to consider ancillaries a second output of the physician's practice, complementing direct patient contacts. Physicians may or may not internalize ancillary services.[11] If they do not, no financial benefit derives from ordering tests and procedures unless illicit kickbacks are being paid. Where physicians do produce ancillaries in their offices, they have a direct financial interest in the allowed charges of third-party payers and in production costs. For each visit, such physicians receive two fees, one for the visit itself and a second for any ancillaries, resulting in the total visit price. The effect of internalizing ancillaries is to shift final visit demand outward, resulting in provision of more private visits (assuming positively sloped supply curves). The marginal physician who internalizes ancillaries has less need or desire to enter the Medicaid market, since marginal revenues per private visit are higher. Physicians with very strong income preferences, however, may feel freer to order additional tests for their Medicaid patients who incur no out-of-pocket cost, a behavior typifying Medicaid mills [28] but not large Medicaid practices in general [29]. For these physicians, the decision to internalize ancillaries and to see large numbers of Medicaid patients is jointly determined.

Other differences in practice style—e.g., time spent with patients, use of support personnel, and amenities—can be characterized as supply shifts. Physicians who see patients on an assembly-line basis and who skimp on auxiliary personnel can certainly see more patients per hour at lower incurred costs. The higher net incomes enjoyed, however, come primarily at the patients' expense and are not condoned by the majority of medical professionals. It is difficult in practice, however, to distinguish between the true quality minimizer and the simply more efficient practitioner.

Data Sources

The primary data base for this analysis is the 1977 physician survey conducted by the National Opinion Research Center (NORC) for the Health Care Financing Administration (HCFA). This survey was a nationally representative sample of 3,482 physicians in 15 specialties. The sample was then reduced to 1,796 physicians in the 5 primary care specialties: general and family practitioners, general surgeons, obstetrician-gynecologists, pediatricians, and internists. All physicians were in private practice, and the vast majority were office based (95.8 percent). Physicians in group practices with ten or more physicians were excluded. All empirical work is based on the individual physician as the unit of analysis, with a prorating of group data where necessary.

An extensive questionnaire was administered to all physicians, primarily by telephone, covering practice costs, work effort, size and type of practice, physician income, and fees. All information was based on physician self-reports. The size distribution of Medicaid practices was calculated from the individual physician's response to the following question: "About what percentage of your patients have Medicaid?"[12]

Measurement error may be present if physicians refused to participate in the survey, or if they reported inaccurate or incomplete information during the interview. Because the dependent variable is dichotomous, less error should exist than if continuous participation rates were used. Analysis of the 1976 physician survey found that nonrespondent physicians did not differ from cooperating physicians along characteristics believed to be associated with large Medicaid practices, such as specialty, board certification, and FMG status [7]. Weights associated with the 1977 sample include adjustments for nonresponse. A downward bias in the number of LMPs undoubtedly remains, as true physician "mills" are likely to have refused the interview. How much this affected the results is unknown.

Three additional data sources were merged with the physician survey for this analysis. Biographical information on individual survey physicians was obtained from the *AMA Masterfile*, including such data as physician age, board certification, and medical school. Variables describing the physician's county, such as demographic characteristics, were drawn from the Area Resource File. Two community variables, per capita income and physician-population ratios, were obtained from a more current source: the American Medical Association's *Physician Distribution and Medical Licensure in the U.S., 1976*.

EMPIRICAL SPECIFICATION

DEPENDENT VARIABLE

The dependent variable is specified as a dichotomous variable in which "one" signifies that the physician runs a large Medicaid practice, and "zero," a small Medicaid practice. Since the purpose of this analysis was to distinguish solely between large and small Medicaid practices, nonparticipants were omitted. (See [7,12] for a continuous participation *rate* analysis.) This alters, in definite ways, the prediction and interpretation of causal variables. For example, outward shifts in private demand should unequivocally reduce the percentage of LMPs in the *total* practice population (including nonparticipants). Whether such a shift has the same effect on the *mix* of SMPs and LMPs, however, is generally ambiguous, because nonparticipants have been dropped in the calculation of LMP probabilities and nonparticipation is correlated with income. High-income areas should have fewer LMPs; they may not have fewer SMPs. The ultimate effect on mix will depend on the distribution of practices around the drop-out kink and the arbitrary definition of an LMP.

To test the sensitivity of parameter estimates to the definition of an LMP, the dependent variable assumes two variants: (1) LMPs are defined as practices with 30 percent or more Medicaid patients (*LMP30*), and (2) LMPs are restricted to those practices with at least one-half of their patients on Medicaid (*LMP50* or *ELMP*). These cutoffs roughly correspond to one and two standard deviations above the mean participation rate of 13.3 percent, respectively. Nonparticipants were 22 percent of the primary care sample, while *LMP30* and *LMP50* constituted 20 and 6 percent of participants, respectively.

INDEPENDENT VARIABLES[13]

Fee Schedules. Two variables were included to measure the influence of relative fee schedules on the physician's decision to run a large Medicaid practice: the Medicaid fee for a routine office visit (*MCDFEE*) and Blue Shield's allowed fee for the same procedure (*BSFEE*). Both variables are defined for the physician's state or plan area. The Blue Shield fee was used as a measure of the relative generosity of private third-party payers, although coverage is rather limited for office care. Fees, as well as all other monetary variables, were adjusted for area cost-of-living differences. Without knowing precisely the distribution of supply in an area, it is impossible to predict *a priori* the effects of raising Medicaid fees on the probability of observing an LMP.

Physician Credentials. Physician credentials include specialty, board certification in a specialty, and FMG status. Specialists have undergone more years of professional training than have general practitioners and thus are less likely to accept large numbers of low-marginal-revenue Medicaid patients. The dummy variables, *GS, IM, OB,* and *PED*, represent general surgeons, internists, obstetrician-gynecologists, and pediatricians, respectively. General practitioners represent the omitted category.

Because board-certified physicians and U.S. medical graduates both are generally considered to have higher technical expertise, they enjoy a greater demand for their services. As a result, they are hypothesized to be less likely to run large Medicaid practices. *BOARD* and *FMG* each assume the value *one* if the physician is board certified, or if he is a Third-World foreign medical graduate, respectively. A Third-World FMG is defined as a graduate of a medical school in a non-English speaking, non-Western European country. (An exception is made for graduates of Mexican medical schools, many of whom are U.S. citizens who studied there. Presumably, they will experience less difficulty in building a practice and obtaining referrals than noncitizens.)

Physician Age. The older physician is likely to face a drop in demand for his services in the fee-setting market, as patients and referring physicians increasingly opt for younger physicians more fully acquainted with the latest medical techniques. If so, he may begin to supply more services in the price-taking (Medicaid) market, and be more likely to run a large Medicaid practice. Conversely, if older physicians wish to reduce their workloads, they may drop low-marginal revenue patients first. Competition versus the work effort effects of age must be tested empirically. Physician age is specified as a dummy variable (*MDAGE*) which assumes the value *one* if the physician is 60 years of age or older. This provides a sharper test of the age hypothesis than a continuous specification.

Community Demand. The demand for physician visits is influenced, *inter alia*, by the ability to pay of the patient population in the physician's county. Two variables measure ability to pay: per capita income (*Y*) of private patients and Medicaid coverage (*MCAID*) for poor patients in the county. *MCAID* measures Medicaid recipients as a percentage of county population, based on the distribution of state poor.[14]

As the physician-population ratio rises, demand per physician falls in the fee-setting market, encouraging higher levels of Medicaid participation. Like fees, income, and other variables that affect private demand, physician density is ambiguously related to the probability of observing a large Medicaid practice. *MDPOP* is defined as the number of office-based patient-care physicians per 1,000 county population.

Practice Costs. When wage rates rise for nonphysician personnel, it is less likely that the Medicaid-allowed fee will provide sufficient marginal revenue to cover increased practice costs. High wage rates should discourage Medicaid participation—though possibly more for the marginal participant. The variable *WAGE* is a county index of wage rates of nonphysician personnel.

Geographic Regions. Regional effects, including variations in supply characteristics, Medicaid program generosity, charity, and discrimination, are proxied by geographic location. *NEAST, SOUTH,* and *WEST* represent the Northeast, South, and West census regions, respectively. The North Central region constitutes the omitted category. *Ceteris paribus*, LMPs should be more prevalent in the South because of higher physician nonparticipation in public benefit programs generally (possibly due to discrimination or conservative political attitudes).[15]

Estimation Methods

With a qualitative, zero-one, dependent variable (SMP = 0, LMP = 1), ordinary least-squares methods are inefficient because of the concentration of values at two extremes [30]. Multivariate probit analysis is preferred because it constrains the predicted values of the dependent variable to the unit (0,1) interval. In the probit model, the conditional expectation is given by:

$$E\left[y_i \mid \hat{I}_i \right] = prob\left[y_i = 1 \mid \hat{I}_i \right] = F(\hat{I}_i)$$

where $F(\hat{I}_i)$ = ordinate of the cumulative normal distribution, which forms an *S*-shaped curve in the unit interval.

The predicted probit index, $\hat{I}_i$, is calculated by multiplying the estimated maximum likelihood coefficients times the appropriate values of the independent variables. The conditional probability of the practice being an LMP (i.e., $prob[Y_i = 1]$) can then be determined by looking up values of $\hat{I}_i$ in a cumulative normal distribution table.

Interpretation of probit results, therefore, is a two-step process, unlike OLS estimates, which have direct implications (e.g., the coefficient of income in a consumption function is the marginal propensity to consume). Estimates must first be converted using the cumulative normal distribution before impacts on conditional probabilities (or elasticities) can be determined. Signs of coefficients and statistical significance do give the *direction* of effects on probabilities, however.

FINDINGS

Two probit regression equations along with the means for the dependent and all explanatory variables are displayed in Table 1. Because the probit coefficients are not directly interpretable, a set of marginal impacts of selected, statistically significant variables is provided in Table 2. Elasticities are calculated for continuous variables from the expectational formula given above, while marginal effects of 0,1 differences are given for the discrete, dummy variables. For example, a 1 percent increase in the size of the Medicaid pool (*MCAID*) results in a 0.49 percent increase in the probability that the practice is 30 percent Medicaid rather than an SMP. Marginal effects simply give the absolute change in the probability of observing an LMP associated with positive values of the discrete independent variables. Thus, being board certified reduces the probability that a practice is an LMP by 8.6 percentage points (around a mean of 20 percent).

Table 1: Regression Results for Large Versus Small Medicaid Practices

	*Probit Maximum Likelihood Estimates**		
Variables	*LMP30*	*LMP50*	*Means*
LMP30	—	—	0.20
LMP50	—	—	0.06
MCDFEE	-0.88	1.40	8.49
BSFEE	-3.01†	-0.08	12.24
IM	33.20‖	-50.54‖	0.22
GS	11.54	-50.62‖	0.21
OB	18.10	-49.01‡	0.09
PED	24.71†	-12.30	0.08
BOARD	-44.24‖	-68.79	0.40
FMG	31.20‡	-147.02‖	0.60
MDAGE	8.79	25.81‡	0.30
Y	-0.02‡	-0.00	5,285.70
MCAID	579.98‖	399.75	0.05
MDPOP	24.19‡	43.83‖	1.09
WAGE	1.41	3.01	4.61
NEAST	2.47	77.11‖	0.28
SOUTH	36.87‖	39.64‡	0.27
WEST	65.50‖	3.00	0.22
CONSTANT	-53.21	-240.83‖	

*Coefficients are multiplied by 100.
†Significant at 10 percent level.
‡Significant at 5 percent level.
‖ Significant at 1 percent level.

The fee schedule variables are generally insignificant.[16] Evidently, the incentive to expand Medicaid caseloads with more generous fees is offset by the entrance of previous nonparticipants (see [12] for direct evidence on the 0,1 participation decision), leaving the mix of SMPs and LMPs unaffected. Higher Blue Shield fees, reflecting an outward shift in private demand, reduces the likelihood of observing an LMP among participants, but only for the 30 percent cutoff point.[17]

Variations in public and private demand have the expected impacts on physician participation levels. In higher-income areas, physicians supply more private visits and thus maintain smaller Medicaid practices. When public demand is high, on the other hand, as measured by a large Medicaid-eligible pool, physicians are willing to supply more Medicaid visits and operate larger Medicaid practices. Neither of these variables (*Y* and *MCAID*) are significant when the "extra-large" definition of LMP is used, suggesting that these demand variations are more important predictors at lower Medicaid participation levels.[18] A large Medicaid program, in other words, will encourage LMPs but mostly in the range of 30–50 percent Medicaid.

The probability that a physician will run a large Medicaid practice is greatly increased in physician-dense areas, however, as shown by the significant, positive *MDPOP* coefficient in both equations. This is particularly important for policy purposes, for it suggests that already participating physicians will respond to increased competition in the private market by supplying more and more visits to Medicaid patients, offsetting the equalizing effects of new participants.

It was hypothesized that specialists face a higher private demand for their services than do general practitioners, and hence are less likely to operate LMPs of whatever size. Yet the specialty parameter estimates appear to be highly sensitive to the definition of LMP used. When defined as practices with 30 percent or more Medicaid patients, the four specialties are *more* likely to run LMPs, internists and pediatricians significantly so. Using a 50 percent cutoff, on the other hand, three specialist groups (internists, general surgeons, and obstetrician-gynecologists) are significantly *less* likely to be found in *ELMP*s. Although specialists can command higher fees for their services, their demand also is more inelastic. Thus, it may be impossible for them to concentrate solely on non-Medicaid patients. Because of their scarce talents, they may also feel morally bound to treat a certain number of sicker Medicaid patients. Hence, we find a surprisingly large percentage of specialists running reasonably large Medicaid practices (between 30 and 50 percent Medicaid). However, we do not find many specialists concentrating exclusively on Medicaid patients either.[19] The need for their specialized skills is not there, and certainly the low Medicaid fees make serving the market unattractive at the margin.

What kinds of specialists are seeing large numbers of Medicaid patients? Apparently those who are less often board certified. They are also more likely to be FMGs, although this depends on the cutoff used. Why FMGs are significantly less likely to be running an *ELMP* is unknown. Possibly it has to do with the intraregional distribution of FMGs. They may locate in large cities where private demand is significant relative to the Medicaid population. They may be seeing all of the Medicaid patients they can, but this only raises their participation to 30–50 percent. If private demand and the Medicaid population were well measured, this hypothesis could not be maintained, but knowing the error in the proxies used, it is quite possible the FMG dummy contains some residual locational information as well.

The *MDAGE* coefficient is positive in both probit equations, and significant with *LMP50* specification. Older physicians appear more than willing to offset falling private demand with increased supplies of Medicaid visits.

Table 2: Impact of Independent Variables on Large Medicaid Practices

Variable	*LMP30*	*LMP50*
*Elasticities**		
MCDFEE	–‡	–
BSFEE	-0.60	–
Y	-1.65	–
MCAID	0.49	–
MDPOP	0.46	1.10
WAGE	–	–
Marginal Effects†		
IM	7.5	-2.9
GS	–	-2.9
OB	–	-2.5
PED	5.6	–
BOARD	-8.6	-4.6
FMG	7.3	-3.9
MDAGE	–	2.1
NEAST	–	7.9
SOUTH	8.2	3.4
WEST	16.2	–

*Based on a 10 percent increase.
†Measured in percentage points (0–100).
‡Independent variable was insignificant.

The *WAGE* coefficient was not significant in either equation, suggesting that labor costs do not affect the decision to run an LMP. Theory had predicted a negative relationship—i.e., that physicians in high-wage areas would decline to see large numbers of Medicaid patients.

Finally, the regional dummy variables indicate strong geographic variations in LMPs above and beyond those captured by other variables such as *MDPOP* and *MCAID*. Physicians in the South and West are more likely to devote 30 percent or more of their practice to Medicaid patients. Using the 50 percent LMP definition, the probability of running an LMP is higher in both the South and Northeast. To the extent that private demand, the Medicaid pool, and the distribution of physician supply are held constant, geographic region may be a proxy for variations in nonmaximizing behaviors, such as discrimination. Also, dislike for government programs or Medicaid patients may lead to greater inequalities in Medicaid practice size in certain areas, such as the South. In particular, physician nonparticipation rates will be higher, leaving large numbers of Medicaid patients to be served by a smaller number of participating physicians.

DISCUSSION

From a policy perspective, the most important finding of this study is the null impact that higher Medicaid fee schedules have on the expected likelihood of patient treatment in large Medicaid practices. Where Medicaid fees are higher, roughly as many physicians opt into the program as expand their Medicaid caseloads to exceptional levels, leaving unchanged the overall probability that a Medicaid-eligible patient will be treated in an LMP. Absolute access has clearly increased, however, with the emergence of new "Medicaid" physicians.

The average Medicaid fee in our 1977 sample was only 70 percent of Blue Shield's, clearly making Medicaid participation financially unattractive. Simply raising Medicaid fees could be frustrated by insurer competition, however, as Blue Shield and others raise fees in order to maintain good provider access for their beneficiaries. Thus, while it is important to know that higher public fees will not exacerbate the Medicaid access/quality problem even more, program cost considerations may discourage states from being more generous.[20]

Other findings further suggest a less-than-optimistic picture of patient access. First, where the number of Medicaid eligibles is large relative to the number of physicians, many are relegated to LMPs (or hospital clinics and emergency rooms) for care. Also, where physician competition is greater, Medicaid patients are more maldistributed. If physician participation rates were higher, this presumably would be less of a problem, although local physician shortages would inevitably remain.

Second, not only are patients in large programs more likely to be treated in Medicaid-dominated practices, but these practices are run, more often than not, by an older, non–board-certified general practitioner [3,29].

Finally, definite regional effects may be symptomatic of a conscious or unconscious mismatch between the Medicaid poor and office-based physicians. Higher nonparticipation in the South may reflect a distaste for Medicaid patients, a dislike for government-sponsored programs, or both. Only 13 percent of Southern physicians in another study (versus a mean of 20 percent overall) agreed strongly with the statement that it was society's responsibility to provide health care regardless of ability to pay [32]. But why, then, are very large Medicaid practices much more prevalent in the Northeast as well as the South? A more sophisticated explanation than overt discrimination against Medicaid eligibles would consider the scarcity of office-based physicians in the poorest urban ghettos and rural areas. The few large Medicaid practices that can be considered "mills" are able to exist and prosper, in part, precisely because of a lack of competition from reputable physicians.

The answer, as we have already seen, of course, is not just to increase physician supplies in an area, but rather to entice those already in the area to participate more fully by making the program more attractive. Raising Medicaid fees would definitely help if other insurer payments could somehow be controlled, say, through health maintenance organizations. Even more attractive might be shorter payment delays and less billing confusion, both of which have been found to encourage nonparticipants to enter the program [9,11,12].

NOTES

1. A more nearly complete exposition of the two-market demand model, including a comparative statics analysis of changes in exogenous demand and supply variables, can be found in Sloan, Mitchell, Cromwell [12]. Furthermore, the "physician" and the "practice" are treated synonymously in the text. As most physicians continue to practice alone, distinguishing between the two seems unnecessary. Nor should it make any difference in the theory. All empirical findings regarding group-practice physicians pertain only to the individual physician.

2. For a monopolist facing a downward sloping demand curve, marginal revenue would be below the demand curve. If the physician were a perfect price discriminator, however, marginal revenue and demand curves would coincide. The relevant marginal revenue curve, therefore, will be closer to the demand curve the more the physician price discriminates. While the extent of price discrimination certainly influences how soon a physician will enter the Medicaid market, it does not basically alter the model, only the empirics.
3. While the total Medicaid pool would more than fill the caseload of any individual physician, limited access implies a finite *potential* pool that a physician could realistically serve. This may or may not exhaust the rest of his patient-contact hours.
4. This assumes no demand inducement, or that people living in physician-rich areas differ from residents of other areas in ways which increase their demand for services. If physicians can protect themselves against competition by arbitrarily shifting private demand, then more physicians in an area would not necessarily lead to fewer private visits per physician—and the corollary, more Medicaid visits. Perceived disadvantages to serving Medicaid patients (e.g., payment delays, discrimination) may actually encourage some physicians to induce private demand rather than entering the public market. Recent proinducement literature includes Fuchs [16], and Mitchell and Cromwell [17]. Anti-inducement literature includes Sloan [18] and Lee and Hadley [19].
5. According to the 1975 HCFA physician survey, 77 percent of nonparticipants did not feel that the absence of Medicaid eligibles explained their nonparticipation. Other factors like low fee schedules were emphasized [12, p. 225].
6. While d_i is usually defined in terms of subjective preferences, real physician costs associated with the Medicaid program which lower net returns (e.g., complicated forms, payment delays) are comingled with preferences and are very difficult to disentangle.
7. Actually, all physicians would receive f_m if no specialty or physician-specific differences in allowable fees existed. Medicaid programs do make specialty distinctions. In addition, many use UCR reimbursement techniques based on individual physician profiles [21,22].
8. For a mathematical treatment of losses due to discrimination in the context of employer discrimination, see Thurow [23, p. 115].
9. This point is clearly arbitrary. In the empirical work that follows point L, where an SMP becomes an LMP has been defined as either 30 or 50 percent of visits Medicaid. This percentage was determined based on inspection of the size distribution of Medicaid participation.
10. Within the five primary care specialties in our sample, for example, the number of weekly visits varied from 191 for general practitioners down to 145 for internists and OB-GYNs.
11. For reasons why they might or might not, including such variables as practice size and specialty, see Ernst [27].
12. Data on the actual number of *visits* rendered to Medicaid patients are not available from the 1977 survey. If physicians provided disproportionately more services to their non-Medicaid patients, however, the extent of physician participation in Medicaid programs would be overestimated. A

t-test of means using 1976 data showed no significant differences, however, supporting our use of "patients treated" as an unbiased estimate of Medicaid practice size.

13. Unfortunately, the 1976 survey did not collect data on two important categories of explanatory variables: (1) measures of the administrative costs incurred in collecting from Medicaid; and (2) physicians' political attitudes. Both sets of variables were significant predictors of Medicaid participation in Sloan, Mitchell, and Cromwell [12]. These variables were less powerful in participants-only equations, however, suggesting that they are more important in explaining the decision to participate, rather than the level of participation once the decision is made.
14. No data on Medicaid enrollments are available below the state level, but data on the percentage of population below poverty are available by county from the 1970 U.S. Census. Taking each state's mean poverty proportion as 1.0, we developed a poverty index for counties in that state. This index, multiplied by state estimates of Medicaid patients as a percentage of population, yielded our Medicaid coverage variable (*MCAID*).
15. The Medicaid nonparticipation rate in the South was nearly 28 percent compared to 21.5, 21.4, and 13.4 percent in the North Central, North East, and West regions, respectively.
16. Null findings can always be attributed to measurement error, but the fact that these same fee variables have successfully predicted absolute participation levels elsewhere [10,12] reinforces our confidence in their accuracy—at least in relative terms.
17. The Medicaid and Blue Shield fees were correlated .43, implying significant collinearity, but probably not enough to account for the generally insignificant fee effects.
18. *Y* and *MCAID* were correlated −.37, so collinearity was not as serious as might be expected.
19. Over 60 percent of LMP30 practices are run by general surgeons, internists, and OB-GYNs, but the percentage drops to less than 30 percent when the LMP50 criterion is used. See [29, Table 2].
20. See [31] for a fuller discussion of insurer competition and the drawbacks associated with unilateral fee increases in public programs.

REFERENCES

1. U.S. Senate Special Committee on Aging. *Fraud and Abuse Among Practitioners Participating in the Medicaid Program.* Washington, DC: Government Printing Office, 1976.
2. Kavaler, F. Medicaid in New York: Utopianism and bare knuckles in public health, IV. People, providers and payment telling it how it is, *American Journal of Public Health* 59:820–25, May 1969.
3. Mitchell, J. B., and J. Cromwell. Medicaid mills: Fact or fiction, *Health Care Financing Review* 37–49, Summer 1980.
4. Jones, M. W., and B. Hamburger. A survey of physician participation in and dissatisfaction with the Medi-Cal program, *The Western Journal of Medicine* 124:75–83, January 1976.

5. Bloom, L. S., *et al.* Medicaid in Cook County: Present status and future prospects, *Inquiry* 5:13–23, June 1968.
6. Studnicki, J., *et al.* Foreign medical graduates and Maryland Medicaid, *New England Journal of Medicine* 294:1153–57, May 20, 1976.
7. Sloan, F., J. Cromwell, and J. B. Mitchell. *Private Physicians and Public Programs*. Lexington, MA: D.C. Heath, 1978.
8. Hadley, J. Physician participation in Medicaid: Evidence from California, *Health Services Research* 14:266–80, Winter 1979.
9. Davidson, S. M., and J. Perloff. Factors Affecting Physician Participation in Medicaid. Paper presented at the APHA annual meeting, October 22, 1980.
10. Mitchell, J. B., J. Cromwell and R. Schurman. Physician Participation in Public Programs. DHHS/HCFA/ORDS, Grant No. 18-P-97723/1-01, September 1981.
11. Cromwell, J., and J. B. Mitchell. The Origins and Impact of Medicaid Reimbursement and Eligibility Policies on Physician Participation. Final Report, DHHS/HCFA/ORDS, Contract No. 500-78-0051, October 1981.
12. Sloan, F., J. B. Mitchell, and J. Cromwell. Physician participation in state Medicaid programs, *Journal of Human Resources* XVIII:Supplement, 211–46, 1978.
13. Bellin, L. E., and F. Kavaler. Medicaid practitioner abuses and excuses versus counterstrategy of the New York City Health Department, *American Journal of Public Health* 61:2001–10, November 1971.
14. Feldstein, M. S. The rising price of physicians' services, *The Review of Economics and Statistics*, 52:121–33, May 1970.
15. Newhouse, J., and C. E. Phelps. New Estimates of Price and Income Elasticities of Medical Care Services. In R. Rosett (ed.). *The Role of Health Insurance in the Health Services Sector.* New York: National Bureau of Economic Research, 1976, pp. 261–320.
16. Fuchs, V. The supply of surgeons and the demand for operations, *Journal of Human Resources* XVIII:Supplement, 35–56, 1978.
17. Mitchell, J. B., and J. Cromwell. Physician-induced Demand for Surgical Operations, Final Report, DHHS/HCFA/ORDS, Grant No. 95-P-97245/2-01, December 1980.
18. Sloan, F. Analysis of Survey Data on Physician Practice Costs and Incomes: Physicians' Fees and Length of Visit, Chapter 3, Final Report, DHHS/HCFA/ORDS, 500–78–0018, April 1981.
19. Lee, R., and J. Hadley. Physicians' fees and public medical care programs, *Health Services Research* 16:185–203, Summer 1981.
20. Becker, G. *The Economics of Discrimination*. Chicago: University of Chicago Press, 1957.
21. Davidson, S. Variations in state Medicaid programs, *Journal of Health Politics, Policy and Law* 55–70, Spring 1978.
22. Mitchell, J. B., and J. Cromwell. Large Medicaid Practices: Are They Medicaid Mills? Health Care Financing Grants and Contracts Report No. 500-78-0051, March 1980.
23. Thurow, L. *Poverty and Discrimination*. Washington, D.C.: The Brookings Institution, 1969.

24. Reinhardt, U. *Physician Productivity and the Demand for Health Manpower.* Cambridge, MA: Ballinger Publishing Co., 1975.
25. Sloan, F. A. A Microanalysis of Physicians' Hours of Work Decisions. In M. Perlman (ed.). *The Economics of Health and Medical Care*, London: MacMillan, 1974, pp. 302–25.
26. Sloan, F. A. Physician supply in the short run, *Industrial and Labor Relations Review* 28:549–69, 1975.
27. Ernst, R. Ancillary production and the size of physicians' practices, *Inquiry* 13:371–81, December 1976.
28. Moss, F. E. Through the Medicaid Mills. In A. D. Spiegel (ed.). *The Medicaid Experience.* Germantown, MD: Aspen Systems, 1979, pp. 387–92.
29. Mitchell, J. B., and J. Cromwell. Large Medicaid practices and Medicaid mills, *Journal of the American Medical Association* 24:33–37, November 28, 1980.
30. Goldberger, A. S. *Econometric Theory.* New York: John Wiley and Sons, Inc., 1964.
31. Mitchell, J. B., and J. Cromwell. Access to Private Physicians for Public Patients: Participation in Medicaid and Medicare, In President's Commission for the Study of Ethical Problems in Medicine and Biomedical and Behavioral Research. *Securing Access to Health Care, Vol. 3,* pp. 105–30, January 1982.
32. Cromwell, J., J. B. Mitchell, and R. Schurman. Physician Political Attitudes. Working paper produced under HCFA Grant No. 18-P-97723/1-02.

Section Three

Modeling Clinical Decision Making

CHAPTER ELEVEN

Weighted Least-Squares Regression in Clinical Decision Analysis

The recent concern over practice variations and the differential effects of procedures and treatments on health outcomes has focused attention on the clinical decision-making process. Decision analysis is a recognized approach to the exploration of why and how certain choices are made, a technique that assigns probabilities to each branch of the decision tree. Decision processes are modeled both to explain why certain choices are made and to develop better criteria for future choices. Mark Young and his colleagues recognized that, among clinicians, a range of assessments takes place at each level of the decision-making process, but that no way has been devised to summarize those differences in a way that helps explain the differences.

Using a weighted least-squares regression model that accounts for the range of decision latitude, the authors show that groups of clinicians have much wider differences than had been thought in their assessment of the threshold at which to treat or perform a procedure for a patient. In their first article, they use data from groups of cardiologists and family physicians to demonstrate the utility of the method. In their second article, they demonstrate that there are significant differences in decision thresholds between two larger groups of similar practitioners. These differences are especially important in the case of an expensive diagnostic procedure like coronary arteriography. The result of the analysis, that family physicians are much more likely to recommend this procedure than cardiologists, is an important predictive result. Using this technique makes it possible to predict significant practice variations before they actually appear, as well as to understand variations that do occur.

The statistical approach uses a relatively unique combination of methods to explore a problem that might otherwise suggest a simpler, but misleading, approach. The key aspect of the analysis is the attention given to the distributions of the data rather than to their central tendencies. The analysis of variance, rather than centrality, may prove to be much more useful in exploring problems that focus on clinical decisions since such decisions have an inherent variability.

Comparing Aggregate Estimates of Derived Thresholds for Clinical Decisions

Mark J. Young, John M. Eisenberg, Sankey V. Williams, and John C. Hershey

Thresholds for medical decision making are the probabilities of disease at which clinicians choose to initiate testing or therapy. A descriptive analysis of clinicians' decision making can derive their test and test-treatment thresholds and has the potential to explain variations in test utilization. A previously described method summarizes thresholds for a group of clinicians by determining the range of probability which includes the maximum number of clinicians' individual thresholds. However, there is no statistical procedure to compare the summary measure of thresholds that is derived from the distribution of clinicians' thresholds. We describe two alternative methods of developing a summary measure of the thresholds for a group of clinicians. These alternative methods enable the analyst to apply standard statistical tests when analyzing the decision-making behavior of groups of clinicians. For the "Unweighted Mean of the Midpoints" method, confidence limits of means and standard t*-tests can be used to compare different groups. For the "Weighted Mean of the Midpoints" method, a weighted standard error of the mean can be calculated to determine confidence intervals, and a weighted* t*-test or weighted regression can be used to compare weighted means of the midpoints of threshold ranges.*

Supported in part by the National Center for Health Services Research (Grant #HS 04953) and the National Science Foundation (Grant #SES–8218565).

Address correspondence and requests for reprints to Mark J. Young, M.D., Division Chief, General Medicine, Medical College of Wisconsin, 8700 West Wisconsin, Milwaukee, WI 53226. At the time of the research reported in this article, Dr. Young and Sankey V. Williams, M.D. were Henry J. Kaiser Family Foundation Faculty Scholars in General Internal Medicine at The University of Pennsylvania. John M. Eisenberg, M.D. is Section Chief and Sol Katz Professor of General Internal Medicine at the Hospital of The University of Pennsylvania; Dr. Williams is Director, Robert Wood Johnson Foundation Clinical Scholars Program and Associate Professor of Medicine, The University of Pennsylvania; and John C. Hershey, Ph.D. is Professor of Decision Sciences, The Wharton School and Director of Research, The Leonard Davis Institute of Health Economics, The University of Pennsylvania.

In models of medical decision making, clinicians decide to order diagnostic tests or to begin therapy at specific probabilities of disease, which are called thresholds. Below the "test threshold," which is the threshold for testing, the clinician perceives the probability of disease to be too low to justify the risk or cost of the diagnostic test. Above the "test-treatment threshold," which is the threshold for treatment, the clinician perceives the probability of disease to be high enough to initiate treatment without further diagnostic testing. If the probability of disease is above the test threshold but below the test-treatment threshold, the clinician will order the diagnostic test. These concepts are shown graphically in Figure 1.

Methods have been proposed to calculate and prescribe optimal thresholds for decision making, using decision-analytic techniques [1,2]. The decision-analytic threshold incorporates the probabilities of chance events and the values a patient or clinician assigns to risks and benefits. Decision analysis has the advantage of explicitly identifying decision components that should be considered. This method has been limited by the difficulties inherent in eliciting and quantifying values for outcomes such as morbidity and mortality. Even though it may be difficult to quantify risk and assign values to morbidity and mortality, clinicians must make decisions in their daily practice. We have previously reported methods that can be used to derive the thresholds that clinicians actually use to guide their decisions [3,4]. These methods yield, for each clinician, a range of probabilities within which the test

Figure 1: The Threshold Model of Decision Making

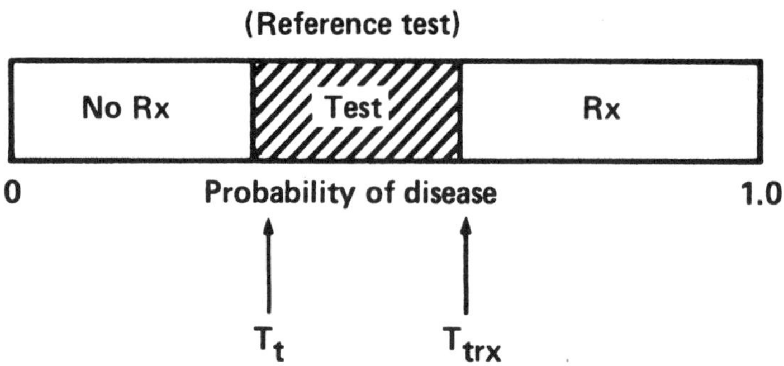

Note: *RX* refers to treatment; T_t and T_{trx} refer to the threshold for testing and the threshold for treatment. (Redrawn from Reference 2; reprinted with permission from *The New England Journal of Medicine* 302 (1980), p. 1111.)

threshold lies and another range of probabilities within which the test-treatment threshold lies.

A descriptive approach to thresholds for decision making may allow researchers to have a better understanding of differences in test utilization by clinicians. One could compare the thresholds of groups of clinicians who differ in training, site-of-practice, or other characteristics. Also, one could compare an individual clinician's aggregate threshold for one group of patients with the same clinician's aggregate threshold for another group of patients. In addition, a descriptive method for deriving thresholds offers the opportunity to compare intuitive decisions with prescriptive decisions, the latter based on the quantitative techniques of decision analysis.

These comparisons require methods for analyzing differences in thresholds. In this article, we describe three methods for aggregating threshold estimates of groups of clinicians. For two of these three methods, we also describe procedures for determining confidence intervals and for performing hypothesis tests of group differences.

We illustrate the methods with an example evaluation of clinicians' decisions in managing patients with suspected ischemic heart disease. Our goal is to describe statistical methods that can be used to aggregate threshold estimates for individual clinicians and to compare the derived thresholds of different groups of clinicians.

METHODS

PATIENT MANAGEMENT QUESTIONNAIRES

To illustrate these analytic methods, this article shows how the test threshold for coronary arteriography can be derived. This test threshold represents the probability of coronary artery disease above which clinicians would recommend arteriography. These testing thresholds were obtained by analyzing responses from clinicians to patient-management problems. In setting forth the problems, we assumed that clinicians believe that there is a subset of patients with coronary artery disease whose lives would be prolonged by coronary artery bypass grafting. We also assumed that determining the appropriateness and feasibility of surgery requires coronary arteriography. The scenarios were designed to represent realistic clinical situations in which the physician is evaluating patients with suspected coronary artery disease. In each scenario, we provided the results of exercise electrocardiographic testing to allow us to establish a range within which the threshold for coronary arteriography must lie.

In order to derive the test threshold for coronary arteriography, the responding clinicians are asked to indicate (1) their estimate of the probability of coronary disease after they read the scenario but before knowing the results of the exercise electrocardiogram; (2) their preference for performing or not performing arteriography at that time (assuming that the exercise test was not available); (3) their revised estimate of the probability of coronary disease after learning the results of the exercise electrocardiogram; and (4) their new preference for performing or not performing arteriography after knowing the exercise test results. Therefore, the clinicians' responses to the scenarios provided a means of obtaining the four basic components needed to derive thresholds (perceived pretest probability, pretest management, perceived posttest probability, and posttest management). See Figures 2 and 3. Examples of the scenarios and an interactive microcomputer program for creating new scenarios on the IBM-PC are available from one of the authors (Eisenberg).

Figure 2: General Information Needed to Derive a Clinician's Decision-Making Threshold

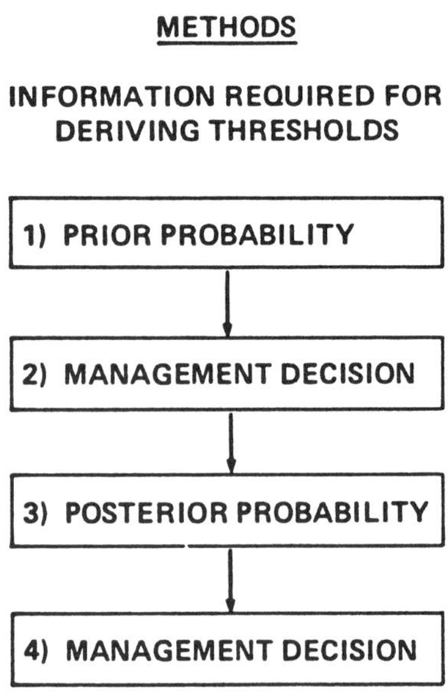

Figure 3: Test Thresholds for Coronary Arteriography

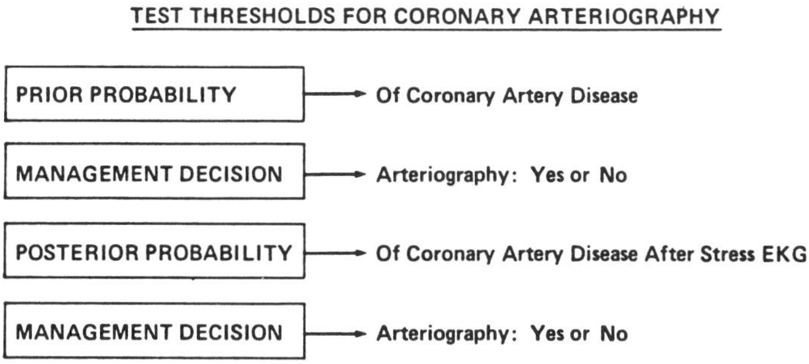

Note: Patient management problems were designed to elicit this information.

DERIVING THRESHOLDS–ONE CLINICIAN MANAGING ONE PATIENT

The threshold for recommending a test (in this case, coronary arteriography) is derived by analyzing the clinicians' estimates of prior and posterior probability and their decisions to recommend or not recommend the test based on the probability of disease. We illustrate the derivation of the feasible threshold range for a given clinician in Figure 4 by examining three possible combinations of responses to the patient scenarios. In this example, we are assuming that the test result is positive, thus yielding a posterior probability that is higher than the prior probability. An analogous procedure is used to determine the feasible threshold range for each of the three possible combinations of responses when the test result is negative.

Bar graph A in Figure 4 illustrates the first situation. In this case, the clinician would not recommend arteriography before knowing the results of the exercise test (based on his estimated prior probability), but would recommend arteriography after finding the exercise test to be abnormal (based on an estimated posterior probability that is higher). Therefore, the threshold for arteriography must lie between the prior probability and the posterior probability. (The reader should note that this method does not derive the test threshold for performing an exercise electrocardiogram. We would expect its threshold to be lower than the threshold for arteriography, which we did derive.)

A second set of hypothetical responses is illustrated by bar graph B in Figure 4. In this case, the clinician does not recommend the test

Figure 4: Method for Deriving Feasible Threshold Ranges from Three Clinicians

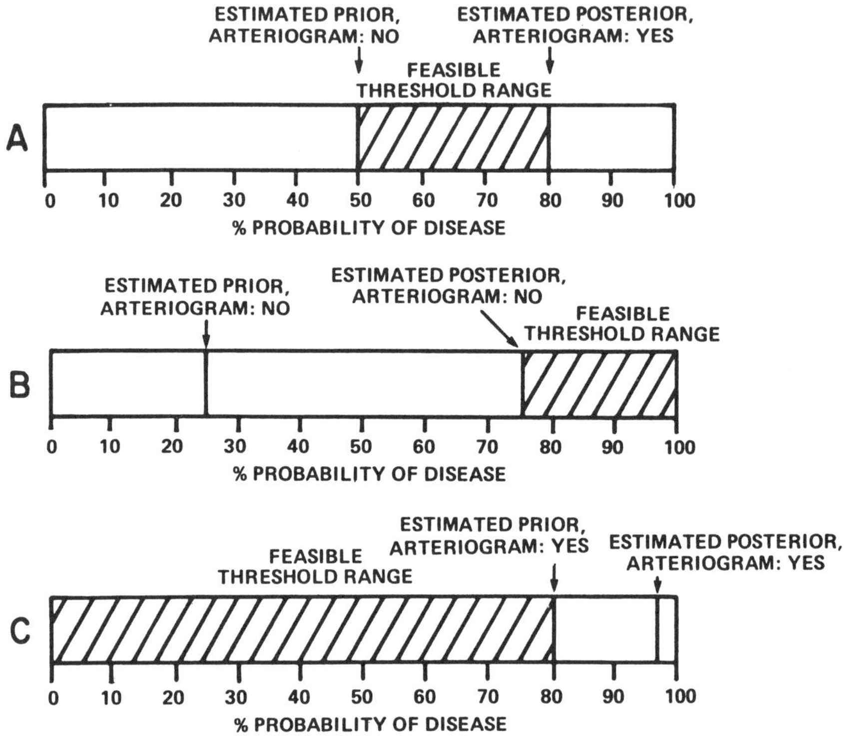

Note: For each clinician, the probability of coronary artery disease (before and after an exercise electrocardiogram) and the management decision to recommend or not recommend coronary arteriography are elicited. This information allows one to infer the feasible threshold range for each clinician.

(arteriography) either before or after the results of the exercise test are known, even though the exercise test is positive (causing the posterior probability to be higher than the prior probability). Therefore, the threshold must lie in the range between the posterior probability and 100 percent.

Finally, bar graph C in Figure 4 shows that, if the clinician recommends arteriography for both the prior probability and a higher posterior probability, the threshold lies in the range between 0 percent and the prior probability.

This clinical situation—deciding whether or not to perform arteriography after learning the results of the exercise test—is an example of the generic situation in which a clinician receives additional clinical information. Whether this additional information is from the history, the physical examination, or another diagnostic test, it would cause him to revise his estimate of the probability of disease.

AGGREGATING THE DERIVED THRESHOLDS OF INDIVIDUAL CLINICIANS

Using the method described above, we can obtain a group of probability ranges, each of which includes the feasible range for the testing threshold of one clinician for a single scenario. As an example, suppose the hypothetical responses in Figure 4 actually came from three different clinicians responding to one patient scenario. The hatched area on each bar is the feasible threshold range for that clinician. There are three ways to develop a measure that represents the derived testing threshold for the group of physicians: Modal Distribution, Unweighted Mean of the Midpoints, and Weighted Mean of the Midpoints.

Modal Distribution. In this method, the clinicians' feasible threshold ranges are displayed as in Figure 5. To determine the aggregate threshold range for the group, find the range that includes the maximum number of the individual clinicians' feasible threshold ranges. In the example shown in Figure 5, this group range would be 75–80 percent. In this instance, all three cases are included in this narrowest range. This method has been described elsewhere [3,4]. The modal distribution provides a graphic display of threshold ranges.

Unweighted Mean of the Midpoints. In this method, the midpoint of each clinician's feasible threshold range is calculated (Figure 6). To determine the aggregate threshold for the group, calculate the arithmetic mean of the individual midpoints. Standard parametric statistical testing can be used to compare the thresholds of groups of clinicians. (Of course, nonparametric tests which assume an ordinal level of measurement could also be used to compare medians or to compare the entire distributions of responses from each group.)

Weighted Mean of the Midpoints. In this method, the midpoint of each clinician's feasible threshold is calculated, as in the previous method. To determine the aggregate threshold for the group, two additional steps are required (Figure 7). First, multiply each individual midpoint by a weighting factor which is equal to one divided by the feasible threshold range squared. Second, use the weighted midpoints

Figure 5: Aggregating Thresholds—Modal Distribution

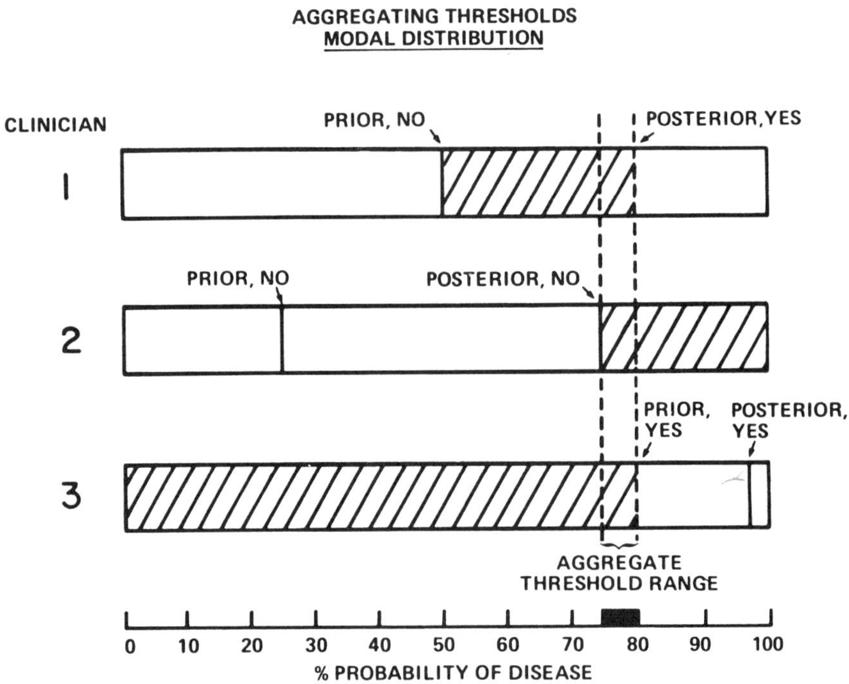

Note: In this method, the feasible threshold range is obtained from each of three clinicians. The summary measure of their threshold for coronary arteriography is the range of probability within which is encompassed the maximum number of feasible threshold ranges (which was 75–80 percent for the sample illustrated here).

in a weighted, linear-regression analysis to calculate the weighted mean and other statistical properties. The principal advantage of this method is that it gives greater weight to individual ranges that are narrow and less weight to broad ranges.

The selection of this particular weighting factor is based on the following considerations. We have obtained data that allow us to infer a range of probabilities within which the test threshold lies. Since any single value in the feasible range for the threshold is equally likely to be the threshold a clinician actually uses, one can assume that the probability density function is uniform over the range. It is desirable to give more weight to the midpoint estimate of a relatively narrow probability range than to a relatively wide one, because we are more confident that

Figure 6: Aggregating Thresholds—Unweighted Midpoints

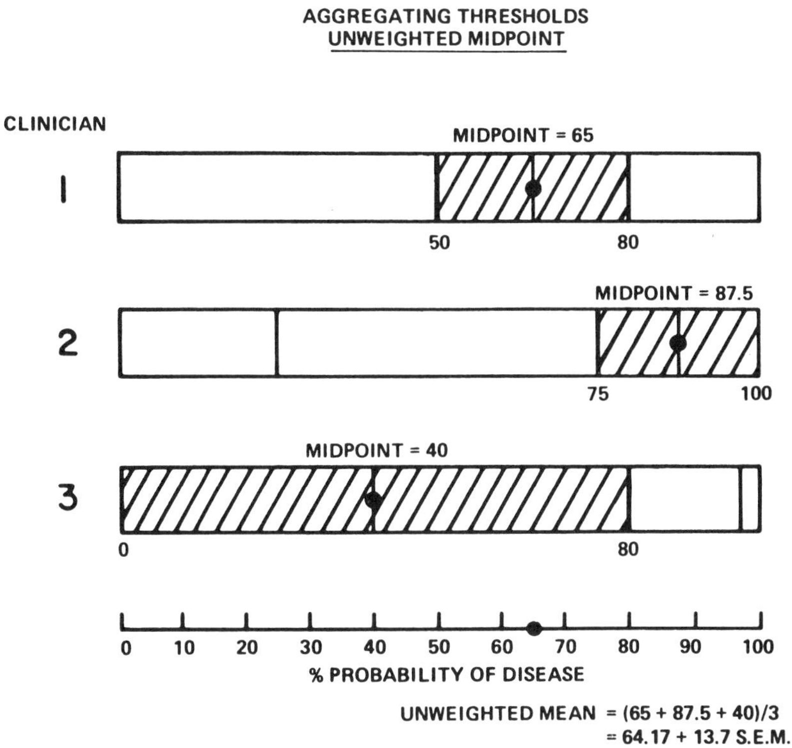

Note: In this method, the feasible threshold range is obtained from each of three clinicians. The summary measure of their threshold for coronary arteriography is the simple arithmetic mean of the midpoints of each feasible threshold range.

the midpoint of a narrow range is closer to the clinician's actual threshold. By way of illustration, Figure 8 shows the three uniform density functions corresponding to the responses of the three clinicians discussed above. A standard technique is available that assigns more weight to narrow ranges and utilizes the statistical properties of the uniform distribution. The weight applied is proportional to the square of the inverse of the range. The weights can be incorporated into standard statistical analyses to determine a measure of central tendency (the weighted mean), a measure of spread (the weighted standard error of the mean), and the significance of group differences [5–7].

Figure 7: Aggregating Thresholds—Weighted Midpoints

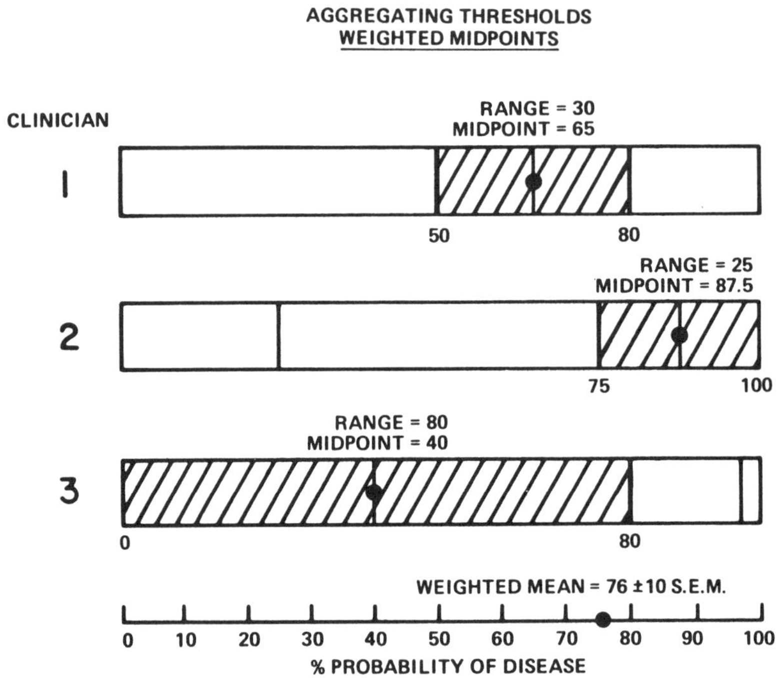

Note: In this method, the feasible threshold range is obtained from each of three clinicians. The summary measure of their threshold for coronary arteriography is the weighted mean of the midpoints of each feasible threshold range.

This weighting procedure is expressly designed for statistical analyses in which the usual assumption of equal variance (homoscedasticity) does not apply. The sample observations in the present study represent an ideal basis for applying weighted analysis, since these observations are ranges, rather than point estimates with their associated variances. Further details are provided in the Appendix.

ILLUSTRATION

The statistical properties of the threshold measurement can be illustrated by considering the responses of 36 family physicians and 20 cardiologists who replied to a written case-management problem—the patient with suspected coronary artery disease—using the format described earlier in this article. An analysis of the responses is shown in

Figure 8: Probability Density Functions for Three Clinicians Based on Uniform Distributions

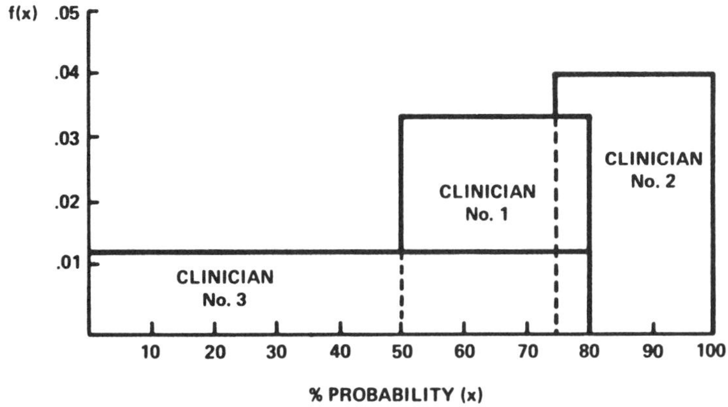

Table 1. In this example, there were striking differences between the two groups of clinicians when the weighted analysis was used. The absolute difference in the thresholds between groups changed substantially and the statistical significance of the difference went from borderline significance to unequivocal statistical significance.

In addition to deriving and comparing thresholds for groups of clinicians, this method can derive and compare thresholds for testing or treating different groups of patients. For example, the threshold for coronary arteriography might be higher for patients who would be poor operative candidates. To evaluate this possibility, the decisions of clinicians about a group of high-risk patients could be compared with decisions of these same clinicians about a group of patients with average operative risk. The means of the midpoints of the threshold ranges would be calculated for each group of patients, and the methods described in this article would be used to compare the means.

Discussion

Each of the three methods described here for analyzing derived thresholds has advantages and disadvantages. The method based on Modal Distribution can be graphically displayed in a straightforward manner. However, since this summary measure does not have an accompanying

Table 1: Comparison of Group Thresholds Using Unweighted and Weighted Methods

	Analysis	
	Unweighted Analysis	*Weighted Analysis*
Cardiologists' (N = 20) mean threshold	57%	66%
Family physicians' (N = 36) mean threshold	47%	37%
Difference between specialists	10%	29%
t-value	1.57	4.45
p-value	0.12	0.00004

measure of variance, it is not possible to apply standard statistical hypothesis testing to the modal thresholds of groups of clinicians.

The Unweighted Mean of Midpoints method provides sample means and standard deviations, and allows application of routine statistical tests. However, the method does not distinguish between narrow and wide threshold ranges. For example, if the derived threshold range for one clinician is 10–90 percent and for another clinician is 45–55 percent, the midpoint is 50 percent in both cases. However, it is more likely that the actual threshold is close to the 50 percent value when the threshold range is narrow than when it is wide.

The Weighted Mean of Midpoints analysis provides increased weight to midpoints of threshold ranges that are relatively narrow. Furthermore, there are statistics that can be applied to weighted data. However, the magnitude of the effect of weighting narrow threshold ranges is troubling. For the example above, in which one threshold range is 80 percent and the other is 10 percent, the narrow range is given 64 times more weight than the wide range. On intuitive grounds we prefer the weighted analysis, but there is no reference standard for objective evaluation in selecting the preferable method.

The potential importance of heavily weighted, narrow threshold ranges is evident in Table 1. The thresholds for recommending coronary arteriography were obtained from a group of cardiologists and family physicians. The distribution of ranges explains the marked differences between the weighted and unweighted analyses. For cardiologists, more responses with narrow ranges were above this group's simple mean, which led to a higher weighted mean threshold for cardiologists in the weighted analysis. For family physicians, more responses with narrow ranges were below this group's simple mean, which led to a lower weighted mean for the threshold of family physicians for prescribing coronary arteriography in the weighted analysis. These data should not be misinterpreted. We use them only as an example of the statistics. They were obtained from convenience samples of clinicians and are not generalizable to larger groups.

A major question about the methods of deriving thresholds is whether they will improve our understanding of clinicians' decision making. Our methods may be limited by clinicians' inability to give accurate estimates of probability. The weighted method gives increased weight to narrow ranges of thresholds. Therefore, it would be important to note whether one group of clinicians systematically revises probability to a lesser degree than the other group. We have described methods for determining measures of central tendency, but one may question whether or not this is a meaningful measure in analyzing clinicians' decision making. In many clinical situations there is likely to be a broad range of opinion on what constitutes the best management strategy. Rather than focusing on differences in central tendency between groups of clinicians, it may be more informative to characterize the clinicians whose responses are substantially different from the central tendency. Moreover, one might wonder how much validity there is in a method that appears dependent on simulated case-management scenarios, which cannot perfectly represent all the factors that influence decision making in actual practice. Because of this problem, we have begun using information from actual clinicians' decisions about real patients to derive thresholds for the decision about arteriography in suspected coronary artery disease.

Perhaps the most interesting application of these methods is the opportunity to contrast derived thresholds with prescriptive thresholds obtained by decision analysis. Such analyses may enable researchers to measure to what extent decision analysis does not capture all of the relevant information used by clinicians and to determine if systematic errors occur in intuitive decision making.

APPENDIX

A METHOD FOR COMPARING DERIVED THRESHOLDS USING WEIGHTED-LEAST-SQUARES REGRESSION

Each physician in each of two groups answers a series of questions that allow us to infer a range of probabilities within which the test threshold lies. Since no value within a given physician's range is any more or less likely than any other value, we assume a uniform probability distribution for the true value of the test threshold over each range.

This appendix describes a set of statistical procedures designed to summarize the data and perform tests of hypotheses. The procedures give more weight to relatively narrow probability ranges than to relatively wide ones. This is desirable because, in the former case, more information can be inferred about the true value of the test threshold. The relative contributions are expressed in terms of weights, which we show to be proportional to the inverse of the variance of each range. We describe procedures for calculating the weighted mean and weighted standard error of the mean for each of the two groups, and we give the t-test statistic which can be used to test whether the difference in the weighted means of the two groups is significant.

Let Y_i be the midpoint of each range, where $i = 1, 2, \ldots, n$. Let r_i be the range for each observation, where $i = 1, 2, \ldots, n$.

Y_i, the midpoint of each range, is also the expected value for each physician's threshold, since we are assuming a uniform distribution. The variance of such a distribution is $r_i^2/12$ [5].

If all of the variances were identical, standard regression analysis procedures could be used to calculate all of the summary measures and the t-test statistic described above. However, in the present situation, the assumption of variance homogeneity which is required for using standard regression analysis does not hold. The weighted-least-squares method of analysis is a modification of standard regression analysis which can be used for dealing with variance heterogeneity [6].

The methodology involves determining the regression coefficients $\hat{a}'$ and $\hat{b}'$ which minimize the expression

$$\sum_{i=1}^{n} w_i(Y_i - \hat{a}' - \hat{b}'X_i)^2$$

where the "weight" w_i for the ith midpoint is $1/\sigma_i^2 = 12/r_i^2$, and x_i is equal to 0 if the physician is a member of group 1 and is equal to 1 if the physician is a member of group 2. When the expression is minimized, $\hat{a}'$ will be the weighted mean for group 1 and $\hat{a}' + \hat{b}'$ will be the weighted mean for group 2.

For our application of weighted-least-squares regression, a' and b' are found as follows:

$$\hat{b}' = \frac{\sum_{i=1}^{n} (X_i - \overline{X}')(Y_i - \overline{Y}')/r_i^2}{\sum_{i=1}^{n} (X_i - \overline{X}')^2/r_i^2}$$

and

$$\hat{a}' = \overline{Y}' - \hat{b}'\overline{X}'$$

where

$$\overline{Y}' = \frac{\sum_{i=1}^{n} Y_i /r_i^2}{\sum_{i=1}^{n} 1/r_i^2}$$

and

$$\overline{X}' = \frac{\sum_{i=1}^{n} X_i /r_i^2}{\sum_{i=1}^{n} 1/r_i^2}$$

Under the usual normality assumption on the Y variable, the following test statistic may be used to test the null hypothesis that $\hat{b}' = 0$ (see [6]):

$$t = \frac{\hat{b}' - 0}{S'_{Y|X}/(S'_X\sqrt{n-1})} \sim t_{n-2} \text{ under } H_o, \tag{1}$$

where, in our application,

$$S'^2_{Y|X} = \frac{1}{n-2}\sum_{i=1}^{n}(Y_i - \hat{a}' - \hat{b}'X_i)^2/r_i^2$$

and

$$S'^2_X = \frac{1}{n-1}\sum_{i=1}^{n}(X_i - \overline{X}')^2/r_i^2$$

Since $\hat{b}'$ is the estimated difference in means, this is equivalent to testing the null hypothesis that the two populations have the same mean.

This procedure is equivalent to introducing weights to the more standard approach for carrying out the t-test. To see this, it is helpful, first, to redefine some variables.

Let Y_{ij} be the midpoint of each range, $i = 1, 2$
$j = 1, 2, \ldots, n_1$ for $i = 1$
$j = 1, 2, \ldots, n_2$ for $i = 2$.

Let r_{ij} be the range for each observation, i and j as above.

The sample mean for group i is:

$$\overline{Y}'_i = \frac{\sum_{j=1}^{n_i} Y_{ij} / r_{ij}^2}{\sum_{j=1}^{n_i} 1/r_{ij}^2}$$

The estimated standard error of the mean for group i is:

$$S'_{\overline{Y}_i} = \left\{ \frac{\sum_{j=1}^{n_i} (Y_{ij} - \overline{Y}'_i)^2 / r_{ij}^2}{(n_i - 1) \sum_{j=1}^{n_i} 1/r_{ij}^2} \right\}^{1/2}$$

The sample mean and the estimated standard error of the mean can be used in the typical manner for providing summary statistics about a given population. General procedures for hypothesis testing and for finding confidence intervals also apply. For example, confidence limits for the population mean for group 1, using the t-distribution, would be:

$$Y'_1 \pm t \cdot S'_{\overline{Y}'_1}$$

where t is determined for $n - 1$ degrees of freedom.

To carry out a t-test for the difference between sample means, one must assume equal population variances. To test the null hypothesis that the difference in population means is zero, we use the t-statistic:

$$t = \frac{\overline{Y}'_2 - \overline{Y}'_1}{S'_{\overline{Y}'_2 - \overline{Y}'_1}} \tag{2}$$

where $S'_{\overline{Y}'_2 - \overline{Y}'_1}$, the estimated standard error of the difference between the two means, is:

$$S'_{\overline{Y}'_2-\overline{Y}'_1} = \left\{ \frac{\sum_{i=1}^{2}\sum_{j=1}^{n_i}(Y_{ij}-\overline{Y}'_i)^2/r_{ij}^2}{n_1+n_2-2} \right\}^{1/2} \left\{ \sum_{i=1}^{2} \frac{1}{\sum_{j=1}^{n_i} 1/r_{ij}^2} \right\}^{1/2} \quad (3)$$

It can be shown that formula (2) for t is equivalent to formula (1) above. The first term in (3) is equivalent to $S'_{Y|X}$ in formula (1); the second term in (3) is equivalent to $1/(S'_X\sqrt{n-1})$ in formula (1) (proof not shown). Computational assistance is available in standard statistical packages, for instance, the weighted regression procedure in BMDP [7].

To illustrate the calculations, using the second method, we provide the following example (where group 2 represents the group of three physicians shown in Figure 3):

Group 1		*Group 2*	
Y_{1j}	r_{1j}	Y_{2j}	r_{2j}
30	40	65	30
50	20	40	80
75	50	87.5	25
55	35		

$$\overline{Y}'_1 = \frac{30/1600 + 50/400 + 75/2500 + 55/1225}{1/1600 + 1/400 + 1/2500 + 1/1225} = 50.36$$

$$S'_{\overline{Y}'_1} = \left\{ \frac{(-20.36)^2/1600 + (-.36)^2/400 + (24.64)^2/2500 + (4.64)^2/1225}{(3)(1/1600 + 1/400 + 1/2500 + 1/1225)} \right\}^{1/2} = 6.32$$

$$\overline{Y}'_2 = \frac{65/900 + 40/6400 + 87.5/625}{1/900 + 1/6400 + 1/625} = 76.19$$

$$S'_{\overline{Y}'_2} = \left\{ \frac{(-11.19)^2/900 + (-.36.19)^2/6400 + (11.31)^2/625}{(2)(1/900 + 1/6400 + 1/625)} \right\}^{1/2} = 9.78$$

$$t = \frac{25.83}{\left\{\frac{1.0683}{5}\right\}^{1/2} \left\{\frac{1}{.00434} + \frac{1}{.00287}\right\}^{1/2}} = 2.32$$

ACKNOWLEDGMENT

We thank Gary Pickens, Ph.D. for his help in developing the statistical methods in this article.

REFERENCES

1. Pauker, S. G., and J. P. Kassirer. Therapeutic decision making: A cost-benefit analysis. *New England Journal of Medicine* 293(5):229-34, 1975.
2. Pauker, S. G., and J. P. Kassirer. The threshold approach to clinical decision making. *New England Journal of Medicine* 302(20):1109-17, 1980.
3. Eisenberg, J. M., and J. C. Hershey. Derived thresholds: Determining the diagnostic probabilities at which clinicians initiate testing and treatment. *Medical Decision Making* 3(2):155-64, 1983.
4. Eisenberg, J. M., et al. Usefulness of synovial fluid analysis in the evaluation of joint effusions: Use of threshold analysis and likelihood ratios to assess a diagnostic test. *Archives of Internal Medicine* 144(4):715-19, 1984.
5. Lindgren, B. W. *Statistical Theory*. New York: McMillan Co., 1962, p. 81.
6. Kleinbaum, D. G., and L. L. Kupper. *Applied Regression Analysis and Other Multivariable Methods*. North Scituate, MA: Duxbury Press, 1978, p. 243.
7. *BMDP Statistical Software*. Berkeley: University of California Press, 1983, pp. 236-237.

Do Cardiologists Have Higher Thresholds for Recommending Coronary Arteriography than Family Physicians?

Mark J. Young, Lisbeth S. Fried, John Eisenberg, John Hershey, and Sankey Williams

The purpose of this study was to use a new model of decision making to understand variability in physicians' utilization of diagnostic tests. We studied physicians' recommendations for coronary arteriography in hypothetical patients with chest pain by analyzing responses of 235 cardiologists and family physicians. Thresholds for testing were derived by obtaining estimates of the probability of disease and recommendations for coronary arteriography before and after an exercise test. We found that cardiologists compared with family practitioners had a significantly higher decision threshold and recommended coronary arteriography in fewer patients. These findings suggest that analyzing physicians' decision-making thresholds may be used to characterize differences in the practice behavior of groups of physicians.

Recent work in medical decision making has identified the importance of decision thresholds, which are probabilities of disease at which clini-

---

This study was supported under Grant No. HS 04953 from the National Center for Health Services Research.

Address correspondence and requests for reprints to Mark J. Young, M.D., Division Chief, General Medicine, Medical College of Wisconsin, 8700 West Wisconsin, Milwaukee, WI 53226. Lisbeth S. Fried, Ph.D. is Research Investigator in the Division of General Internal Medicine, University of Michigan Medical Center, Ann Arbor; John Eisenberg, M.D. is Section Chief and Sol Katz Professor of General Internal Medicine at the Hospital of the University of Pennsylvania; John Hershey, Ph.D. is Professor of Decision Sciences, The Wharton School and Director of Research, The Leonard Davis Institute of Health Economics, The University of Pennsylvania; and Sankey Williams, M.D. is Director, Robert Wood Johnson Foundation Clinical Scholars Program and Associate Professor of Medicine, The University of Pennsylvania.

cians change the way they manage their patients. Below the threshold probability for testing, a doctor does not do a test, but if the probability of disease is just above the threshold, the test is ordered. If the probability of disease is high enough, the test may not be ordered—or treatment may be started without waiting for the test result.

Pauker and Kassirer have used decision analysis to calculate normative values for these test and test-treatment thresholds [1, 2]. These decision analytic thresholds use explicit risks and benefits of performing a diagnostic test or recommending treatment in an individual patient and define the optimum probability at which the threshold should lie. In contrast to the thresholds calculated using decision analysis (i.e., the thresholds clinicians *should* use), it is possible to characterize decision-making thresholds that *are* used by analyzing the decisions that physicians make [3]. We have previously reported the theoretical framework and the statistical methods for characterizing the decision-making thresholds of physicians [4–6].

The purpose of this study was to use descriptive thresholds to understand physicians' utilization of diagnostic tests. The reasons for variation in physicians' use of diagnostic tests are unknown but, at least in part, variation may be related to differences in physicians' decision thresholds. Since recent literature has demonstrated differences in practice style among medical specialties, our specific objective was to determine if there is a difference in the threshold for recommending coronary arteriography between family physicians and cardiologists. We studied physicians' recommendations for coronary arteriography in patients with suspected chest pain because of the clinical and economic importance of coronary artery disease [7–15] and because of the extensive efforts being made to clarify the role of probability of disease in managing patients with coronary artery disease [16–22].

METHODS

The overall design of this study was (1) to develop patient management problems describing patients with chest pain, (2) to administer the problems to a group of family physicians and cardiologists, (3) to use the information to derive the thresholds for recommending coronary arteriography, and (4) to determine if there are differences in thresholds for coronary arteriography between family physicians and cardiologists.

DERIVING THE THRESHOLDS

The detailed explanation of the methods for deriving and analyzing decision-making thresholds has been published previously [4–6]. In brief, the test threshold for recommending coronary arteriography can be calculated after obtaining four pieces of information: (1) an estimate of the pretest probability and (2) the clinician's management decision, followed by (3) the posttest probability and (4) the revised management decision after the test results have been considered. These four pieces of information are used to determine the range of probability within which the decision-making threshold must lie. For example, consider a clinician who estimates the probability of coronary artery disease as .30 based on available clinical information, but who will not recommend coronary arteriography for that probability of disease. However, after acquiring the results of a positive stress electrocardiogram he revises his probability of disease to .70 and at this point will recommend arteriography. This information allows us to infer that the threshold for arteriography must lie between the prior probability and the posterior probability. In this case, the threshold is between .30 and .70. A similar procedure enables us to derive the feasible range for the threshold for any combination of probability estimates and management decisions. The aggregate threshold for a group of clinicians can be calculated using a simple average of the midpoints of the threshold ranges or by performing a weighted regression that gives increased weight to observations in which the feasible range for the threshold is narrow [6].

Consider, as an example, the feasible ranges of the threshold that had been obtained from three clinicians. For clinician A, the range was between .50 and .80; for clinician B, the range was between .75 and 1.00; and for clinician C, the range was between .0 and .80. A summary measure of the threshold for these three different clinicians can be obtained by averaging the midpoints of the ranges. The arithmetic mean would be $(.65 + .875 + .4)/3 = .641$. The weighted regression technique gives a mean threshold of .76. This value is higher than the unweighted threshold and reflects the increased confidence that the midpoint obtained from a narrow range represents the true threshold.

PATIENT MANAGEMENT PROBLEMS

We wrote four scenarios that described patients with chest pain. The physicians were asked to manage the patients as they would in their own practices. The patients in each case were similar in age, sex, and socioeconomic status but differed in pattern of chest pain and results of exercise testing. The scenarios stated that the patient would consider coronary artery surgery if the physicians felt surgery was indicated. The data of Diamond and Forrester [21] were used to design the scenarios and to estimate the probability of coronary artery disease. Each scenario was written to include a different range of probability.

The scenarios were designed to represent realistic clinical situations. The scenarios first gave a brief description of a patient's history, physical examination, and initial laboratory tests. Next, the doctor was asked to estimate the probability of coronary artery disease (50 percent or greater obstruction of at least one coronary artery) and to decide whether or not to recommend coronary arteriography. Finally, the results of an exercise stress electrocardiogram were given, and the doctor was asked to revise the probability of disease and the decision for arteriography. The scenarios were pilot-tested with practicing physicians and were found to be clinically plausible. An example of the scenarios is included in the appendix; complete copies of the patient management problems are available upon request.

SUBJECTS

Subjects consisted of 400 physicians from Pennsylvania and Michigan, 100 cardiologists and 100 family practitioners from each state. Cardiologists were randomly selected from the directory of the American College of Physicians and family practitioners from the directory of the American Academy of Family Practice. A letter explaining the project was sent with the patient management problems to each subject selected for participation. Subjects were asked to complete the questions in the four scenarios and to provide demographic information about their practices, their patients, and themselves.

STATISTICS

Standard *t*-tests and Fisher's exact tests were used to analyze the demographic variables and the proportion of doctors who recommended coronary arteriography. The thresholds were measured using an arithmetic mean and a weighted analysis [6]. Since each subject's threshold was derived from each of four scenarios, repeated measures analysis of variance was used to compare differences in thresholds between cardiologists and family physicians. Finally, multiple regression was used to examine the influence of demographic variables on the thresholds. All analyses were performed using BMDP statistical software [23].

RESULTS

DESCRIPTION OF RESPONDENTS

Of the 400 physicians sampled, 21 had retired, moved, or died; responses were obtained from 235 of the 371 remaining, a 62 percent response rate. The nonrespondents were similar to the respondents in age, sex, and board certification. Of the total respondents, 123 were from Michigan (52 cardiologists, 67 family practitioners, and 4 of unknown specialty) and 112 were from Pennsylvania (57 cardiologists, 52 family practitioners, and 3 with unknown specialty).

The two sites did not differ in the proportion of female respondents (4.2 percent in Michigan and 4.5 percent in Pennsylvania), in the proportion of respondents who were board certified (83 percent in Michigan and 79 percent in Pennsylvania), or in the number of patients seen each week (92.9 in Michigan and 92.6 in Pennsylvania). However, the respondents from Pennsylvania were slightly older than those from Michigan (53.3 years versus 47.6 years, $p < .001$).

The respondents in the two specialties did differ noticeably from each other. Cardiologists were more likely than family practitioners to be board certified (90.7 percent versus 72.4 percent, $p < .001$), to see fewer patients each week (68.8 versus 117.5, $p < .001$), and to see more patients each week with suspected coronary artery disease (36.6 versus 18.0, $p < .001$). The two specialties did not differ significantly in the proportion of female physicians in each (1.8 percent among the cardiologists responding and 6.8 percent among the family practitioners, $p = .07$).

THRESHOLDS FOR CORONARY ARTERIOGRAPHY

Figure 1 shows the average threshold for recommending coronary arteriography for the two types of specialists. Results were unchanged when weighted analyses were performed. The data are shown separately for each scenario. Since responses to all four scenarios were obtained from each clinician, we used a repeated measures analysis of variance to test for a significant main effect of specialty, geographic site, or scenario type. We found that cardiologists had a higher threshold than family physicians for recommending coronary arteriography in all four scenarios ($p < .001$). That is, the cardiologists required a higher probability of coronary artery disease before recommending invasive testing. There was no statistically significant effect of site on threshold: the average threshold in Michigan was .50; in Pennsylvania it was .44.

Figure 1: Thresholds for Recommending Coronary Arteriography

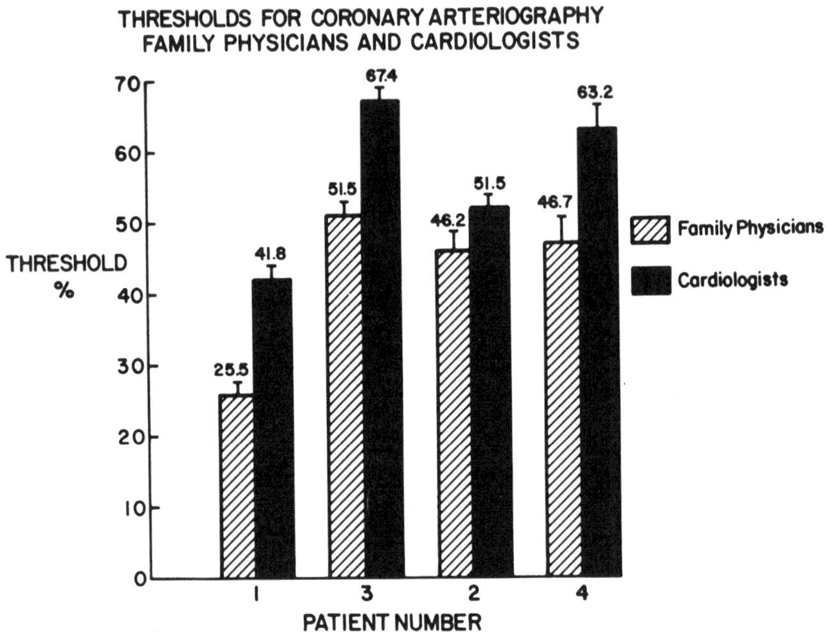

The SEM is shown for each threshold. The overall differences between the thresholds of family physicians and cardiologists was significant, $p < 0.001$ by repeated measures analysis of variance.

Even though the patient's age, sex, and socioeconomic status were held constant, the scenario to which the physician was responding exerted a large main effect on the derived threshold ($p < .001$).

EFFECT OF ADDITIONAL INDEPENDENT VARIABLES ON THE DERIVED THRESHOLD

Because the doctor's age, sex, number of patients per week, number of patients with coronary artery disease, and board certification might influence the derived threshold, these variables along with specialty and site were regressed against the midpoint of each threshold range. This analysis revealed that, in addition to specialty, physicians' age was a significant predictor of their decision thresholds. There was a negative correlation between age and threshold, indicating that the younger physicians compared to older physicians have a higher threshold for recommending catheterization. No other independent variable correlated with physician threshold after controlling for age and specialty.

PROBABILITY ESTIMATES

Table 1 shows the probability of coronary artery disease based on Diamond and Forrester's data for the different scenarios and the estimates of the physicians. The estimates of the pretest probabilities are of special interest in that no consistent difference between specialties was reported. Cardiologists as compared with family physicians assigned higher probabilities for patients with typical angina but equal or lower probabilities for patients with atypical angina.

PROPORTION OF PHYSICIANS WHO WOULD RECOMMEND CATHETERIZATION

Figure 2 presents the proportion of physicians in each group who recommended catheterization for each patient problem. In each case, fewer cardiologists than family practitioners recommended catheterization. In three out of four scenarios, the difference was significant (by Fisher's exact test, $p < .05$). This result was found in both states. Therefore, the proportion of physicians recommending catheterization was consistent with the conclusion that cardiologists had higher thresholds than did family practitioners.

Table 1: Probability Estimates (N = 109 Cardiologists and 119 Family Physicians)

		Source of Probability Estimate		
Scenario	*Type of Probability*	*Diamond and Forrester**	*Cardiologists (± SEM)**	*Family Physicians (± SEM)**
1	Pretest	.22	.23 (.02)†	.23 (.01)
	Posttest	.39	.66 (.02)	.57 (.02)
2	Pretest	.70	.61 (.02)	.44 (.02)
	Posttest	.96	.80 (.02)	.75 (.02)
3	Pretest	.22	.19 (.01)	.31 (.02)
	Posttest	.06	.13 (.01)	.11 (.01)
4	Pretest	.70	.65 (.02)	.46 (.02)
	Posttest	.26	.40 (.02)	.36 (.02)

*Probability estimates include results based on Diamond and Forrester's data, estimates made by cardiologists, and estimates made by family physicians.

†Numbers in parentheses are the SEM for the probability estimates.

Figure 2: Proportion of Physicians Recommending Arteriography for Each Scenario

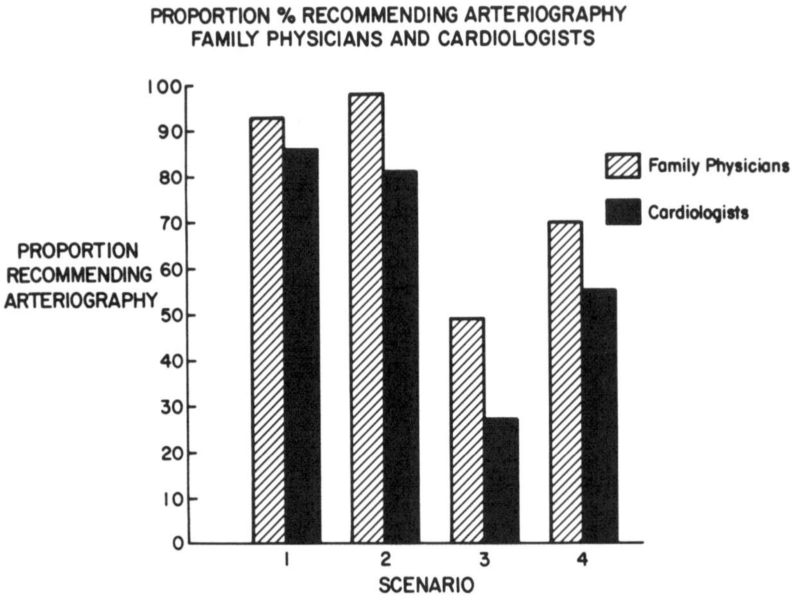

Cardiologists less frequently recommended arteriography than did family physicians. The difference in proportion was significant at $p < .02$ for scenarios 2–4 and $p = .06$ for scenario 1.

DISCUSSION

This study attempted to determine whether family physicians and cardiologists differ in the probability of coronary artery disease at which they recommend coronary arteriography. It used a new method of deriving physicians' thresholds and comparing the thresholds of different groups of physicians. Because some investigators [24–28] have found that family physicians use fewer diagnostic tests than internists, we anticipated similar findings for their recommending coronary arteriography. Instead, family physicians recommended coronary arteriography more often and at a lower probability of disease than did cardiologists.

There may be several explanations for this finding. Since family physicians do not actually perform arteriography, they may look upon the decision as one in which they will merely seek an opinion from a cardiologist. For them, the decision is really to refer, not to perform the test. Further work needs to be done to clarify the consultative versus the technical-service role of cardiologists when their practice styles are being evaluated. Are subspecialists generally asked for an opinion about management or simply for performance of a procedure that the referring physician wants?

Since family physicians are likely to see patients whose chest pain is not of cardiac origin, family physicians might simply give systematically lower estimates of probability of coronary artery disease than do cardiologists. Since our method uses these estimates of probability, the differences in thresholds could have been due to a difference in estimates of probability. Our results show that cardiologists did not consistently give higher estimates of disease than family physicians. Furthermore, we examined the number of instances in which the physicians recommended coronary arteriography. The family physicians more frequently recommended the test than did cardiologists, even though the scenarios were the same for both groups.

Another explanation for the difference in thresholds may relate to the different specialists' opinions of the importance of defining the anatomy in managing patients with coronary artery disease. For instance, if the clinician felt that a large portion of patients with coronary artery disease need coronary artery bypass grafting to prolong their lives, the threshold for coronary arteriography was lower. Cardiologists may have been aware that the most recent studies of coronary artery surgery suggest that relatively few patients need surgery to prolong their survival [29]. In addition, the cardiologists may have been more skeptical of the role of arteriography in deciding on the need for surgery [30, 31].

Finally, the differences in decision-making thresholds between the two specialty groups are based only on simulated patients. It is possible that the case summaries were more realistic for the cardiologists to interpret. It is also possible that the physicians were influenced by concerns that they were being evaluated. Family physicians might request catheterization to avoid missing coronary artery disease; cardiologists might avoid catheterization to avoid being perceived as over-ordering or excessively reliant on technology. There is legitimate concern about the validity of generalizing results from artificial tasks to the real world [32, 33]. We are currently applying threshold analyses to actual decision making in the exercise electrocardiogram laboratories of our institutions.

One other unexpected finding in this study was the effect of age on the threshold for recommending coronary arteriography. Contrary to other studies [34], older physicians more frequently recommended testing than did younger physicians. The fact that younger physicians had a higher testing threshold than older physicians suggests that familiarity with the technical aspects of the test and with the recent literature may be influential in their greater reluctance to order the test.

This study, in showing that cardiologists have higher thresholds for recommending coronary arteriography than family physicians demonstrates the importance of understanding the underlying reasons for variation among physicians' practice patterns. The method of deriving thresholds described in this article offers one probe into medical decision making as a means of exploring interphysician variation.

APPENDIX

The following is an example of the case scenarios that were used to determine the decision-making thresholds. The design enabled us to obtain the four pieces of information necessary for deriving the threshold for coronary arteriography: (1) pretest probability of disease, (2) pretest management decision, (3) posttest probability of disease, and (4) posttest management decision.

CASE ONE

The patient is a 37-year-old man who complains of persistent burping. He works as a travel agent. Three years ago he was admitted to another hospital for chest pain of unknown etiology. A mycardial infarction was ruled out by enzymes and ECG. No further evaluation was undertaken at that time. In the last three years, he has had no symptoms that could be attributed to his cardiovascular system until two months ago. Then he noted the onset of "burping" with exertion without any chest tightness or discomfort or any associated shortness of breath, paroxysmal nocturnal dyspnea, orthopnea, dizziness, syncope, or palpitations. An upper gastrointestinal series was negative. Since then his burping has continued. Although the patient said that he had tried nitroglycerin tablets, they gave him such a bad headache he could not tell if they improved his burping sensation. He smoked cigarettes in high school but none since then. His past medical history and review of systems are unremarkable. His family history shows that both parents are well; his 42-year-old brother is also healthy. His current medications include cimetidine, 300 mg., q.i.d., and liquid antacid p.r.n.

On physical examination he is 5 feet, 9 inches tall and weighs 165 pounds. He has a blood pressure of 115/70 in the right arm standing and his resting heart rate is 65 and regular. His physical examination is completely within normal limits, including his cardiovascular examination.

His electrocardiogram is remarkable for sinus bradycardia at a rate of 60 with minor nonspecific repolarization abnormalities. An echocardiogram reveals only slight dilatation of the left atrium with normal left ventricular dimensions. Results of a chest film, urinalysis, complete blood count, and multiphasic biochemical screen are all within normal limits.

Questions

1. If you were to see 100 patients exactly like this one, in how many of them would you expect to find significant (> 50 percent of at least one vessel) coronary obstruction when coronary arteriography is performed?

2. Assuming the patient would accept surgery if indicated, would you recommend coronary arteriography?

   An exercise test is performed using Bruce's multistage maximal treadmill protocol. The treadmill time is 3 minutes and 21 seconds with a maximal speed of 2.5 mph and maximal grade of 12 percent. Fifty-one percent of the predicted maximal heart rate is achieved. The test is stopped because the patient develops frequent burping at a heart rate of 80 with mild substernal pressure. 1.3 millimeters of horizontal to downward sloping ST segment depression appear at the same time and persist for five minutes. There is a rise in post-exercise blood pressure to 170/100. On the report you receive, this is interpreted as a positive test.

3. Now if you were to see 100 patients with the clinical information and exercise test result of the patient in this scenario, in how many of them would you expect to find significant (> 50 percent of at least one vessel) coronary obstruction when coronary arteriography is performed?

4. Assuming the patient would accept surgery if indicated, would you recommend coronary arteriography?

REFERENCES

1. Pauker, S. G., and J. P. Kassirer. Therapeutic decision making: A cost-benefit analysis. *New England Journal of Medicine* 293:229–34, 1975.
2. Pauker, S. G., and J. P. Kassirer. The threshold approach to clinical decision making. *New England Journal of Medicine* 302:1109–17, 1980.
3. Allman, R. M., et al. Physician tolerance for uncertainty: Use of liver-spleen scans to detect metastases. *Journal of the American Medical Association* 254:246–48, 1985.
4. Eisenberg, J. M., and J. C. Hershey. Derived thresholds: Determining the diagnostic probabilities at which clinicians initiate testing and treatment. *Medical Decision Making* 3:155–64, 1983.
5. Eisenberg, J. M., et al. Usefulness of synovial fluid analysis in the evaluation of joint effusions: Use of threshold analysis and likelihood ratios to assess a diagnostic test. *Archives of Internal Medicine* 144:715–19, 1984.
6. Young, M. J., et al. Comparing aggregate estimates of derived thresholds for clinical decisions. *Health Services Research* 20(6):763–80, February 1986.
7. Goldman, L., and E. F. Cook. The decline in ischemic heart disease mortality rates. *Annals of Internal Medicine* 101:825–36, 1984.
8. Hansing, C. E. The risk and cost of coronary angiography: I. Cost of coronary angiography in Washington State. *Journal of the American Medical Association* 242:731–34, 1979.
9. Hansing, C. E. The risk and cost of coronary angiography: II. The risk of coronary angiography in Washington State. *Journal of the American Medical Association* 242(8):735–38, 1979.
10. Levin, D. C. Invasive evaluation (coronary arteriography) of the coronary artery disease patient: Clinical, economic and social issues. *Circulation* 66(5):71–79, 1982.
11. Epstein, S. E., S. T. Palmeri, and R. E. Patterson. Current concepts: Evaluation of patients after acute myocardial infarction: Indications for cardiac catheterization and surgical intervention. *New England Journal of Medicine* 307:1487–92, 1982.
12. Silverman, K. J., and W. Grossman. Angina pectoris: Natural history and strategies for evaluation and management. *New England Journal of Medicine* 310:1712–17, 1984.
13. Kennedy, R. H., et al. Use of the cardiac-catheterization laboratory in a defined population. *New England Journal of Medicine* 303:1273–77, 1980.
14. Kennedy, R. H., et al. Cardiac-catheterization and cardiac-surgical facilities: Use, trends, and future requirements. *New England Journal of Medicine* 307:986–93, 1982.
15. Schwartz, W. B., and P. L. Joskow. Duplicated hospital facilities: How much can we save by consolidating them? *New England Journal of Medicine* 303(25):1449–57, 1980.
16. Pauker, S. G. Coronary artery surgery: The use of decision analysis. *Annals of Internal Medicine* 85:8–18, 1976.
17. Pauker, S. G., and J. P. Kassirer. Clinical decision analysis by personal computer. *Archives of Internal Medicine* 141:1831–37, 1981.
18. Pliskin, J. S., et al. Coronary artery bypass graft surgery: Clinical decision making and cost-effective analysis. *Medical Decision Making* 1(1):10–27, 1981.

19. Li, T. C., et al. The selective impact of a cardiology data bank on physicians' therapeutic recommendations. *Medical Decision Making* 4:165–76, 1984.
20. Sisson, J. C. What promise the preliminary tests of coronary artery disease? *Journal of Nuclear Medicine* 22:303–08, 1981.
21. Diamond, G. A., and J. S. Forrester. Analysis of probability as an aid in the clinical diagnosis of coronary-artery disease. *New England Journal of Medicine* 300:1350–58, 1979.
22. Rifkin, R. D., and W. B. Hood, Jr. Bayesian analysis of electrocardiographic exercise stress testing. *New England Journal of Medicine* 297:681–86, 1977.
23. BMDP Statistical Software. University of California Press, Berkeley, 1983.
24. Weiss, B. D. Family physicians in university hospital intensive care units. *Journal of Family Practice* 17:693–96, 1983.
25. Bennett, M. D., et al. Comparison of family medicine and internal medicine: Charges for continuing ambulatory care. *Medical Care* 21:830–39, 1983.
26. Hamburger, S., P. Barjenbruch, and A. Soffer. Treatment of diabetic ketoacidosis by internists and family physicians: A comparative study. *Journal of Family Practice* 14:719–22, 1982.
27. Noren, J., et al. Ambulatory medical care: A comparison of internists and family-general practitioners. *New England Journal of Medicine* 302:11–16, 1980.
28. Scherger, J. E., et al. Comparison of diagnostic methods of family practice and internal medicine residents. *Journal of Family Practice* 10:95–101, 1980.
29. Braunwald, E. Effects of coronary artery bypass grafting on survival. *New England Journal of Medicine* 309:1181–84, 1983.
30. White, C. W., et al. Does visual interpretation of the coronary arteriogram predict the physiologic importance of a coronary stenosis? *New England Journal of Medicine* 310:819–24, 1984.
31. Wahl, J. M., A. H. Hakki, and A. S. Iskandrian. Prognostic implications of normal exercise thallium 201 images. *Archives of Internal Medicine* 145:253, 1985.
32. Goran, M. G., J. W. Williamson, and J. S. Gonnella. The validity of patient management problems. *Journal of Medical Education* 48:171–77, 1973.
33. Leaper, D. J., et al. Clinical diagnostic process: An analysis. *British Medical Journal* 3:569–74, 1973.
34. Charap, M. H., R. I. Levin, and J. Weinglas. Physician choices in the treatment of angina pectoris. *American Journal of Medicine* 79:461–66, 1985.

Section Four

Health Program Evaluation

CHAPTER TWELVE

Time-Reversed Crossover Design for Policy Analysis and Program Evaluation

Experimental design, though the most elegant and preferred approach to health policy and health services research, cannot be executed in some situations. In most cases, assessments are done retrospectively or through the prospective study of so-called "natural experiments," where health programs are introduced to some populations but not made available to others. The problem in such evaluations is to find methods of minimizing threats to internal validity that would bias the results of such studies, thus compromising the external validity and generalizability of the findings in a larger policy context.

The article by Sollecito and Gillings illustrates a quasi-experimental method for assessment of the effects of a change in a health program or policy affecting a large population where data on relevant outcome variables are available for periods before and after the introduction of the policy change. Such methods are particularly applicable to situations, like the one described here, where a major change is made in the provisions of a health insurance scheme for a population whose health services utilization behavior has been a matter of record over the period from the time before the change occurred to the time when its effects have taken place.

The United Mine Workers Health and Retirement Funds introduced a cost-sharing provision as part of their health benefits program in 1977. Sollecito and Gillings undertook to determine whether significant changes occurred in the health care utilization of mine workers and their families within the six-month period following the introduction of this change in the plan. The study design they chose, the time-reversed crossover design, is particularly well suited to this kind of evaluation study. Its unique feature is the use of separate sampling and analysis strategies, which acts to improve external validity through stratification on outcomes in the process of sample selection and corrects for internal validity problems associated with selection biases and regression effects. The technique has limitations—most importantly, that it should not be used when significant historical events (like a sudden secular economic downturn) might have occurred during the study period. Such factors cannot be controlled using this technique, and other quasi-experimental designs may be preferred.

The time-reversed crossover design is a particularly useful method for evaluating the effects of a change in policy or program within a defined population in situations where prospective random assignment to experimental and control groups is not possible.

The Assessment of Health Policy Changes Using the Time-Reversed Crossover Design

William A. Sollecito and Dennis B. Gillings

The time-reversed crossover design is a quasi-experimental design which can be applied to evaluate the impact of a change in health policy on a large population. This design makes use of separate sampling and analysis strategies to improve the validity of conclusions drawn from such an evaluation. The properties of the time-reversed crossover design are presented including the use of stratification on outcome in the sampling stage, which is intended to improve external validity. It is demonstrated that, although this feature of the design introduces internal validity threats due to regression toward the mean in extreme-outcome strata, these effects can be measured and eliminated from the test of significance of treatment effects. Methods for within- and across-stratum estimation and hypothesis-testing are presented which are similar to those which have been developed for the traditional two-period crossover design widely used in clinical trials. The procedures are illustrated using data derived from a study conducted by the United Mine Workers of America Health and Retirement Funds to measure the impact of cost-sharing on health care utilization among members of its health plan.

Assessment of the impact of health policy changes should be carried out with the same exactitude as any controlled clinical trial. Whenever possible, true experimental designs, which make use of randomization to assign subjects to treatment or control groups, should be used to carry out such assessments. However, when dealing with situations in which the impact of a change in health policy on a large population is to

---

This research was supported by Grant #R03-HS04201 from the National Center for Health Services Research, and by the U. S. Bureau of the Census (JSA-84.1).

Address correspondence and requests for reprints to William A. Sollecito, Dr. P.H., Vice President for Operations, Quintiles, Inc., 1000 Franklin Square, 1829 East Franklin Street, Chapel Hill, NC 27514. Dennis B. Gillings, Ph.D. is President of Quintiles, Inc.

be evaluated, it is sometimes impossible to meet the randomization and other requirements of a true experimental design. A rare example of the case in which a true experimental design was applied to carry out a health policy evaluation for a large population is the health insurance experiment which was undertaken by Newhouse et al. [1]. But more typically, changes in health policy are assessed in retrospect, using service statistics which have been collected routinely for other purposes. Denniston and Rosenstock [2] discuss several health services studies in which true experimental designs were not applied and point out various sources of invalidity which threaten conclusions from such studies. These are the situations in which quasi-experimental designs can be used to provide some degree of control over the "experiment" and to improve the validity of inferences to be made.

The application of these designs is discussed at length by Campbell and Stanley [3] and, more recently, by Cook and Campbell [4]. These authors define the term *quasi-experimental design* to refer to situations in which random assignment of subjects to equivalent groups is not feasible but where other strategies are introduced to compensate for lack of randomization and thus to improve the validity of conclusions.

The time-reversed crossover design is a quasi-experimental design applicable specifically to the retrospective evaluation of the effects of policy changes which have occurred over time, i.e., natural experiments in time. This design, which was first introduced by Gillings et al. [5], uses separate sampling and analysis strategies to minimize threats to validity which may be present in such natural experiments in time. These include threats to internal validity, external validity, and statistical conclusion validity.

The time-reversed crossover design uses a sampling methodology based on stratification on outcome as a way of improving both external and internal validity. The analysis methodology, which is based on the traditional two-period crossover design, enhances internal validity and statistical conclusion validity.

The time-reversed crossover design can be applied to any natural experiment occurring over a period of time during which some change in social or health policy (the treatment effect to be evaluated) has occurred. In order to apply this design, data must be available—preferably on a computerized file—both before and after the "treatment" to be evaluated has occurred; and the analysis must be carried out retrospectively.

SAMPLING METHODOLOGY

In a health policy evaluation study, if data are available for a large population over a period of time during which some policy change has occurred, it may be desirable to analyze a sample of the available data even though the entire population is on computerized files. The main reasons for this lie in the expense of manipulating vast arrays of data. Further, local computers otherwise dedicated to routine processing may get diverted to do statistical analysis, and management may not judge this to be in the company's best interests. An example would be a large health insurance company in which a change in benefits is to be assessed to determine its impact on utilization or length of stay in hospitals.

Another reason for using a sampling approach is that the sample design chosen can be used to induce a quasi-experimental design on the data to be analyzed. Various sample designs can be used which allow for precise estimates of the effects to be studied and the elimination of effects which are not of interest.

If an entire community is followed over time to evaluate the effect of a policy change such as the addition of a community health program, the change can be thought of as the "treatment" of interest; furthermore, if the evaluation is to be carried out after the change has occurred, the data can be analyzed retrospectively and several different sampling approaches can be used to evaluate the effect of this "treatment."

The simplest approach is one in which a simple random sample is taken from the population before and after the change in policy or "treatment" was implemented. This yields a quasi-experimental design which Campbell and Stanley [3] call "the separate sample pretest-posttest design."

A second sampling approach is to identify a subpopulation which was present in the periods both before and after treatment, and then to select a simple random sample from the period before the treatment. Data on these persons would be collected by following them forward into the after-treatment period. This approach yields a pre-experimental design which Campbell and Stanley call the "one group pretest-posttest design" (equivalent to that which many authors refer to as a "panel study").

Campbell and Stanley [3] and Cook and Campbell [4] discuss both of these designs at length regarding their susceptibility to sources of invalidity. Both of these designs have several weaknesses, but the second—the one group pretest-posttest design—is especially to be avoided since it is subject to several major threats to validity which include history effects, maturation effects, and statistical regression effects.

Another sampling approach which can be used in this situation allows for a crossover design to be simulated on the observed data set. This sampling approach, which allows for the time-reversed crossover design to be implemented, can be illustrated best through showing its recent implementation in a health services application. This example, used throughout this article, can be described as follows.

THE FUNDS STUDY

Prior to July 1977, the United Mine Workers of America Health and Retirement Funds (the FUNDS) provided first dollar coverage for medical care for all union members and their families. However, financial exigencies made it necessary to impose a cost-sharing program to help reduce expenditures. Therefore, beginning on July 1, 1977, union members and their families were required to pay at least part of the cost of each medical visit. It was of interest to determine the effect of the imposition of cost-sharing on overall utilization of the health plan by members. Since utilization data were routinely available on computerized claims payment files both for the period before and the period after cost-sharing was imposed, this situation could be viewed as a naturally occurring experiment in time, and these data could be used to evaluate the impact of cost-sharing. In order to do this, a study period was defined which represented 6 months before and 6 months after the imposition of cost-sharing, and the time-reversed crossover design was applied by selecting a sample of families covered by the health plan during the study period. Utilization data were then collected on these families for the period before and after the imposition of cost-sharing.

TIME-REVERSED CROSSOVER SAMPLING METHODOLOGY

The sampling methodology of the time-reversed crossover design, illustrated in Figure 1, was used by the FUNDS in selecting families for study in evaluating the impact of cost-sharing.

The first step in the FUNDS sampling procedure was to subdivide the population present (eligible for benefits) during the study period into two groups: those who were present before (P1) and those present after (P2), the imposition of cost-sharing. Next, the population was

Figure 1: Time-Reversed Crossover Design—FUNDS Sampling Methodology

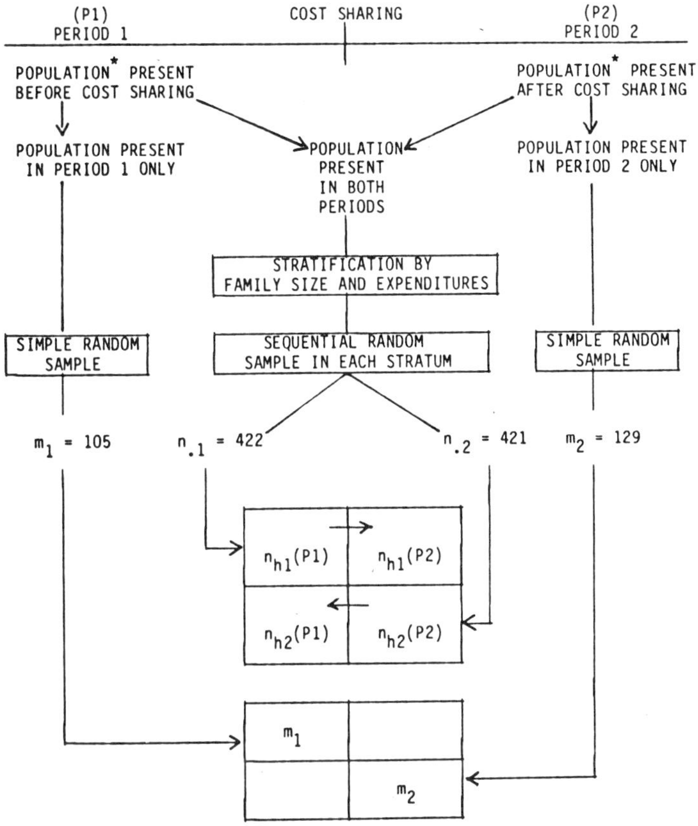

*Actually represents 10% of population of active miners as of January 1977.

further subdivided into those who were present in both P1 and P2 versus those present only in P1 or only in P2. The population that was present in both periods, which is the main focus of the time-reversed crossover design, was then stratified according to two types of variables, one based on outcome and one based on an "independent" or explanatory variable. In the case of the FUNDS study, the outcome variable used was total health care expenditures. Since the main focus of the study was on changes in utilization, a dependent variable highly correlated with utilization was chosen as an outcome variable (rather than using an outcome measure based on health status). Since the family was to be the main unit of analysis, the independent stratification variable chosen was family size. Therefore, each family that was eligible for benefits during both periods was first stratified according to family size and level of health care expenditures in the period before cost-sharing and then again in the period after cost-sharing. Family size strata were defined in five levels: 1, 2, 3, 4, and 5 + . Because all analyses were carried out retrospectively, definitions of outcome strata were easily determined using five levels of expenditures ranging from zero to very high, based on the relative frequency distribution of expenditures within each period (e.g., the very high expenditures stratum represents the upper fifth percentile of the distribution in each period). Therefore, each family was classified into two different expenditure strata (one in each period).

Stratification on outcome is an important step in the sampling process—and a unique feature of the time-reversed crossover design. The use of total family health expenditures as the outcome measure for stratification was based on convenience; other outcome measures which might have been used were total utilization or total services. Stratification on any of these outcome measures is intended to produce improvements in both internal and external validity. These improvements result from creating groups within each stratum which are guaranteed to be homogeneous at each point in time relative to outcome; this also allows for better estimates of changes over time. Stratification on outcome also creates groups which are fairly homogeneous relative to important predictors of outcome; thus this step lessens the need to control for the effect of these "independent" variables by means of regression procedures or other linear modeling techniques.

After subdividing the population into family size and expenditure strata, samples were then selected from each stratum using a sequential procedure in which families were alternately selected from each period. For example, for any given stratum the first family chosen in the sample was randomly selected from the P1 subpopulation and the second family was chosen at random from the P2 subpopulation in that same stratum; then the third family was chosen randomly from P1. The process was repeated in this manner until a prespecified number of families was selected from each stratum. As each family was selected, a check was made to ensure that it had not been selected in the other period's sample, if it had, the family was treated as a "blank" and discarded. Using these procedures, 422 families were selected in the period before cost-sharing and 421 families in the period after cost-sharing. For each family chosen, utilization data were collected (abstracted from claims files) in both periods. Therefore, each family selected can be viewed as having been selected in one of two sequence groups: those selected in P1 and followed forward in time to P2 and those who were selected based on their level of health care expenditures in P2 and followed backward in time to P1. Furthermore, because of the sample selection procedures and the small sampling fraction (approximately .3 percent), the families selected can be considered to be independent of each other both within and between sequence groups.

In regard to the two subpopulations who were not present in both periods, two separate simple random samples were selected; 105 families were chosen in P1 and 129 families in P2. No further results based on these components will be presented here; however, details on the analysis methods which are applicable to these groups are given by Sollecito [6].

ANALYSIS METHODOLOGY

The two most important features of the FUNDS sampling method which characterize it as representative of the time-reversed crossover design are the use of stratification on outcome to identify families with known levels of outcome in the selection period and the identification of two separate sequence groups which are independent of each other and which are followed either forward or backward in time. As described by Sollecito [6], several analysis methods can be used when data are selected in this manner. However, the most efficient method is one based on the traditional two-period crossover design which has been widely used in clinical trials and has been described by Grizzle [7] (parametric analysis), Koch [8] (nonparametric analysis), and several others.

Estimation and hypothesis testing methods can be derived for the time-reversed crossover design based on the traditional two-period crossover methodology. These methods, briefly summarized here, will be illustrated using data from the FUNDS study. The Appendix presents a detailed specification of a mathematical model to represent the value of any outcome measure (y_{hijk}) in the time-reversed crossover design. This model specification is similar to that for the traditional crossover design. A further simplification of this model can be achieved by representing the expected value of any outcome measure using the following shorthand or "*P*-notation."

Figure 2: Time-Reversed Crossover Design Representation of Outcome Measure Within Any Stratum Using *P*-Notation

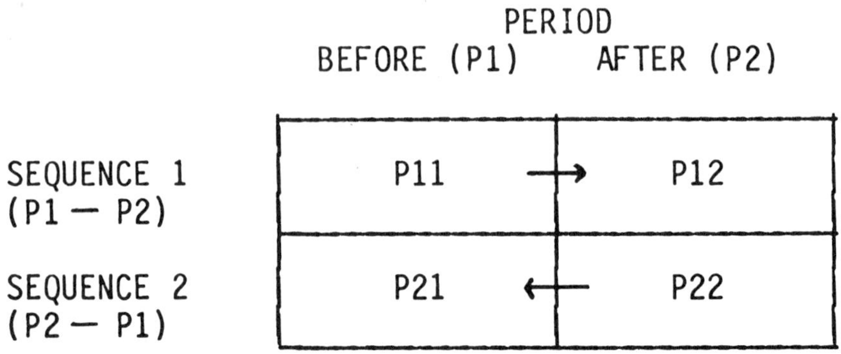

Figure 2 presents a simple schematic diagram of the data configuration resulting from the application of the time-reversed crossover sampling method. Within any given stratum, the expected value of any observation can be represented by *Pik*, where *i* represents the sequence group (and period) in which each family was selected and *k* represents the period in which data were collected. Using this "*P*-notation," estimates and hypothesis tests of effects of interest within each stratum can be represented as follows.

ESTIMATION OF EFFECTS

The first effect of interest is the time-order effect, which is a measure of effects due to the sample selection method and in particular due to stratification on outcome. This effect measures the presence of threats to internal validity which are related to follow-up over time; the main component is changes in outcome which may be due to regression toward the mean resulting from selection based on extreme levels of outcome. This effect, which is similar to a residual or carryover effect in the traditional two-period crossover design described by Grizzle [7], is estimated by finding the difference in outcome between the sample selection period and the follow-up period for each sequence group and then forming an unweighted average of these differences across sequence groups. Using the *P*-notation described in Figure 1, the time-order effect for the *h*th stratum, denoted r_h, can be described as follows:

$$r_h = 1/2[(P12 - P11) + (P21 - P22)] \qquad (1)$$

The treatment effect of interest, i.e., the cost-sharing effect in the FUNDS study, can be estimated using two different methods; both of these are based on the difference in outcome between the period before and the period after cost-sharing. The first estimate is unadjusted for the presence of time-order effects and makes use of data from all four cells (see figure 2). This effect, denoted t_h, is found by forming the before/after difference in outcome within each sequence group and then averaging these differences across sequence groups. For the *h*th stratum this is expressed:

$$t_h = 1/2[(P12 - P11) + (P22 - P21)] \tag{2}$$

Since the presence of time-order effects may bias this estimate, an estimate of the treatment effect which is adjusted for time-order effects can be found based only on the two sample selection periods (i.e., P11 and P22). Therefore, the adjusted treatment effect within the *h*th stratum can be represented by:

$$t_h^* = (P22 - P11) \tag{3}$$

The treatment estimate and the adjusted treatment estimate will be positively correlated; the degree to which these two estimates differ is directly proportional to the size of time-order effects which are present. This is expected since the adjusted treatment effect differs from the (unadjusted) treatment effect only in that it is free of time-order effects which would be present only in the follow-up periods.

Because of the correlation between these two measures of treatment effect, it is not necessary to compute both. Instead, is is recommended that conclusions be based on the unadjusted treatment effect alone, unless there is strong evidence of unequal time-order effects, in which case then only the adjusted treatment effect should be used to derive conclusions.

In order to form overall estimates of effects, the within-stratum estimates described above are combined across strata using weighted formulas which are similar to those described by Kish [9] for finding estimates from stratified random samples. In the case of the FUNDS data, the proportion of the population in each stratum was used as a weighting factor in finding overall estimates.

GRAPHIC REPRESENTATION OF EFFECTS

The following procedure can be used in a time-reversed crossover design to assess outcome patterns graphically in each stratum and to compare patterns across strata to assess overall effect.

Several expected patterns of response can be described which provide important information regarding effects that may be detected in the time-reversed crossover design. This procedure involves plotting the mean value of each outcome variable by period and sequence separately for each stratum. However, instead of plotting outcome in the correct order, the first mean value plotted in each sequence refers to the period in which each family was sampled and the second mean value plotted refers to the follow-up period. This procedure is illustrated in Figure 3.

The points on the horizontal axis are such that the sample selection point represents P1 data for the sequence group selected in the first period and P2 data for the sequence group selected in the second period; likewise, points plotted for the follow-up period represent P2 data for the group selected in the first period and P1 data for the group selected in the second period. As in the traditional crossover design, when outcome is plotted in this fashion, the presence of a substantial treatment effect in conjunction with a lack of a residual effect would be indicated by a distinct crisscrossing pattern similar to that which is illustrated in part (a) of Figure 3.

Once again, using the FUNDS study of cost-sharing as an example, the plots in Figure 3 will be used to illustrate this methodology and the various effects which can be detected in a time-reversed crossover model. For simplicity of presentation, it will be assumed that all plots in Figure 3 represent total utilization of health services for families who were selected in the stratum defined by high health care expenditures. Since the expected effect of cost-sharing is to lower utilization, and likewise expenditure, the mean level of utilization in P2 should be lower than P1 for each sequence if there has been a substantial cost-sharing effect. Furthermore, since the definition of each expenditure stratum is based on the relative frequency distribution of all expenditures in each period, the definition of high expenditures is expected to vary for each period. Specifically, the value which defines the high-expenditures stratum is expected to be lower for those selected in P2 than in P1. Therefore, these expectations yield the crisscrossing pattern, described in Figure 3(a), which represents a substantial cost-sharing effect and no time-order effect. In Figure 3(a) those identified in P1 and followed forward to P2 exhibit a decreasing slope (utilization decreased over time); those identified as high utilizers in P2 and followed backward in time exhibit an increasing slope (utilization was even higher in P1). The plot in Figure 3(a) is an example of a pattern which is characteristic of a strong cost-sharing effect, since the difference between P1 and P2 mean utilization within a sequence is large—

Figure 3: Crossover Plots of Total Health Care Utilization Per Family by Period.* Examples of Possible Effects Within High-Expenditure Stratum

(a) Evidence of substantial cost sharing effect with no time order effects:

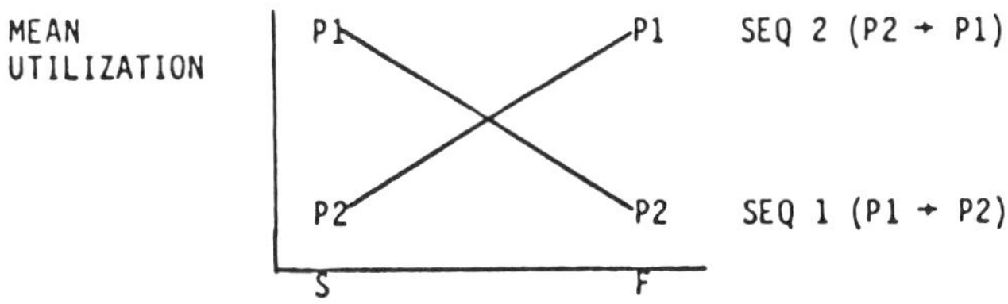

(b) Evidence of selection effect:

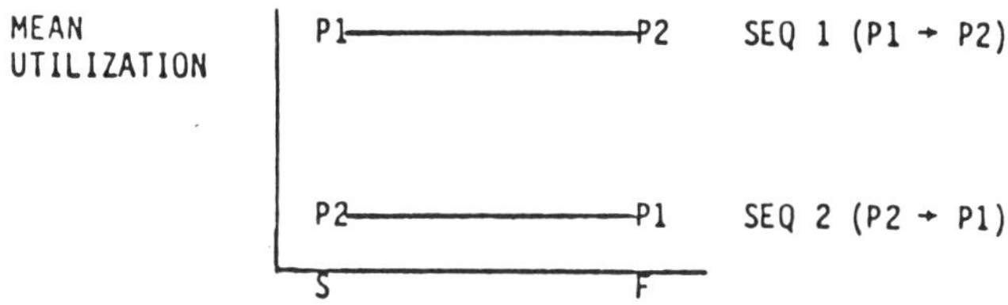

(c) Evidence of regression effect:

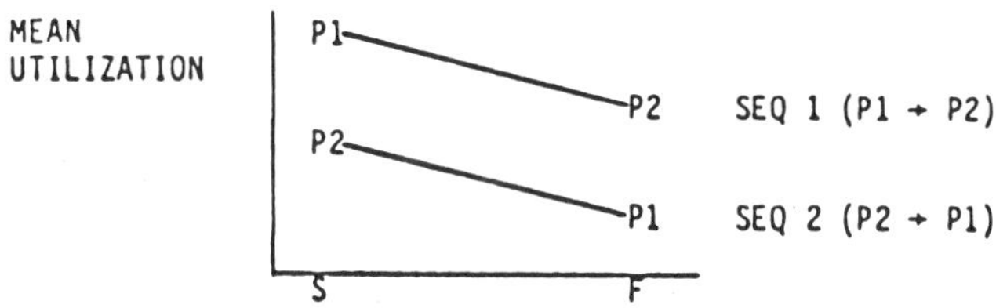

(d) Evidence of combined selection and regression effects:

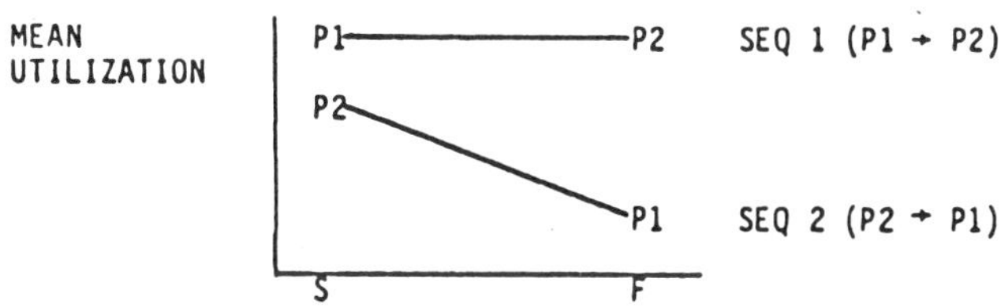

*In all plots, "*S*" represents period in which sample was selected, "*F*" represents follow-up period.

and is exactly equal to the difference between P1 and P2 utilization between sequences. In most cases, actual data cannot be expected to yield this kind of a clear-cut pattern; however, the closeness of an actual pattern to this expected cost-sharing pattern will provide first evidence of a possibly significant cost-sharing effect.

The presence of time-order effects will distort the cost-sharing patterns described above. Figures 3(b) and 3(c) present the pattern expected to result when the two most extreme forms of time-order effects are present. Figure 3(b) illustrates the pattern of response expected when substantial selection effects are present. This is indicated by the fact that within each sequence the P1 and P2 utilization means are exactly the same; that is, the utilization level in the sample selection period completely determines utilization in the follow-up period for each sequence.

Figure 3(c) illustrates the pattern of response expected when substantial regression effects are present. Since the data depicted in this plot are assumed to represent the high-expenditures stratum, it is implied that each family in this stratum had a high value of health expenditures in the sample selection period and, thus, that a regression effect would cause outcome to decrease from the sampling period to the follow-up period. In Figure 3(c), both sequence groups exhibit a decreasing slope when plotted in this manner. When viewed by itself, the outcome pattern for the group selected in P1 and followed to P2 does not automatically imply that a regression effect is present, since the decreasing slope is consistent with the presence of a cost-sharing effect. However, when viewed in conjunction with the decreasing slope of the second sequence group, there is strong evidence that the differences observed within each sequence are due to regression effects. The decreasing slope for those who were identified in P2 and followed backward to P1 indicates that utilization was substantially higher in the period after cost-sharing than before—the opposite of what is expected as a result of cost-sharing. Therefore, this may be completely due to the fact that this group was selected as high utilizers in P2 and had lower utilization in P1 due to regression toward the mean.

Figure 3(d) presents another pattern which is an indicator of a time-order effect, but which cannot be neatly classified in terms of the source of the effect. This plot is but a single illustration among a wide variety of possible patterns which represent various combinations of selection effects and regression effects occurring simultaneously in the same stratum. In Figure 3(d), the first sequence group—selected in P1 and followed in P2—exhibits a selection effect, since there is no change in utilization from P1 to P2; the second sequence group—P2 to P1—

Figure 4: Within-Stratum Significance-Testing Procedures—Across-Period Functions for Each Sequence Group To Be Used To Test Effects of Interest

	Within Family Function for Comparison of		
Significance Test	**Sequence 1**	vs.	**Sequence 2**
Equality of time-order effect in each sequence	(P11 + P12)	vs.	(P21 + P22)
Significance of cost-sharing effect	(P12 - P11)	vs.	(P21 - P22)
Significance of adjusted cost-sharing effect	P11	vs.	P22

exhibits a regression effect since utilization was higher in P2 than P1. It is quite clear that this particular pattern is not more likely to appear than any other in which time-order effects are present; however, together with Figures 3(b) and 3(c), it illustrates the various forms of time-order effects which can be detected using crossover plots of this type.

The one characteristic which is common to the plots in Figures 3(b), (c), and (d) is the lack of a crisscrossing pattern; this is an indication of unequal residual effects in a crossover experiment (either traditional or time reversed). Both the direction and the magnitude of the slopes in these plots provide evidence to help determine the strength and the nature of time-order effects.

TESTS OF SIGNIFICANCE

Because they involve the fewest assumptions and thus lessen threats to statistical conclusion validity, nonparametric methods are recommended in performing significance tests for the time-reversed crossover design. These methods, which are based on nonparametric procedures presented by Koch [8] for the traditional two-period crossover design, involve forming within-subject (family) functions across periods for each sequence group and then performing nonparametric hypothesis tests to compare these functions between the two (independent) sequence groups. Therefore, in regard to the FUNDS data, each test of significance is based on a comparison of families in sequence 1 versus sequence 2 after first forming the across-period function which is appropriate for each effect to be tested. The across-period functions related to each significance test of interest are listed in Figure 4. These are further described in the Appendix.

In carrying out these significance-testing procedures for the FUNDS cost-sharing study, each of the within-family functions was first formed based on dependent variables of interest; then the Wilcoxon Rank Sum test [10] was applied to carry out each of the comparisons described in Figure 4. It is important to note that the test of time-order effects described in Figure 4 is not directed at the presence or absence of time-order effects but rather at the equality of time-order effects between sequence groups. The test of equality of time-order effects is of primary interest, because, if time-order effects are found to differ significantly between sequence groups, then only the test of the adjusted treatment effect should be used to evaluate the impact of cost-sharing. However, if time-order effects are not found to be significantly different, then the test of the unadjusted treatment effect should be used to evaluate the effect of cost-sharing. This is similar to the procedure used in the traditional crossover design for testing the significance of the difference between carryover effects prior to testing the significance of treatment effects.

The significance-testing methods just described allow for within-stratum tests of each effect to be carried out. Sollecito [6] describes several methods for performing across-stratum significance tests in the time-reversed crossover design. One method which can be used and which has been applied to the data to be presented here is van Elteren's test [11]. This procedure combines Wilcoxon rank sum statistics across various experimental blocks or strata by forming a weighted average using the inverse of the number of subjects in each stratum (plus one) as a weighting factor.

RESULTS

As part of a larger study [12], the time-reversed crossover design, as described here, was applied to selected data from the FUNDS data set. The following results briefly describe some of these findings and provide an illustration of the time-reversed crossover analysis methodology.

Table 1 and Figure 5 present results based on total physician services per family in the period before and after the imposition of cost-sharing. Total physician services, which is considered to be a measure of both the quantity and quality of care, is computed by multiplying the number of encounters with a physician times the number of services per encounter. This measure is expected to decrease after the imposition of cost-sharing.

The data in Table 1 are based on 290 families selected in two (of six) regions of the FUNDS population which had a totally computer-

Table 1: FUNDS Sample of Families—Comparison of Total Physician Services per Family in the 6-Month Period Before and After the Imposition of Cost-Sharing, for Strata Defined by Family Size and Health Expenditures

Family Size and Health Expenditures Stratum	Sample Seq.†	N*	Mean (S.E.) No. of Services P1	P2	Estimate of Effects (S.E.) Time-Order Effect	Cost-Sharing Effect	Adj. Cost-Sharing Effect	Significance Test p-Values Time-Order Equality‡	Cost-Sharing Effect§	Adj. Cost-Sharing Effect§
Size 1–3										
Low expenditures	P1–P2	44	1.8 (0.31)	2.9 (0.56)						
	P2–P1	41	3.9 (0.83)	1.4 (0.33)	1.77 (0.47)	-0.69 (0.47)	-0.43 (0.45)	.819	.322	.254
High expenditures	P1–P2	59	17.8 (2.39)	9.9 (1.63)						
	P2–P1	32	16.2 (3.19)	16.1 (3.65)	-3.90 (1.49)	-4.00 (1.49)	-1.65 (4.36)	.547	.001	.374
Size 4 +										
Low expenditures	P1–P2	19	4.9 (1.21)	5.8 (1.43)						
	P2–P1	27	9.0 (1.90)	1.5 (0.38)	4.19 (1.25)	-3.33 (1.25)	-3.38 (1.27)	.884	.020	.004
High expenditures	P1–P2	40	22.8 (3.09)	12.0 (1.93)						
	P2–P1	28	24.2 (4.42)	18.8 (3.43)	-2.66 (2.45)	-8.05 (2.45)	-3.97 (4.62)	.443	.001	.383
All Strata Combined	P1–P2	162	13.2 (1.34)	8.0 (0.84)						
	P2–P1	128	12.5 (1.49)	8.9 (1.37)	-0.54 (0.80)	-4.11 (0.80)	-2.81 (1.69)	.440	<.001	.007

*Data include families from only two regions of the total FUNDS population.
†Actual study period after cost-sharing includes less than 6 months. All data have been adjusted to make both periods equal to 6 months.
‡Test of equality of size of time-order effect in each sequence group (two-tail test).
§Test whether average effect is significantly different from zero (two-tail test).

ized claims payment system during the entire study period. The mean and standard error of the number of services per family are presented for each sequence group in the period before and after cost-sharing in each of the family size/health expenditure strata which have been collapsed into two levels each (or four combined strata). Strata have been collapsed to reduce the effect of regression toward the mean in extreme strata and to maximize the sample size in each stratum. It can be noted that the mean number of services per family is correlated with both family size and level of health expenditures; the smallest mean (1.4) is found among families of size 1 to 3 with low expenditures, and the largest mean (24.2) is observed for families of size 4 or more with high expenditures. The overall mean, computed using the proportion of the population in each stratum as a weighting factor, decreases from approximately 13 services per family in the period before cost-sharing to approximately 9 services per family in the period after cost-sharing.

The middle columns of Table 1 present estimates and standard errors of the effects described. The estimated time-order effects in each stratum exhibit a pattern indicative of regression toward the mean. That is, for both of the low-expenditure strata, the time-order effect is positive and fairly large (relative to its standard error). This can be interpreted to mean that families who were selected as low utilizers (indicated by their expenditures) had higher levels of utilization (indicated by total physician services) in the follow-up period. Similarly, both of the high-expenditures groups had negative time-order effects indicating a decrease (toward the mean) from the selection to the follow-up period. These patterns, which are also depicted in Figure 5, indicate that the presence of regression effects must be considered as a possible threat to validity of conclusions from these data.

Both the unadjusted and the adjusted cost-sharing effects were consistently negative in all four strata and provide strong evidence of a decrease in total physician services after the imposition of cost-sharing. The consistency of the adjusted cost-sharing effect with the unadjusted effect indicates that the presence of some evidence of regression toward the mean is not large enough to outweigh the presence of cost-sharing effects. This conclusion is also supported by the clear crisscrossing pattern exhibited in each stratum in Figure 5; as previously noted, this is expected when there are substantial cost-sharing effects. However, because there is evidence of regression toward the mean, it is worthwhile to review both of the measures of cost-sharing effects and to note any inconsistencies between the two.

Overall estimates of effects for all strata combined were computed using the population proportion in each stratum as a weighting factor.

Figure 5: Crossover Plot of Mean Number of Total Physician Services for Strata Defined by Family Size and Health Expenditures

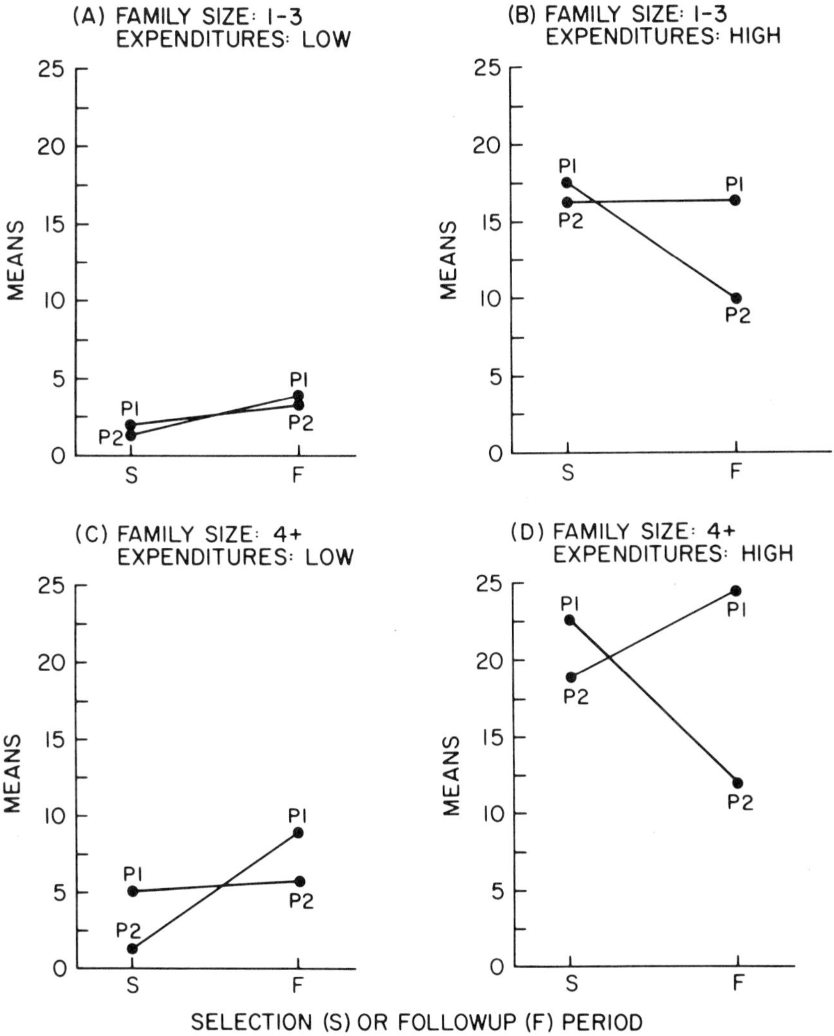

It can be noted that there is a counterbalancing of time-order effects across all strata and that the positive and negative effects within each stratum tend to cancel out and produce a fairly small overall time-order effect (which is equal to -.54 with a standard error of .80). On the other hand, the cost-sharing effects are quite consistent across strata and produce overall effects which are fairly large relative to their standard errors and relative to the size of the time-order effects. The overall weighted estimates of the adjusted (-2.8) and unadjusted (-4.1) cost-sharing effects indicate that after the imposition of cost-sharing there was a decrease of between three and four physician services per family.

Significance-testing procedures described above have also been applied and are presented in the far right-hand columns of Table 1. The test of equality of time-order effects yields highly nonsignificant p-values in all four strata, with the smallest (most significant) being equal to only .443. Thus, although there is evidence of regression effects, these effects are equally dispersed between the two sequence groups and can be ignored for the purposes of testing the significance of cost-sharing effects.

Since time-order effects do not differ significantly, conclusions should be based on the unadjusted cost-sharing effect alone; however, for comparative purposes, both the cost-sharing and adjusted cost-sharing effect are used to test the significance of the imposition of cost-sharing here. A test of the unadjusted cost-sharing effect yielded significant ($p \leq .050$) p-values in three of four strata with the most highly significant p-values observed in the two high-expenditure strata; the p-value equals .001 for both strata. The only stratum which did not yield a statistically significant cost-sharing effect was family size 1–3 with low expenditures ($p = .322$).

Based on the test of the adjusted cost-sharing effect, only one of the four strata yielded statistical significance—the stratum defined by family size 4+ with low expenditures ($p = .004$).

The difference in significance levels for the two measures of cost-sharing effect is due to the fact that the adjusted cost-sharing effect is based on data from only the two sample selection periods and is considered to be a less powerful test than that based on the unadjusted cost-sharing effect which makes use of data from all four cells.

When combined across strata using van Elteren's test [11], the test of equality of time-order effect continues to be highly nonsignificant ($p = .440$); however, both the cost-sharing ($p < .001$) and adjusted cost-sharing effect ($p = .007$) are found to be highly significant. It is interesting to note that despite the fact that the adjusted cost-sharing effect is statistically significant in only one out of four strata, it is highly significant overall. This is due in part to the consistency in the direction of the effect in all four strata, which tends to enhance the power of van Elteren's test.

Therefore, based on these findings, it can be noted that total physician services per family have decreased since the imposition of cost-sharing and that, based on a sample of 290 families, this decrease is indicative of a highly significant cost-sharing effect.

ANALYSES BASED ON STRATA DEFINED BY EXPENDITURES ALONE

An important feature of the time-reversed crossover method is the use of outcome to define sampling strata; in the example of the FUNDS study, outcome strata were defined using total health care expenditures. It is expected that due to regression toward the mean, substantial time-order effects would be present if these analyses were also based on expenditure strata alone; it is for this reason that all analyses in Table 1 are based on combined family size and expenditure levels combined into four categories. Table 2 and Figure 6 are presented to illustrate the sensitivity of the time-reversed crossover model in detecting time-order effects and the impact of these effects on tests of treatment effects.

Table 2 and Figure 6 present the results for total physician services based on strata defined by the level of health expenditures in which each family was classified in the sample selection period.

Significant differences in time-order effects ($p \leq .05$) between sequence groups can be noted in Table 2 in strata which represent zero expenditures and high expenditures in the sample selection period; these results can be attributed primarily to regression toward the mean in extreme strata.

It is worth noting that the medium-expenditures stratum, which is not expected to be influenced by regression toward the mean, had the smallest time-order effect (.29) and the least significant time-order difference ($p = .880$). It is also interesting to note that the very high expenditure stratum did not yield significantly different time-order effects despite having the largest estimated time-order effect (–9.36). Due to the extreme definition of this stratum, this result might be considered contrary to expectations. However, this result is due to the very small differences in time-order effects between sequence groups. This pattern clearly illustrates the important point that the test of equality of time-order effects is carried out only as a preliminary step to testing cost-sharing effects and that, for these purposes, it is not the size of the time-order effects but rather the equality of time-order effects

Table 2: FUNDS Sample of Families—Comparison of Total Physician Services per Family in the 6-Month Period Before and After the Imposition of Cost-Sharing for Strata Defined by Health Expenditures Alone

			Mean (S.E.) No. of Services		Estimate of Effects (S.E.)			Significance Test p-Values		
Health Expenditures	*Sample Seq.*†	N*	*P1*	*P2*	*Time-Order Effect*	*Cost-Sharing Effect*	*Adj. Cost-Sharing Effect*	*Time-Order Equality*‡	*Cost-Sharing Effect*§	*Adj. Cost-Sharing Effect*§
Zero expenditures	P1–P2	22	0.00 (0.00)	0.88 (0.45)						
	P2–P1	37	4.73 (1.19)	0.00 (0.00)	2.80 (0.63)	-1.93 (0.63)	0.00 (0.00)	.014	.014	–
Low expenditures	P1–P2	41	4.22 (0.58)	5.30 (0.79)						
	P2–P1	31	7.32 (1.50)	3.16 (0.35)	2.62 (0.88)	-1.54 (0.88)	-1.06 (0.68)	.750	.193	.340
Medium expenditures	P1–P2	46	12.83 (1.17)	8.27 (1.34)						
	P2–P1	28	15.18 (3.73)	10.04 (0.90)	0.29 (1.88)	-4.84 (1.88)	-2.78 (1.45)	.880	.001	.103
High expenditures	P1–P2	28	17.61 (3.17)	6.25 (1.43)						
	P2–P1	19	25.42 (4.78)	22.11 (5.19)	-4.02 (2.37)	-7.33 (2.37)	4.50 (6.08)	.013	.001	.422
Very high expenditures	P1–P2	25	35.00 (5.24)	20.31 (3.33)						
	P2–P1	13	22.15 (6.30)	26.18 (7.78)	-9.36 (3.15)	-5.33 (3.15)	-8.82 (9.38)	.451	.088	.180

All strata combined	P1–P2	162	13.15	8.03						
			(1.34)	(0.84)						
	P2–P1	128	12.48	8.90	−0.77	-4.36	-4.25			
			(1.49)	(1.37)	(0.77)	(0.77)	(1.92)	.047	< .001	.105
Low, medium,	P1–P2	112	14.63	9.87						
and very high			(1.67)	(1.10)						
expenditure	P2–P1	72	13.06	9.99	−0.85	-3.91	-4.63	.973	< .001	.026
strata			(2.03)	(1.71)	(1.07)	(1.07)	(2.40)			

*Data include families from only two regions of the total FUNDS population.

†Actual study period after cost-sharing includes less than 6 months. All data have been adjusted to make both periods equal to 6 months.

‡Test of equality of size of time-order effect in each sequence group (two-tail test).

§Test whether average effect is significantly different from zero (two-tail test).

between sequence groups that is of concern. Therefore, although the use of stratification on outcome in the sample selection period may have introduced fairly substantial regression effects in extreme strata, this will have little impact on significance tests for cost-sharing effects if these effects are equal in each sequence group.

Due to the significantly different time-order effects in Table 2, tests of significance based on cost-sharing effects must be interpreted with care. Although the cost-sharing effect in the zero- and high-expenditure stratum is significant ($p \leq 0.05$), the inequality of time-order effects in these strata invalidate these results. Therefore, the adjusted cost-sharing effect alone must be used to determine significance. For those families in the high-expenditure stratum, the adjusted cost-sharing effect was nonsignificant ($p = .422$). Among families in the zero-expenditure stratum, no determination of the effect of cost-sharing can be made; the unadjusted cost-sharing effect is invalid, and the adjusted cost-sharing effect cannot be computed because, by definition, the mean of both sample selection periods is equal to zero for all families in this stratum. This presents a clear example of why the use of stratum definitions which are too extreme can be counterproductive—why it can lead to spurious results. It provides another clear example of why time-order effects must be considered prior to performing tests of cost-sharing effects.

Among the three strata in which there are no significant differences between time-order effects, only the medium-expenditures stratum presents clear evidence of significant cost-sharing effects. Among families in this stratum, the unadjusted cost-sharing effect was −4.84 and the test of significance yielded a p-value of .001; thus, total physician services decreased significantly.

These findings are substantiated by the patterns illustrated in the crossover plots presented in Figure 6. The plots which correspond to the zero- and high-expenditure strata do not exhibit the crisscrossing pattern which is expected when time-order effects are absent (see Figures 6(a) and 6(d)). Both plots depict horizontal V-shaped patterns which are indicative of both regression and selection effects.

The hypothesized causes for the time-order patterns observed in the zero- and high-expenditures stratum cannot be verified in these data. It is clear that these examples illustrate why the presence of time-order effects complicates results in the time-reversed crossover design. It is also clear that the data from the follow-up periods which are subject to the joint effects of time-order and cost-sharing effects cannot be used to make conclusions when time-order effects differ between sequence groups.

Figure 6: Crossover Plot of Mean Number of Total Physician Services by Expenditures Stratum

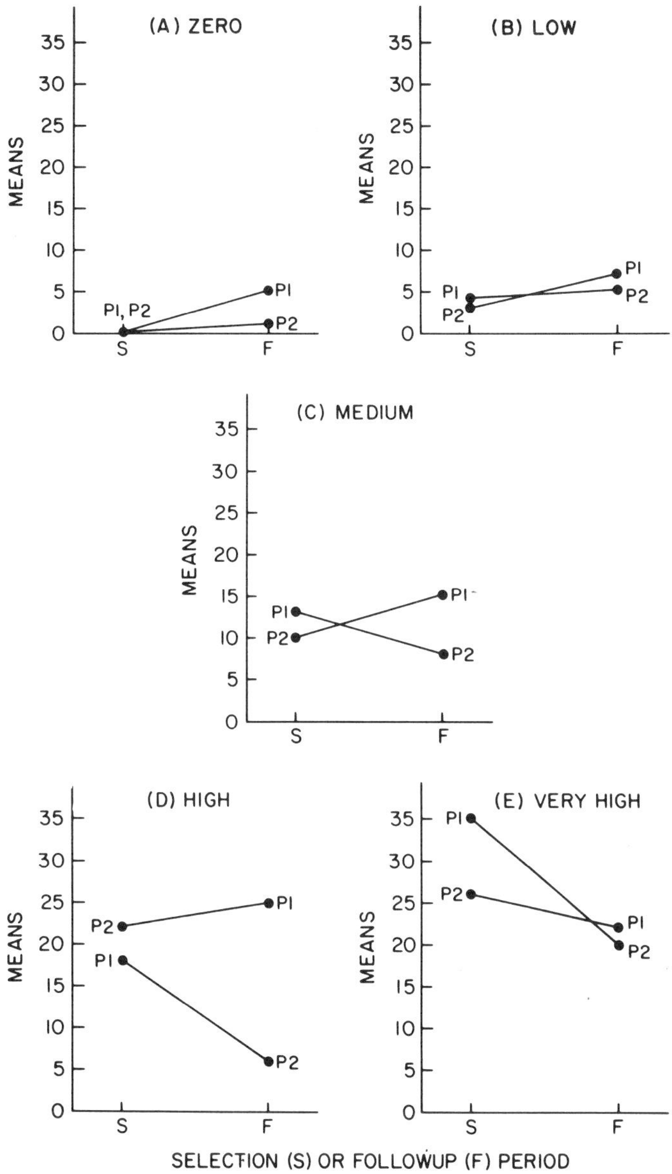

Among strata which are not found to have significant time-order differences, Figure 6 also illustrates that the expected crisscrossing pattern is obtained. The best example of this pattern is the medium-expenditure stratum which, by definition, should be free of any regression effects. For this stratum, which is described in Figure 6(c), the expected crossover pattern is noted with mean outcome lower in the period after cost-sharing than before. The nonsignificance of the adjusted cost-sharing effect in this stratum is due in part to the smaller difference between sequence groups in the sample selection period than in the follow-up period.

Overall hypothesis tests based on strata defined by expenditures alone are also complicated by the significance of time-order effects within strata. Furthermore, the overall hypothesis test of the equality of time-order effect averaged across all five expenditure strata yielded a statistically significant p-value ($p = .047$). In addition, the significance of this effect in two out of the five expenditure strata makes the overall estimate of the (unadjusted) cost-sharing effect questionable if it is based on all five strata. This is due to the fact that if any of the within-stratum tests are not valid due to the inequality of time-order effects within that stratum, then these should not be included in the test of overall effect.

In this type of situation, two separate strategies can be considered to provide an overall test of the cost-sharing effect. The first, most conservative, approach is to base the overall test on the adjusted cost-sharing effect alone, since this effect is free of any possible differences in time-order effects between sequence groups. Using this approach, the adjusted cost-sharing effect based on total physician services is not statistically significant ($p = .105$). The power of this test is weakened by exclusion of data from the zero-expenditure stratum and, as noted in Table 2, by substantial inconsistency among strata in the sign and size of the adjusted cost-sharing effect.

A second approach which can be considered is to carry out two separate hypothesis tests—one based on the unadjusted cost-sharing effect only for those strata in which the equality of time-order effects is highly nonsignificant ($p > .15$), and the other based on the adjusted cost-sharing effect for the strata in which time-order effects are significantly different between strata. The zero-expenditure stratum must be excluded from all analyses due to the inequality of time-order effects and the lack of data to provide an adjusted cost-sharing effect. Therefore, the within-stratum test of the adjusted cost-sharing effect in the high-expenditure stratum serves as the only significance test which can be performed for strata in which unequal time-order effects are noted.

The two-tailed p-values based on the test of average partial association across the three strata (low, medium, and very high expenditures) in which time-order effects were not significantly different are presented in the bottom row of Table 2. Based on these strata, the overall time-order effect is highly nonsignificant (p = .973). Likewise, the (unadjusted) cost-sharing effect is highly significant ($p < .001$); the adjusted cost-sharing effect is also significant (p = .026). Since the sign of the difference between sequence groups is negative in all three strata, this provides an indication that services have decreased significantly from the period before to the period after cost-sharing. This result also illustrates once again that although there is variation in the degree of the cost-sharing effects within each stratum, both the cost-sharing and adjusted cost-sharing effects are consistent in terms of the direction of effects across strata. The overall estimates indicate a decrease of between four and five services per family in the 6-month period after the imposition of cost sharing.

SUMMARY AND CONCLUSIONS

The time-reversed crossover design has been reviewed with emphasis on two main features, a sampling component and an analysis component. An application of the time-reversed crossover design to evaluate the impact of cost-sharing on utilization among members of the United Mine Workers health plan has been illustrated. Based on the time-reversed crossover analysis methodology, this analysis indicated a significant decrease in the number of physician services per family in the 6-month period after the imposition of cost-sharing. Furthermore, this analysis illustrated the measurement and elimination of time-order effects (which include selection and regression effects) from the test of cost-sharing effect.

An evaluation of the sensitivity of these methods for detecting varying degrees of effects was carried out informally by reanalyzing the FUNDS data using alternative stratum definitions. In particular, the use of strata defined by total health expenditures alone yielded significant differences between sequence groups for time-order effects in extreme strata. However, overall cost-sharing effects did not vary substantially from the results which were found based on strata defined by family size and health expenditures combined. As a result of the significant differences (between sequence groups) of within-stratum time-order effects, alternative methods of finding overall estimates of cost-sharing effects were illustrated based on adjusted cost-sharing effects and then based on unadjusted cost-sharing effects combined only across strata in which time-order effects were not significantly different. Both methods yielded overall results which supported the conclusions previously noted regarding a significant decrease in physician services after the imposition of cost-sharing.

These results, based on strata defined by expenditures alone, conform with expectations (both in regard to the significance and lack of significance of various effects) and provide some evidence to support the overall validity of the time-reversed crossover methods. It is also noteworthy that both sets of results are quite consistent with regard to the significance of the cost-sharing effects observed in these data. This can be attributed in part to the robustness of the time-reversed crossover analysis methodology, but also in part (as is recognized) to the substantial cost-sharing effect observed in the FUNDS data.

In describing these findings, it is important to note that because these results are not based on a true experimental design, any method of analysis will be subject to question. As previously noted, a true experimental design should be applied whenever feasible to gain advantages from the use of randomization in assigning subjects to treatment groups.

Whenever a true experimental design is not possible, then an assessment should be made of the advantages and disadvantages of each of the applicable quasi-experimental designs. Figure 7 presents a list of the advantages and disadvantages of the time-reversed crossover design in comparison to the "one group pretest-posttest design," the "separate sample pretest-posttest design," and other applicable quasi-experimental designs described by Campbell and Stanley [3].

The primary disadvantage of the time-reversed crossover design is that it does not include a control group; thus, it is susceptible to threats to validity due to history effects. History effects can only be assessed indirectly by evaluating factors, other than the treatment of interest, which may have caused changes in outcome. For example, the possibility of a general turndown in the economy could lead to decreases in health expenditures. If history effects are suspected, then it is not recommended that the time-reversed crossover design be applied; instead, a quasi-experimental design which eliminates history effects would be more applicable.

Other possible disadvantages which should be considered prior to applying the time-reversed crossover design are listed in Figure 7.

Among the advantages listed are gains in precision and improvements in statistical conclusion validity resulting from the use of the crossover approach to carry out estimation and hypothesis-testing pro-

Figure 7: Summary of Advantages and Disadvantages of the Time-Reserved Crossover Design

ADVANTAGES

Due to Design and Sampling Method:

A. Lower cost due to sample instead of entire population analysis
B. Inducement of design on naturally occurring data set
C. Stratification on outcome and independent variables
   1. Improvement in external validity due to representation of selected strata of interest
   2. Improvement in statistical conclusion validity by creating homogeneous groups within each stratum
      a. Elimination of needs for further adjustment via regression methods
      b. Provision of improved estimates of change over time
   3. Improvement in statistical conclusion validity by allowing for analysis of consistency of effects across strata
D. Separate before/after sampling method
   1. Improvement in external validity due to representation of both populations before and after policy change
   2. Improvement in internal and statistical conclusion validity by allowing for analysis methodology based on crossover model

Due to Analysis Methodology:

A. Flexibility regarding analysis methodology which permits evaluation based on simpler designs
B. Evaluation via time-reversed crossover model
   1. Improvement in internal and statistical conclusion validity due to measurement and elimination of time-order effects
   2. Improvement in statistical conclusion validity due to gains in precision which are similar to traditional crossover model
   3. Allowance for separate estimates and tests of treatment effects whether or not time-order effects are present
   4. Relative simplicity of methods based on existing theory to carry out within and across stratum analyses

DISADVANTAGES

Due to Design and Sampling Method:

A. Design possibly more costly and difficult to apply than designs using simple random sample
B. Possible threats to internal and statistical conclusion validity due to regression effects in extreme-outcome strata
C. Inability to eliminate threats to internal validity due to history effects

Due to Analysis Methodology:

A. Threats to internal validity due to confounding of period and treatment effects
B. Possible threat to statistical conclusion validity due to lack of power of test for equality of time-order effects

cedures. As noted by Sollecito [6], these advantages are similar to those described, by Grizzle [7] and others, as resulting from the use of the traditional crossover design.

Other important advantages of the time-reversed crossover design are the improvements in internal and external validity resulting from stratification on outcome and the separate sampling of populations who were present before and after change has occurred in the health policy to be evaluated. As illustrated by the examples presented here, stratification on outcome can also result in a potential disadvantage: too narrow definitions of strata can cause the presence of regression effects. However, as demonstrated by the FUNDS data, this can be overcome by combining strata in a way that minimizes the impact of regression toward the mean. Another related advantage of this design, which was shown using the FUNDS data, is the ability to use it in measuring the magnitude and equality of regression and other time-order effects; furthermore, it was demonstrated that valid hypothesis tests of treatment effects can be carried out regardless of the presence or absence of significant time-order effects. This implies another advantage of the analysis methodology. The estimates of adjusted treatment effects are the same as those which would be found if a "separate-sample pretest-posttest design" had been employed within each stratum. Therefore, this simpler design and its associated analysis methodology is incorporated as part of the time-reversed crossover design.

Further conclusions regarding the advantages and disadvantages of this design are discussed by Sollecito [6] and will continue to be explored through the further application of this design. The use of the time-reversed crossover design in the FUNDS cost-sharing study demonstrates its applicability in assessing the impact of health policy changes on large populations; this design is suggested as a useful tool for carrying out such evaluations in the future.

APPENDIX

TIME-REVERSED CROSSOVER MODEL EQUATION

The time-reversed crossover model, as introduced by Gillings et al. [5], is parameterized in a manner which enhances the similarities between the time-reversed crossover and traditional two-period crossover design.

The statistical model for analysis of the time-reversed crossover design is complicated by the sampling procedures adopted, so an approach consistent with finite population sampling is the correct approach from a theoretical viewpoint. For purposes of this discussion, an approximate model, based on the traditional crossover model as described by Grizzle [7], may be used. This model will be approximate in that finite population corrections will not be included for purposes of computing variances; it is assumed that because sample sizes are small relative to the population size in each stratum, the effect of the finite population corrections will be negligible. The statistical model for the time-reversed crossover design can be described as follows.

For any outcome variable (y) in the hth stratum:

$$y_{hijk} = \mu_h + b_{hij} + \pi_{hk} + \phi_{hk} + \lambda_{hk'} + e_{hijk} \tag{1}$$

such that

h = 1, 2, . . . , q (where q = number of strata).
i = 1, 2 = index of sequence group.
j = i, . . . , n_{hi} (where n_{hi} = number of subjects in the ith sequence in the hth stratum).
k = 1, 2 = index of period.
k' = 1, 2 (1 for sequence 1, 2 for sequence 2).

where

μ_h = overall mean in the hth stratum.
b_{hij} = the random effect of the jth subject within the ith sequence within the hth stratum, assume $E(b_{hij}) = 0$.
π_{hk} = the effect of the kth period within the hth stratum.
ϕ_{hk} = the effect of the kth treatment in the hth stratum, i.e., the effect of cost-sharing in the FUND study.
$\lambda_{hk'}$ = the residual effect of the kth treatment (for the ith sequence in the hth stratum), i.e., the time-order effect.
e_{hijk} = random error, assume $E(e_{hijk}) = 0$.

In the parametric analysis situation, b_{hij} and e_{hijk} are also assumed to be normally distributed as $N(0,\sigma_b^2)$, $N(0,\sigma_e^2)$, and are mutually independent. The covariance between two measures on the same subject is σ_b^2.

Each of the parameters above is defined within the stratum in which each subject is identified, which implies that effects may differ between strata and that all estimates and hypothesis tests will be made separately for each stratum. This is necessitated by the sampling design and has the advantage of providing more precise estimates due to homogeneity of effects within each stratum. It also provides more descriptive information since it allows the estimates in each stratum to be compared across strata.

From the above model equation, the following estimates of effects are derived:

Residual or time-order effects:

$$E(r_h) = \tfrac{1}{2}(\lambda_{h1} + \lambda_{h2})$$

Treatment (and period) effect:

$$\begin{aligned} E(t_h) &= (\phi_{h2} - \phi_{h1}) + (\pi_{h2} - \pi_{h1}) \textit{ iff } \lambda_{h1} = \lambda_{h2} \\ &= \phi_{h2} - \phi_{h1} \textit{ iff } \pi_{h1} = \pi_{h2} \text{ and } \lambda_{h2} = \lambda_{h1} \end{aligned}$$

In describing treatment effects, it is important to make the distinction between effects due to treatment versus those due to period. Any measure of change over time includes effects due to the treatment of interest, e.g., the imposition of cost-sharing, as well as other effects which can be grouped together and called period effects. Period effects measure factors related to the definition of the time frame during which data have been collected, for example, changes due to seasonal variation. The time-reversed crossover model makes the distinction between these two effects since in many applications, the period effect can be adjusted for, e.g., through seasonal adjustments, or can be assumed to be negligible based on external evidence or control, e.g., comparisons based on a narrow time frame in which these factors do not vary. Therefore, although treatment and period are confounded in the model as defined above, control of period effects can often be achieved, thus allowing for treatment effects to be estimated separately from those due to period.

Note that the *P*-notation presented in the body of the article represents the expected values of each outcome measure (y_{hijk}); thus, the above representations of effects from the time-reversed crossover model lead directly to the estimates in terms of *P*-notation. These in turn can be used to derive the contrasts needed to carry out significance tests, as described in Figure 4. For example, assuming that period and time-order effects are negligible and recalling that *Pik* represents estimates for the *i*th sequence and *k*th period, the estimate of treatment effect (t_h) can be derived as follows. Using *P*-notation, the period 1 effect (ϕ_{h1}) is estimated by the average (across sequences) of period 1 results, i.e., ½ ($P11 + P21$). Similarly, the period 2 effect (ϕ_{h2}) is estimated by the expression, ½ ($P12 + P22$), and the overall treatment effect for the *h*th stratum ($\phi_{h2} - \phi_{h1}$) is estimated by:

$$t_h = {}^1\!/\!_2[(P12 + P22) - (P11 + P21)]$$

A significance test for treatment effect can be carried out by computing this estimate and testing whether it is significantly different from zero, or—equivalently—by comparing (across period) contrasts formed within each sequence groups. The appropriate contrast is derived directly from the expression above. The treatment effect can be rewritten:

$$t_h = {}^1\!/\!_2[(P12 - P11) + (P22 - P21)]$$

This expression equals zero if and only if ($P12$ - $P11$) equals ($P21$ - $P22$), which are the sequence-group contrasts presented in Figure 4.

In like manner, each of the other expressions described in Figure 4 can be derived based on the model parameterization described here.

Further details on the model specification and derivations of estimates and hypothesis tests are provided by Gillings et al. [5] and Sollecito [6].

ACKNOWLEDGMENTS

The authors would like to express their appreciation to Dr. Allen Berkowitz for his assistance in obtaining these data from the United Mine Workers of America Health and Retirement Funds, and to Bea O'Quinn for her conscientious typing of the manuscript.

REFERENCES

1. Newhouse, J. P. A design for a health insurance experiment. *Inquiry* 11(1):5–27, 1974.
2. Denniston, O. L., and I. M. Rosenstock. The validity of non-experimental designs for evaluating health services. *Health Services Reports* 88(2):153–64, 1973.
3. Campbell, D. T., and J. C. Stanley. *Experimental and Quasi-Experimental Designs for Research*. Chicago: Rand McNally College Publishing Company, 1963.
4. Cook, T. D., and D. T. Campbell. *Quasi Experimentation: Design and Analysis Issues for Field Settings*. Chicago: Rand McNally College Publishing Company, 1979.
5. Gillings, D. B., W. A. Sollecito, and G. G. Koch. The use of time reversed crossover designs in evaluative research. *Proceedings of the Social Statistics Section of the American Statistical Association*, 336–40, 1980.
6. Sollecito, W. A. The Time Reversed Crossover Design in Health Ser-

vices Research. Doctoral Dissertation, Department of Biostatistics, University of North Carolina at Chapel Hill, 1982.

7. Grizzle, J. E. The two period change-over design and its uses in clinical trials. *Biometrics* 21(2):467–80, 1965. (Corrigenda, *Biometrics* 30(4):727, 1974).
8. Koch, G. G. The use of nonparametric methods in the statistical analysis of the two period change-over design. *Biometrics* 28(2):577–84, 1972.
9. Kish, L. *Survey Sampling*. New York: John Wiley and Sons, Inc., 1965.
10. Wilcoxon, F. Individual comparisons by ranking methods. *Biometrics* 1(1):80–83, 1945.
11. van Elteren, P. H. On the combination of independent two sample tests of Wilcoxon. *Bulletin of the International Statistical Institute* 37(3):351–61, 1960.
12. Research and Statistics Department of the United Mine Workers of America Health and Retirement Funds. Summary Report of a Study of the Effect of Cost Sharing on Beneficiaries of the UMW Health Plan. Unpublished report prepared for the National Center for Health Services Research, Washington, DC, 1982.

Chapter Thirteen

Multiple Regression as a Program Evaluation Strategy

The National Long Term Care Demonstration (Channeling) Project, begun in 1979 with support from the U.S. Department of Health and Human Services, required over six years to plan, implement, and evaluate. The principal results of the demonstration were published in *Health Services Research* in April 1988. The demonstration was intended to test whether the substitution of community-based case management services for nursing home care could reduce long-term care costs and improve the quality of life for elderly persons and their caregiving families. As its name implies, the purpose of the project was to channel health and human services to elderly persons who experience serious deficits in their capacity for self-care. During the period of time the study took place, Weissert (1988) reports that 27 other studies of this question also took place. In none of them, including the Channeling Project, did the results indicate that the substitution of home care for nursing home care is a cost-saving intervention. The costs of home care seem to exceed the small reductions in nursing home costs that might result from serving these persons' needs in noninstitutional settings. Furthermore, the psychosocial and physical benefits of these programs for those who are served seem to be of only negligible importance.

The Channeling Project involved the evaluation of home-based services in ten states. Two different models for providing these services were evaluated. The "basic case management model" tested the effects of case management where managers provided information to clients about a broad spectrum of services available in the community, but had no authority or means of purchasing services directly for clients. This intervention model was essentially one of determining needs, providing information, and coordinating access to services available within the client's community. Some limited funds were available for the purchase of services to fill residual gaps that would have prevented the implementation of a comprehensive care plan for a given individual. But, in general, services available to these clients were those conventionally accessible within the community where they lived. The "financial control model" gave case managers the authority and means to purchase services needed by their clients up to a fixed per person and per program ceiling. In neither plan did the experimental group differ from the control group in the use of nursing home care, hospital care, or services of physicians, nor in mortality or overall cost of care. Clients' functional status and measures of psychosocial well-being were apparently little influenced by these interventions.

The evaluation encountered several methodological problems, which had to be overcome through the use of statistical procedures described in this article by Brown. Most importantly, problems of estimating the intervention effects arose from the differences in the way the data at baseline were collected. In the experimental groups, data were collected by the case managers; in the control groups, the research team collected the data. There were also very high attrition rates, especially among the control groups. The high frequency of use of proxy respondents led to concern that the measures of psychosocial variables were really measures of attitudinal effects among the caregivers and not representative of the elderly clients themselves.

In this article, Brown illustrates the use of regression techniques to estimate channeling impacts and the potential effects of these several types of methodological problems on the evaluation results. His discussion makes a case for the use of regression in preference to simple differences in means as a way of estimating program impacts. Despite the negligible effects of the channeling intervention on the costs and quality of long-term care for the elderly, the demonstration has provided useful methodological guidance for the future of long-term care research, and for all other efforts where the effects of such large-scale demonstrations are to be measured.

REFERENCE

Weissert, William G. "The National Channeling Demonstration: What We Knew, Know Now, and Still Need to Know." *Health Services Research* 23(1), April 1988: 175–87.

The Evaluation of the National Long Term Care Demonstration

2. Estimation Methodology

Randall S. Brown

Channeling effects were estimated by comparing the post-application experience of the treatment and control groups using multiple regression. A variety of potential threats to the validity of the results, including sample composition issues, data issues, and estimation issues, were identified and assessed. Of all the potential problems examined, the only one determined to be likely to cause widespread distortion of program impact estimates was noncomparability of the baseline data. To avoid this distortion, baseline variables judged to be noncomparably measured were excluded from use as control variables in the regression equation. (Where they existed, screen counterparts to these noncomparable baseline variables were used as substitutes.) All of the other potential problems with the sample, data, or regression estimation approach were found to have little or no actual effect on impact estimates or their interpretation. Broad implementation of special procedures, therefore, was not necessary. The study did find that, because of the frequent use of proxy respondents, the estimated effects of channeling on clients' well-being actually may reflect impacts on the well-being of the informal caregiver rather than the client. This and other isolated cases in which there was some evidence of a potential problem for specific outcome variables were identified and examined in detail in technical reports dealing with those outcomes. Where appropriate, alternative estimates were presented.

The key design features of the channeling evaluation described in the previous article (diverse sites, large sample sizes, experimental design, sound data) were intended to ensure that the estimates of program impacts obtained would be valid and credible. The credibility and

---

Randall S. Brown, Ph.D. is a Senior Economist with Mathematica Policy Research. Address correspondence to Randall S. Brown, Mathematica Policy Research, Inc., P.O. Box 2393, Princeton, NJ 08543-2393.

robustness of the estimates of program impacts depend in large part on whether valid estimates can be obtained using straightforward statistical procedures and tests, with little dependence on assumptions that are difficult or impossible to test. This guiding principle was instrumental in the decision to assign randomly all eligible program applicants to either the treatment group or the control group, and to estimate program impacts by comparing the two groups.

Despite the strong design and the emphasis on straightforward estimation, however, a number of features of the evaluation—some affecting nearly all evaluations and others peculiar to this project—created complications for the analysis and may cast doubt on the quality of the estimates that were obtained. The procedures used to estimate channeling impacts and the examinations of potential methodological problems that were conducted are documented in a channeling evaluation technical report (Brown, 1986). This article summarizes that report. Presentation of even a fraction of the estimates examined, however, would have made this article unacceptably long, and selective presentation of exceptions to the general pattern of results may give readers a distorted picture of the overall findings. Readers interested in more detail are referred to the technical report and to other reports cited in this article.

ESTIMATION OF CHANNELING IMPACTS AND HYPOTHESIS TESTING

Given the randomized design, unbiased estimates of channeling impacts could be obtained simply by comparing mean values of outcomes for the treatment and control groups. Note that this approach involves comparison of means for *all* treatment group members in each model, not just program participants, to the means for controls from the sites in which the model was implemented. Clearly, channeling cannot affect the outcome of treatment group members who do not participate; hence, treatment-control differences will understate the impacts on those who actually receive channeling services. Nonetheless, since those who decline to participate after being offered the opportunity may differ in important ways from those who do participate, comparing only the participants to the control group would not yield unbiased estimates. Thus, whatever statistical method is used, estimates of program impacts are based on the comparison of all treatment group members with available data to all available controls.

The approach actually used in the evaluation was ordinary least-squares regression. The regression models used in the evaluation, the types of statistical tests and significance levels employed, and the interpretation of estimates and tests are the topics of this section.

THE REGRESSION MODEL

Regression (or equivalently, analysis of covariance) offers three advantages over simple differences in means as a way of estimating program impacts. First, although the two experimental groups should have very similar average characteristics initially, there may in fact be differences between them, either by chance or because of different patterns of sample attrition for treatment and control groups. If these differences are fully reflected in the observed initial characteristics of the sample, the regression model can control for such differences between the groups. Second, the ratio of treatments to controls differs across sites, ranging from 1:1 to 2:1. If sample members or the health care environment differ across sites, the treatment/control differences in mean outcomes will reflect not only effects of channeling but the different distributions as well. Again, regression will control for these differences. Finally, to the extent that outcomes are related to baseline or screen characteristics, regression can explain some of the variation among individuals, leading to more precise estimates of channeling impacts (that is, estimates with lower standard errors) than are obtained from differences in means.

The regression model used was

$$Y = a_o + a_B T_B + a_F T_F + a_s S + a_x X + e$$

where Y is the outcome variable that is hypothesized to be affected by channeling; T_B and T_F are binary variables equal to one for sample members in the basic (B) and financial (F) sites; S is a set of binary site variables; X is a set of explanatory variables taken from the screen or baseline interviews; e is a disturbance term, and the a's are coefficients to be estimated. The inclusion of binary site variables is exactly equivalent to first transforming all variables (Y and X) into deviations around their site means and then running the regressions; hence, treatment group members are in effect compared only to controls at the same site. Under this model, the coefficients a_B and a_F measure the treatment/control differences in mean outcomes, controlling for any differences that exist between the two groups on baseline explanatory variables. Hence, a_B and a_F are our estimates of impacts for the two channeling models.

The same regression model was used to estimate the impacts of channeling on all outcome measures examined in the evaluation. Although it may seem unlikely that the factors that affect well-being (for example) are exactly the same as the factors that affect nursing home use and other outcomes, there exists a strong justification for this approach. The outcome variables are highly interrelated and depend on each other as well as on many of the same exogenous variables. However, the interrelationship of the outcome variables is complex; trying to model it could lead to biased estimates, since some of the explanatory variables would be endogenous (that is, correlated with the disturbance term *e* in the regression). Furthermore, our principal interest is in the *total*, combined effect of channeling on the outcome variables; that is, taking well-being as our illustrative outcome, we are not particularly concerned with distinguishing the amount of the impact that was indirect (for example, improved well-being of clients resulting from channeling-induced reductions in institutionalization) from the amount of the impact that was direct (such as improved well-being due directly to the services provided by channeling). Therefore, we estimate the "reduced form" equation for the outcome variables. In the reduced form, all explanatory variables must be exogenous (baseline/screen) variables, and any exogenous variable that affects *any* of the interrelated outcome variables of interest is included. Thus, the explanatory variables in the reduced form include any baseline or screen variables that directly or indirectly affect the particular outcome variable being examined.

The explanatory variables that were used in the regression model fell into six categories:

- Sample members' level of need for assistance due to physical or mental disabilities
- The availability of informal caregivers to provide this assistance
- The amount of formal care received by sample members at baseline
- The sample members' ability to pay for additional services or nursing home care
- Binary site variables (reflecting the availability of nursing home beds and all other area-specific factors)
- The sample members' demographic characteristics and outlook on life.

The variables included in the model and their means are given in Table 1. All variables were obtained from the screen or baseline interviews, as designated in the table.

TESTING STRATEGY

The regression procedure described above provides estimates of treatment/control differences in outcomes, controlling for any initial differences between the two groups. These are our best estimates of channeling impacts. However, even if channeling had no impact, the treatment and control groups might have had somewhat different outcomes strictly by chance. Hence, we relied on statistical tests to determine if the estimated differences were large enough to have made chance occurrence unlikely.

Three types of tests were used in the analysis: t-tests on the estimates of a_B and a_F, the estimated treatment/control differences, to determine if they were significantly different from zero; F-tests to test whether or not the estimated impacts in the basic and financial control models differed from each other by more than might have been expected to occur by chance; and multivariate F-tests to test if estimates of channeling impacts on sets of related outcome measures were equal to zero.

The t-tests were two-tailed and conducted at the .05 significance level. For most outcomes examined, the intention was that channeling would have a particular directional effect (for example, reduction in nursing home use). However, for the vast majority of the outcomes, there were plausible reasons why the impact could be in the opposite direction, and for some important outcomes, a high degree of uncertainty existed regarding the direction of channeling impacts to expect (for example, informal caregiving and costs). Since we would clearly not ignore estimates that were of the "wrong" sign but were large and would have been statistically significant had a two-tailed test been conducted, the appropriate test to use is the two-tailed test.

To avoid the appearance of arbitrariness in the selection of tests, and confusion in the minds of readers about the type of test being employed in any given table (particularly in reports covering multiple outcomes), two-tailed tests were used throughout the analysis. (They were used even for those few outcomes where the only plausible hypothesis about channeling's impact is unidirectional.) The use of two-tailed t-tests also should result in greater consistency between these tests and the multivariate F-tests (described below), which are by definition two-tailed. To make it relatively unlikely that chance differences

Table 1: Mean Values of Explanatory Variables Used in Regression Model

Variable	*Mean**
Need for Assistance	
ADL impairment (S)†	
Extremely severe	0.233
Severe	0.348
Moderate impairment	0.223
(Mild or no impairment)‡	0.196
Incontinence (S)	
Incontinent	0.472
Needs help with catheter or colostomy bag	0.102
(Continent)	0.426
Cognitive impairment (S)	
Severe	0.153
(Moderate impairment)	0.318
Mild or no impairment	0.471
Missing data	0.058
Unmet needs (S)	
High unmet needs	0.303
(Moderate unmet needs)	0.340
Low unmet needs	0.302
Missing data	0.054
Whether experienced recent change in health (S)	0.818
Whether death of close friend or relative other than spouse (S)	
Death of close person	0.244
(No death)	0.406
Missing data	0.350
Availability of Informal Care	
Living arrangement (B)	
Lives alone, no informal support	0.073
Lives alone, informal support	0.282
Lives with child	0.251
(Lives with someone other than child)	0.377
Missing information	0.016
Hours of care received per week from visiting informal caregiver (B)	12.0
Demographic Characteristics and Attitudes	
Whether male (B)	0.285
Age (B)	79.6
Ethnicity (S)	
Black	0.223
Hispanic	0.037
(White or other)	0.740
Whether currently married (B)	0.318
Overall satisfaction with life (B)	
Completely	0.117
(Somewhat)	0.248
Not very	0.288
Missing data	0.348
Ability to Pay for Care	
Whether home owner (B)	0.421

Continued

between the two groups would be interpreted as channeling impacts, all t-tests were conducted at the customary 5 percent significance level.

Although these decisions about one-tailed versus two-tailed tests and significance levels were considered the most appropriate, the t-statistics were provided along with the estimates throughout the final technical reports on channeling impacts. From those reports, interested readers can determine for themselves whether and how inferences would change if alternative choices had been made.

In addition to determining whether the basic and financial control models affected specific outcome measures, it was also important to assess whether the models differed from each other in the size of the

Table 1: Continued

Variable	*Mean**	*Variable*	*Mean**
Referral source (S)		Medicaid coverage (B)	
Hospital or nursing home	0.297	Currently eligible	0.226
Home health agency	0.173	Eligible within 3 months	0.304
(Other)	0.531	(Not eligible in 3 months)	0.401
		Missing information	0.069
Number of physician visits in previous two months (B)†	1.7	*Site*	
		Basic	
Whether waitlisted or applied to nursing home (B), or in nursing home at screen	0.097	Baltimore	0.108
		Eastern Kentucky	0.079
		Houston	0.111
Type of respondent at baseline		Middlesex County	0.112
Self-respondent	0.417	(Southern Maine)	0.079
(Mixed proxy/Self-respondent)	0.298	Financial control	
All proxy respondent	0.285	Cleveland	0.093
Receipt of Formal Services		Greater Lynn	0.096
Whether received formal		Miami	0.118
in-home care (B)	0.600	Philadelphia	0.140
		(Rensselaer County)	0.065
Hours of formal in-home care received per week (B)	7.3		
Model			
(Basic)	0.488		
Financial control	0.512		

*Means were computed for the largest analysis sample (N = 5,554) employing these standard control variables.

†Letters in parentheses following variable names indicate whether data used were from the baseline (B) or screen (S) interviews.

‡For variables represented by a set of binary indicators (e.g., ADL), parentheses indicate which category was excluded from the regression equations, although this choice has no bearing on the estimates of program impacts.

impact. It was hypothesized that the greater resources and flexibility of funding available under the financial control model would result in larger impacts for this model. However, differences between the environments into which the two models were introduced could also produce differences in the size of impacts achieved by the alternative models. Simple F-tests of the equivalence of a_B and a_F (from the regression equation) provided the tests of this hypothesis. The tests were conducted at the 5 percent level, consistent with the significance level selected for the t-tests.

The individual tests described above were conducted at a significance level that made it relatively unlikely that, for any particular outcome measure, chance differences between treatment and control groups would be interpreted incorrectly as channeling impacts. However, because so many outcomes were examined (each for two models and three time periods), the probability that such errors would occur in at least a few instances was very high. To lessen the probability of making such errors, multivariate tests were employed that simultaneously tested the hypothesis that channeling impacts on a set of related outcome measures were jointly equal to zero.

Testing to verify that impacts on the set of outcomes being considered jointly were all zero were conducted for the basic model, the financial control model, and both models together. Multivariate tests also were used to determine whether impacts on given sets of outcomes in the basic model were equal to those in the financial control model. In each case, the tests were conducted on related outcome measures, such as alternative measures of well-being or informal care, for a given time period. Because the tests require that the same observations be used in all of the equations for which the coefficients are being tested jointly, outcomes in different time periods were tested separately.

The use of multivariate tests decreases the frequency of erroneously concluding that chance differences between treatment and control groups on some particular outcome measures are due to channeling impacts. However, this increased protection against type I errors raises the probability of making the opposite error, that is, of concluding that channeling had no impact when the program indeed was effective (type II errors).

To decrease the number of both type I and type II errors, we looked, throughout the analysis, not only at the statistical significance of the estimates but also at their magnitudes and patterns. Specifically, to assess whether channeling affected a given outcome, analysts looked for consistency in the direction, size, and statistical significance of estimated impacts on (1) related outcome measures, (2) the same outcome in other time periods, and (3) the same outcome in the other channeling model.

The estimated impact at the site level also was examined to see if the model-level estimate was essentially due to results from one or two particular sites rather than being widespread. Dependence on patterns across model, time period, and site to verify whether impacts exist cannot be rigid, since there are reasons why effects may differ across these dimensions. Nevertheless, if patterns exist they provide evidence that the observed differences were due to channeling rather than to chance.

Finally, the evaluation also drew on theory and results from the process analysis (Carcagno et al., 1986) to assess the likelihood that the estimates obtained represented real impacts rather than chance differences. Awareness of how outcomes interrelate and the process by which channeling was likely to bring about effects on individuals, coupled with knowledge about how the local programs operated, were useful inputs to the assessment of whether impacts existed when the statistical evidence was mixed.

In addition to ascertaining *whether* channeling affected outcomes, the *size* of the estimated impact was also examined. In general, it would make little difference, from a cost-effectiveness perspective, whether channeling impacts in a given area were zero or just very modest in size. To obtain some indication of the proportionate magnitude of impacts, mean values of the outcome variable for the control group were presented, in tables displaying the results, alongside the estimated impacts on these outcomes. The dollar value of the impact also provided a useful way of assessing the importance of a given estimate for some outcome measures.

ESTIMATED IMPACTS FOR SUBGROUPS

In addition to determining whether channeling impacts differed by model, we also tested whether impacts on key outcomes differed across sites and for various subsets of the sample defined by characteristics of the sample members. The baseline and screen characteristics used to form these subsets, described more fully in Grannemann et al. (1986), include:

- Impairment in activities of daily living (extremely severe, severe, moderate, mild/none)
- Continence (incontinent, needs help with catheter or colostomy bag to be continent, continent)
- Unmet needs (high, medium, low)
- Living arrangement (alone without current informal support, alone with current support, with own child(ren), with someone but not with child)
- Health system contact (in nursing home at randomization, on nursing home waiting list, in a hospital or referred to channeling by a hospital or nursing home, referred by a home-health agency, referred by family or other source or self)
- Medicaid eligibility (eligible at baseline, not eligible but would be within three months after entering nursing home, would not be eligible within three months)

—Cognitive impairment (severe, moderate, mild/none)
—Site.

To obtain estimated impacts for the three to five subgroups formed by each of the classifying variables, the standard regression was modified as follows:

$$Y = a_0 + a_T T + a_1 X_1 + a_2 X_2 + a_{T1} T^* X_1 + a_S S + a_{TS} T^* S + e$$

where X_1 is a vector that contains the binary variables representing the characteristics defining the subgroups and X_2 contains the other explanatory variables used in the standard regression model. This equation was estimated separately for the basic and the financial control models, to reduce the number of parameters and simplify the calculation of impacts and standard errors.

The primary tests conducted were to determine whether the estimated impacts differed from each other across the subgroups defined by each of the classifying variables. The hypothesis that no such difference occurred was tested by performing for each classifying characteristic an F-test of whether the coefficients in a_{T1} on the binary variables representing that characteristic (or a_{TS} for tests of equivalence across sites) were equal to zero. Given the large number of such tests, however, we first jointly tested *all* of the coefficients in a_{T1} to determine whether they were equal to zero. Rejection of this hypothesis indicated that channeling impacts on a given outcome did vary with at least one of the classifying characteristics. In such cases, the F-tests for each characteristic were then examined to determine with which of the characteristics channeling impacts varied. More details on the computation and interpretation of these test statistics is given in Grannemann et al. (1986).

Potential Problems with Sample Composition

The randomized design, large sample sizes, and straightforward estimation methodology eliminate the major reasons for questioning the evaluation results. However, two potential problems with the composition of the sample available for analysis could cast doubt on the findings: initial differences between the treatment and control groups due to chance or failure to implement appropriate randomization procedures, and differences between the two groups due to attrition from the sample.

THE EQUIVALENCE OF TREATMENT AND CONTROL GROUPS AT RANDOMIZATION

Because eligible channeling applicants were assigned randomly to either the treatment or the control group, the collective observed and unobserved characteristics of the individuals that comprise the two groups were similar in the preapplication period. Hence, the control group should yield valid estimates of what would have happened to clients in the absence of channeling—and comparison of outcomes for the treatment and control groups therefore should yield unbiased estimates of channeling impacts.

Only two factors (other than measurement error) could cause the mean values of the preapplication characteristics of the full treatment and control groups to differ: deviation from the randomization procedures and normal sampling variability. The names of eligible individuals who applied or were referred to the program were telephoned to Mathematica Policy Research (MPR), where a designated researcher assigned them to the treatment or control group, using carefully developed randomization procedures (Phillips et al., 1986). Hence, deliberate or accidental subversion of this process was deemed extremely unlikely. Furthermore, for the sample sizes available at the model level, differences between the two groups due to sampling variability should be very small. Nevertheless, the implication of large differences between the two groups for estimates of program impacts was so great that it was necessary to verify that in fact the two groups were comparable.

This assessment was carried out by comparing mean values of characteristics for the treatment and control groups in each model, using data from the screening interview and adjusting for the unequal distribution of the two groups across sites (Brown and Harrigan, 1983). The screen, which was used to assess eligibility of applicants and to gather some information on other client characteristics, was administered by site intake workers prior to random assignment. Of the 53 screen variables examined for each model, differences were significantly different from zero at the .05 level for only one characteristic in the basic model and for four in the financial control model. Furthermore, even the significant differences were small in magnitude. Treatment/control comparisons at the site level yielded similar conclusions: the number of statistically significant differences was no larger than would be expected by chance, and no patterns of differences were found to indicate that noncomparable groups were obtained in any site. Thus, the control group should provide a valid measure of what would have happened to the treatment group in the absence of channeling.

THE EFFECTS OF SAMPLE ATTRITION

Although the experience of the control group should provide a reliable estimate of what should have happened to treatment group members in the absence of the demonstration, this may not be the case if the sample available for analysis after attrition was not comparable for the two groups. Regression models were used in the evaluation to control for observable differences between the treatment and control groups that could arise because of attrition, but estimates may still be biased if the two groups differed on unobservable characteristics. Bias in estimates of channeling impacts occurs if three conditions hold: (1) those sample members for whom data are available differ on unobservable characteristics from those for whom data are not available, (2) those unobservable factors also affect outcomes of interest, and (3) rates or patterns of attrition differ for treatment and control groups.

For each of the major areas of analysis in the evaluation, an analysis sample was defined, which included those observations from the full research sample for which the data necessary for that analysis were available (see Table 3 of Carcagno and Kemper, this issue, for a list of the sources of data by subject area). The percent of the full sample included in most of these analysis samples, displayed in Table 2, ranged from over 90 percent to as low as 30 percent at 18 months (due mainly to the death of nearly 40 percent of the sample). The rates varied with the outcome examined, the time period, and the model, but were consistently greater (by 6–14 percentage points) for treatments than for controls, especially in the financial control model. Thus, one of the conditions, which in combination with the other two could lead to bias, was present.

The analysis of the effects of attrition from these samples on estimates of channeling impacts was greatly enhanced by the fact that some pretreatment and follow-up data were available on the entire research sample. Two types of analyses were performed during the evaluation and reported on in Brown et al. (1986)—a heuristic approach and a statistical modeling approach. Under the heuristic approach, Medicare follow-up data, which were available for virtually the entire research sample, were used to construct several variables measuring the amount of Medicare-covered services used, including

Table 2: Percent of Full Sample Included in Analysis Samples

	Basic Model		*Financial Control Model*	
	Treatments	*Controls*	*Treatments*	*Controls*
Number of Observations in Full Sample	1,779	1,345	1,923	1,279
6-month outcomes				
Percent of full sample included in analysis of:				
Hospital/Medical service use	90.4	82.1	93.3	81.9
Nursing home use	72.0	67.1	80.5	67.3
Client quality of life	66.4	62.0	73.1	59.2
Formal and informal care	54.8	51.5	62.3	48.9
12-month outcomes				
Percent of full sample included in analysis of:				
Hospital/Medical service use	90.4	82.1	93.3	81.9
Nursing home use	76.4	69.5	82.0	68.9
Client quality of life	59.1	52.1	63.0	51.4
Formal and informal care	47.1	41.0	50.7	40.7
Number of Observations in 18-Month Cohort	922	697	926	620
18-month outcomes				
Percent of cohort included in analysis of:				
Hospital/Medical service use	89.3	84.9	94.1	80.8
Nursing home use	69.8	68.1	78.8	64.4
Client quality of life	43.8	40.3	50.9	40.2
Formal and informal care	33.6	31.3	38.8	31.5

Note: Percentages differ from 100 because of missing data due to death (the most common reason), interview nonresponse, or missing records data. See Brown et al. (1986) for a breakdown on the reasons for missing data.

hospital days and expenditures, nursing home days and expenditures, and several types of home-health and physician services. Channeling impacts on these Medicare variables were then estimated on the full sample, and again on each the various analysis samples. The estimates were then compared to determine whether limiting the analysis to observations in the analysis samples produced estimates different from those of the full sample.

For the Medicare variables, the impact estimates obtained on the analysis samples rarely differed substantively from those for the full sample. For hospital use, the similarity of the impact estimate for the full and analysis samples provided convincing evidence that attrition did not lead to bias, because over 98 percent of all hospital use by sample members was covered by Medicare. For other outcomes and samples, however, this type of comparison was less compelling: although there were few instances of noteworthy differences between the full and analysis samples in estimated impacts on the Medicare-covered services examined, it was possible that estimated impacts on other outcomes for which Medicare data provided no information or only partial information (for example, nursing home use, well-being, formal care receipt) would be biased by attrition. Alternative procedures were required to determine whether attrition bias for these outcomes was present.

A statistical model developed by Heckman (1979) to control for the nonrandom selection of an analysis sample was used for this purpose. For each analysis sample, a model was estimated to predict which of the full-sample observations were retained in the analysis, as a function of personal characteristics measured on the screening interview. From each estimated sample inclusion model a new variable was constructed for each member of the corresponding analysis sample. This variable was then included as an additional explanatory variable in the impact regression equations to control for the effects of attrition. The coefficient on the constructed attrition bias term was then tested for statistical significance to determine whether the condition necessary for regression estimates to be biased by sample attrition was met.

This procedure was implemented for several key outcome variables in each of the substantive areas of analysis, for each of the three time periods:

Hospital/Nursing Home Use
Whether admitted to hospital
Number of hospital days
Whether admitted to nursing home
Number of nursing home days
Whether residing in community at follow-up

Formal Care
Whether received care from visiting formal caregiver
Hours of formal care
Whether received comprehensive case management

Informal Care
Whether received informal care
Whether received care from visiting informal caregivers

Client Well-Being/Mortality
Satisfaction with life
Number of unmet needs
Number of ADL impairments
Whether deceased at time of follow-up.

The results indicated very little evidence of attrition bias. The estimated correlations between unobserved factors affecting attrition and those affecting a given outcome variable were not large and in only one instance were they significantly different from zero. Impact estimates obtained from the regressions that included the control variable for the effects of attrition were very similar to the impact estimates obtained without this correction term. (Results are presented in Table 3 for a representative subset of the variables examined.) A somewhat more general statistical model, accounting for potential differences between treatments and controls in the relationship of observed and unobserved characteristics to the probability of response, led to the same conclusion: there was no evidence that estimates of channeling impacts were biased by attrition.

By definition, it is never possible to know with certainty what results would have been obtained had no sample attrition occurred. The heuristic and statistical approaches were the best methods available to assess the effects of attrition on our impact estimates, and both approaches provided convincing evidence that the inferences drawn from the analysis samples about the existence and general magnitude of channeling impacts were no different from what would have been drawn had the full sample been available for analysis. Even if the evidence were not so compelling, at worst the study should be viewed as having a very strong quasi-experimental design that compares very favorably with other studies of community care interventions.

POTENTIAL PROBLEMS WITH DATA

Another potential source of erroneous inferences about channeling effects was data that may not be comparably measured for the treatment and control groups. This concern was raised because baseline data were collected by different types of interviewers for the two groups, and because proxy respondents often completed the baseline and follow-up interviews for sample members.

THE COMPARABILITY OF BASELINE DATA FOR TREATMENT AND CONTROL GROUPS

As indicated in the first article of this issue (Carcagno and Kemper), the combination of several factors—conflicts between research needs and good case management practices, data collection costs, and the desire to minimize the burden on sample members—led to the decision

Table 3: Estimation of Channeling Impacts on a Selected Set of Key Outcomes at 12 Months, with and without Corrections for Attrition Bias (t-Statistics in Parentheses)

	Basic Model		*Financial Control Model*		
	Uncorrected Estimate	*Corrected Estimate*	*Uncorrected Estimate*	*Corrected Estimate*	*Correlation*
Number of nursing home days	-1.19 (-0.63)	-2.61 (-1.19)	-2.19 (-1.15)	-4.94 (-1.75)	-0.31 (-1.32)
Number of unmet needs	-0.31** (-3.52)	-0.38** (-3.50)	-0.31** (-3.52)	-0.43** (-3.21)	-0.36 (-1.20)
Percent satisfied with life	2.2 (0.94)	3.5 (1.22)	5.0* (2.07)	7.1* (1.97)	0.24 (0.79)
Number of visits from visiting formal caregivers	0.55** (3.01)	0.71** (3.47)	2.12** (11.56)	2.37** (10.22)	0.40 (1.74)
Number of visits from visiting informal caregivers	0.15 (0.49)	0.33 (0.98)	-0.47 (-1.56)	-0.19 (-0.49)	0.28 (-1.22)

Note: Estimates differ slightly from those presented in later articles of this issue because this methodological analysis was conducted on slightly different samples or variables from those used in the final analysis. The need to investigate potential methodological problems prior to conducting the final analysis occasionally required the use of preliminary outcome measures or somewhat different sets of sample observations.

*Statistically significant at the 5 percent level.

**Statistically significant at the 1 percent level.

that baseline data would be collected by channeling staff for members of the treatment group, and by research interviewers for the control group. For a variety of reasons, this difference in data collection could result in differences between the two groups on observed data for some characteristics, when in fact no real differences exist between the two groups on these baseline characteristics. Estimates of channeling impacts obtained from regression models that use these baseline data as explanatory variables could then be distorted, because these artificial differences between the two groups create spurious correlation between the binary treatment variable and the explanatory variables. The bias is exacerbated if these noncomparable variables are used to create subgroups for which channeling impacts are calculated.

An extensive analysis was conducted (Brown and Mossel, 1984) to determine whether the baseline data for treatments and controls were comparable and, if not, what needed to be done to ensure that regression estimates of channeling impacts would not be biased by such differences. The examination of screen data, described earlier in this article, demonstrated that the treatment and control groups were equivalent at the time of randomization. A similar treatment-control comparison of screen variables restricted to those sample members who completed the baseline interview showed that only very minor differences between the two groups had been introduced by differential attrition from the sample at baseline.

Despite the strong similarity of the two groups on the screen data, which were collected immediately prior to randomization for all sample members, a substantial number of large and statistically significant differences existed between the two groups on baseline variables, including some of the same variables for which no differences were found on the screen. In virtually every case, the observed baseline differences were in the direction that one would expect if they were due to the difference in interviewers. For example, many more unmet needs, much greater impairment on activities of daily living, and lower incomes were reported for the treatment group, even though the *screen* version of each of these variables indicated no treatment-control difference. Although real differences between the two groups (due either to differential attrition or to preexisting differences not detected by screen measures) could not be ruled out entirely, the similarity of the two groups on screen variables provided strong evidence that differential measurement was largely responsible for the observed baseline differences between treatments and controls.

The study then showed how regression estimates of channeling impacts would be affected by the use of noncomparable data items as explanatory variables in the regression. The expressions for bias induced by noncomparable data suggested two types of tests of baseline variables, both designed to determine whether the baseline differences observed were too large to be considered real differences between the groups, given the observed differences on screen variables. One of the two tests was for baseline variables for which similar measures were available on the screen; the other test was for variables that had no such screen counterparts.

The tests showed that among the set of baseline variables then being considered for use in the final analyses, about half were comparably measured. These variables included demographic characteristics such as age, sex, and living arrangement, and objective variables such as hours of formal and informal care received per week. Noncomparable variables tended to be those that were more subjective and those that had more influence on the services that treatment group members would receive from channeling: ability to perform activities of daily living, unmet needs, attitude toward nursing homes, medical conditions, and self-rating of health. These results, in general, were consistent with a priori expectations about the particular variables likely to be affected by noncomparable measurement and the direction of the treatment/control differences. They were also broadly consistent with baseline-reinterview differences observed for a subsample of treatment group members who were given a second baseline by research interviewers.

Only those baseline variables found to be comparable were included as control variables or used to form subgroups in the final channeling analyses. For noncomparable baseline variables with screen counterparts, the screen version was used as a control variable in its place. The other noncomparable baseline variables were excluded from the set of control variables.

The exclusion of the noncomparable variables is not likely to have caused serious problems for the analysis. Analyses showed that dropping the noncomparable variables as control variables did lead to changes in the impact estimates, as expected, but did not lead to a loss of precision (larger standard errors) in these estimates. However, the inability to examine impacts for subgroups defined on potentially important but noncomparable variables, such as medical conditions, mental functioning, attitude toward nursing homes, and instrumental activities of daily living, did weaken the analysis of subgroup effects.

THE EFFECTS ON IMPACT ESTIMATES OF USING PROXY RESPONDENTS

Because of their frailty, many sample members required the help of others (family, friend, nurse, caregiver) to complete the interview. However, proxies' responses to questions may have differed considerably from those that the sample members would have given—especially to questions about attitudes or feelings. This issue raised concerns from the beginning of the evaluation about whether use of proxies at follow-up would distort estimates of channeling impacts.

Rates of proxy use for treatment and control groups were found to be remarkably similar for the two groups at all three follow-up interviews, both in answering specific questions and in overall response to the interview. Overall, about 40–45 percent of the interviews were completed without any assistance from proxies, while another 40–45 percent were completed entirely by proxies. The similarity of rates for the treatment and control groups made it less likely that proxy use distorted estimates of channeling impacts. However, such distortion was still possible, unless proxies (on average) responded no differently from sample members.

To provide an indication of whether impact estimates were affected by proxy use, impacts on the set of key outcomes listed earlier were estimated separately for sample members with proxy respondents and those who responded themselves. Relatively few significant differences in impacts were found between these two groups—but more than would be expected by chance. For 10 of the 90 outcomes examined, impacts for the two groups were significantly different from each other at the .05 level. Seven of these ten cases were scattered across outcome measures and time periods, and exhibited no pattern that could be logically associated with the use of proxy respondents. The other three significant differences were for client global life satisfaction—at 12 months in both models and at 6 months in the financial control model. In each case, the estimates indicated that channeling increased satisfaction with life among those with proxy respondents but had no impact on sample members who completed the interview themselves.

It was unclear from these results if the differences in estimated impacts were due to differences in physical (or cognitive) impairment between the types of clients who required proxy respondents and those who did not, or if they were due to responses by proxy members that were not accurate reflections of responses that the sample members would have given themselves. To distinguish between these two alternative explanations for the differences in impacts between self- and proxy-respondent cases, the regression model used to estimate impacts for the two groups was modified by including additional interaction terms involving treatment status and screen measures of physical and cognitive impairment to control for impact differences due to client impairment. This model was then estimated for life satisfaction at 6 and 12 months and for a few of the other outcome variables for which significant differences in impacts had been observed between proxy- and self-respondent cases. Tests were conducted on the interaction terms involving proxy respondent status and treatment status to determine if impacts varied with the type of respondent.

For nine of the ten variables for which these tests were conducted, the difference in impacts between proxy- and self-respondent cases was not statistically significant. The exception was clients' satisfaction with life at 12 months in the basic model. Furthermore, although the estimated impact on life satisfaction at six months for the basic model and at both follow-ups for the financial control model were no longer significantly different for the two types of respondents, the estimated differences remained quite large. This indicated significant improvements in life satisfaction due to channeling for those with proxy respondents, but not for the self-respondents, even after controlling for disability and cognitive impairment.

We concluded from these studies that, in general, the use of proxy respondents did not lead to distortion of program impact estimates, but that impacts on life satisfaction may have been seriously affected. Since the proxies typically were informal caregivers for the sample member, it may well have been that for the treatment group, proxies' responses reflected their own increased satisfaction rather than that of the sample members for whom they were supposed to be responding. On the other hand, channeling may have increased life satisfaction among sample members requiring proxies at follow-up. In any case, channeling appears to have had an impact on reported life satisfaction. Whether the impact was for a certain set of sample members or for the caregivers of those sample members is unclear.

Potential Problems with Estimation

A multiple regression model was used to estimate program impacts. While the use of this straightforward analytic procedure should produce robust estimates of channeling impacts, three issues had to be addressed in formulating the models and interpreting the results: (1) whether observations could be pooled across sites in estimating impacts; (2) whether there were differences in program effectiveness over calendar time that would distort inferences about how impacts vary with length of time since entering the program; and (3) whether regression could lead to poor estimates of channeling impacts for outcome variables that were skewed, binary, or truncated.

THE VALIDITY OF POOLING OBSERVATIONS

The advantage of pooling is that if the restrictions on regression estimates implied by pooling are true, more precise estimates (estimates with smaller variances) can be obtained because only one estimate is being made for each channeling model rather than one for each site. The disadvantage of pooling is that if the implied restrictions are not true, pooling observations can produce biased and misleading estimates of the model- or site-level impacts.

It was anticipated that impacts for some outcomes might vary across sites; hence, for each substantive area of the evaluation, tests were conducted to determine whether this was the case, using the model with site interactions described in the first section of this article. However, whether or not impacts differed across the five sites implementing a channeling model, there was interest in obtaining overall estimates of impacts for the two channeling models. The methodological issue, then, was whether observations could be pooled in obtaining these model- and site-specific estimates.

The basic question to be addressed was whether differences across sites in either (a) the relationship between outcomes of interest and the explanatory variables in the regression or (b) the effects of channeling were so large that combining all observations in a single regression (such as that presented earlier) would lead to biased estimates of impacts for the two channeling models. To address this question, alternative regression specifications were estimated, and statistical tests of the implied restrictions were conducted (Johnston, 1972). The most restrictive specification was the equation presented in the first section of this article; the least restrictive specification was to estimate an analogous equation separately for each site, and then to compute the average impact across the sites implementing the model.

Tests of the restrictions on regression coefficients implied by pooling were conducted on 45 key dependent variables (the 15 key outcomes listed earlier, each for three time periods). In 11 cases, the implied restrictions on the coefficients of explanatory variables were rejected at the .05 significance level. However, even for these 11 cases, the pooled and unpooled specifications yielded very similar impact estimates at the model level for both the basic and financial control models. Of the 22 model-level impact estimates on these 11 outcomes, there were only three for which the pooled and unpooled estimates differed markedly, and these were for three different outcome measures in three different time periods. The pooled estimates also tended to exhibit greater consistency with the estimates for other time periods and for related outcomes. Furthermore, standard errors from the pooled model were typically 10–20 percent lower than those from the unpooled specification.

Tests of the other restrictions implied by pooling—equivalence of impacts across sites—yielded similar results: the restrictions were rejected in 10 out of 80 tests, but even in these ten cases the model-level impacts obtained from averaging these site-specific estimates were very close to the model-level estimates obtained directly from the regression model given in the first section. Hence, despite the differences across sites in impact estimates and in coefficients on explanatory variables, pooling did not lead to distorted estimates of impacts for the two channeling models.

There was also concern that impact estimates at the *site* level would be distorted if a single regression equation were used, since the relationship between outcomes and explanatory variables could differ across sites and that difference could affect the estimate of channeling impacts. Of the 530 site-specific estimates examined, however, only 17 instances were found in which the unpooled estimate differed substantially from the pooled estimate in terms of size or statistical significance. The lack of evidence that pooling produced distorted or otherwise inferior estimates of channeling impacts at either the model or site level, combined with the smaller standard errors and much greater ease of estimation, led to the decision to use the pooled specification (presented earlier) throughout the evaluation.

DIFFERENCES BETWEEN EARLY AND LATE COHORTS OF SAMPLE MEMBERS

From the outset of the demonstration, it was recognized that the impacts of channeling might vary with the clients' length of time within the program, in line with changes in clients' needs and health status, and as case managers and clients became more familiar to each other. However, comparing estimates of channeling impacts at 18 months to those obtained at 12 months could result in misleading inferences about such changes, because only half of the sample was followed up at 18 months, and time constraints led to defining this group as the half who entered the sample earliest. Erroneous inferences would occur if channeling's effectiveness changed with calendar time (because of specific changes in the operational environment or in the program itself) rather than with the length of time the sample member was in the program. Alternatively, program effectiveness could change if the type of clients served by channeling changed over time. Since the 18-month cohort consists of those enrolling earliest, it was necessary to ensure that any differences between 12- and 18-month results were not due to differences in the calendar period covered by the early and late cohorts or to differences between the cohorts rather than to the length of time spent in channeling.

To distinguish changes in impacts due to length of time in the program from those due to cohort effects such as those just described, estimated impacts on the set of 15 key outcomes at 6 and 12 months for the early cohort were compared to the corresponding estimates for the late cohort. A finding of statistically significant differences between cohorts in impacts during the 1–6- and 7–12-month periods would indicate that 18-month results should be compared to 6- and 12-month results estimated for only the early cohort.

The tests indicated that the estimates at 18 months for the early cohort could be compared to those at 12 months for the full sample with little concern that the comparison would be distorted by differences between the cohorts. The exception to this conclusion was that if such comparisons for formal care outcomes suggested sizable changes in impacts between 12 and 18 months, it would be important to interpret these changes in light of the cohort difference in impacts observed at 12 months. In the final analysis of channeling impacts on use of formal community services, a marked decline in impacts between 12 and 18 months was observed and attributed to this cohort effect (Corson et al., 1986).

THE EFFECTS OF BINARY, TRUNCATED, OR SKEWED OUTCOME VARIABLES ON REGRESSION ESTIMATES OF CHANNELING IMPACTS

Given the random assignment of sample members to treatment and control groups, estimates of channeling impacts obtained by regression are expected to be unbiased. Unbiasedness is not the only desirable property of the estimates, however. When outcome variables are not normally distributed, regression estimates lose some of their other desirable properties and may exhibit characteristics that are undesirable. Two types of channeling outcome variables that had non-normal distributions were those that were binary or truncated at zero, and those that were skewed (that is, had extremely large values for a small number of observations). Analyses were conducted to determine if the regression estimates of impacts on such outcomes were substantively different from estimates obtained using statistical procedures designed specifically to deal with these problems.

Probit and logit models are the estimation procedures most widely used for binary-dependent variables, and Tobit analysis typically is used by economists for truncated variables (Maddala, 1983). In practice, these more complex and expensive estimation procedures typically provide estimates of the effects of explanatory variables on dependent variables which closely resemble in size and significance the estimated effects obtained from least-squares regression (Corson, Long, and Maynard, 1985; Hollister, Kemper, and Maynard, 1984; and Greene, 1983). The much greater ease with which statistical tests can be performed with least-squares regression and the much lower computational cost compared to probit, logit, and Tobit (which require iterative maximum likelihood estimation) led to our strong preference for least-squares as an estimation strategy. However, to ensure that computational ease and cost savings were not achieved at the cost of seriously distorted impact estimates or test statistics, estimates of channeling impacts obtained from regression were compared to estimates obtained from the more complex procedures, using key outcome variables that were binary or truncated at zero.

For binary variables the result was very clear: for both channeling models, the probit and regression impact estimates and *t*-statistics were very similar for all eight of the variables examined. For the truncated variables, comparison of Tobit and regression yielded slightly more ambiguous results. For 3 of the 24 comparisons, differences between the alternative estimates were fairly large and resulted in a change in the statistical significance of the impact estimates. However, the three outcome variables exhibiting such differences, as well as several of the other truncated variables, had distributions that were skewed toward large values as well as truncated at zero. This suggested that a more appropriate estimation procedure was the "two-part model," developed specifically for use on variables with such distributions.

The two-part model involves breaking such service-use variables (measured either in physical units or expenditures) into two separate variables: whether the service is used at all and, for those who use it, the amount of such service (Duan et al., 1983). The expected value of use is the product of the probability of use and the expected amount of use given that some occurred. Thus, a probit model is estimated first for whether any use occurred, as a function of treatment status and other explanatory variables. Then, using only observations that had some service use, a regression model is estimated to predict the amount of use (again dependent on treatment status and other explanatory variables), with the amount being expressed in logarithmic form to reduce the influence of outliers on the estimates. These two equations are then used to obtain predicted probabilities of use and amounts of use by service users for treatments and for controls with the same characteristics. These estimates in turn are used to compute overall expected use for the treatment and the control groups, and the difference between them.

This procedure was used on a set of key hospital and nursing home outcome variables with skewed distributions. The two-part model yielded estimates that differed somewhat from the regression estimates, but not by enough to change the inference about whether channeling affected hospital and nursing home outcomes. The two-part estimates were also generally closer to the least-squares estimates than to the Tobit estimate, especially for the outcomes exhibiting the largest discrepancy between least-squares and Tobit.

These results suggested that the more cumbersome two-part method was not necessary, at least for hospital and nursing home outcomes where outliers were most likely to occur. However, the results from the Tobit analysis suggested that estimates of channeling impacts on hours of formal care received at six months was also affected by outliers. To investigate this, the two-part method was used for this outcome variable as well. Examination of the data showed that the small regression estimate of treatment/control differences was heavily influenced by the receipt of continuous (24 hours per day) formal care by seven control group members (representing 20 percent of total use by the 1,000 controls in the basic model sample), but only two treatment group members. Use of the two-part method dampened the effect of these outliers on the estimated treatment/control difference, and completely reversed the inference about the basic model's effect on the average amount of care received by recipients.

Given the similarity of the two-part estimates to the ordinary least-squares regression estimates for nursing home and hospital days and expenditures, the final reports on these outcomes (and the subsequent articles in this issue) relied upon the regression results. This was done because the standard errors of impacts from the two-part method are more cumbersome to calculate, and multivariate tests would be especially difficult to conduct. For hours of formal care, the effect of outliers was explicitly examined. Impacts were estimated using least-squares regression both with and without the outliers. No other outcome measures appeared to have skewed distributions; hence, no other analyses of the effects of outliers were conducted.

CONCLUSION

Investigation revealed that only one of several potential methodological threats to the validity of channeling impact estimates was likely to cause widespread distortion of the results. This problem, noncomparability of some baseline data items for treatment and control groups, was dealt with by restricting the set of explanatory variables used in regression equations to variables from the prerandomization screening interview and to those baseline variables found to be comparably measured for the two groups. This regression equation was used to obtain the results presented in the rest of this issue. The two instances in which other methodological concerns appeared to affect the impact estimates for a particular outcome measure are documented and dealt with in the appropriate articles.

REFERENCES

Brown, R. S. *Methodological Issues in the Evaluation of the National Long Term Care Demonstration*. Princeton, NJ: Mathematica Policy Research, 1986.

Brown, R. S., and M. Harrigan. *The Comparability of Treatment and Control Groups at Randomization*. Princeton, NJ: Mathematica Policy Research, 1983.

Brown, R. S., and P. A. Mossel. *Examination of the Equivalence of Treatment and Control Groups and the Comparability of Baseline Data*. Princeton, NJ: Mathematica Policy Research, 1984.

Brown, R. S., et al. *Final Report on the Effects of Sample Attrition on Estimates of Channeling's Impacts*. Princeton, NJ: Mathematica Policy Research, 1986.

Carcagno, G. J., and P. Kemper. The evaluation of the National Long Term Care Demonstration: 1. An overview of the channeling demonstration and its evaluation. *Health Services Research* 23(1) (this issue).

Carcagno, G. J., et al. *The Evaluation of the National Long Term Care Demonstration: The Planning and Operational Experience of the Channeling Projects*. Princeton, NJ: Mathematica Policy Research, 1986.

Corson, W., S. Long, and R. Maynard. *An Impact Evaluation of the Buffalo Dislocated Worker Demonstration Program*. Princeton, NJ: Mathematica Policy Research, 1985.

Corson, W., et al. *Channeling Effects on Formal Community Based Services and Housing*. Princeton, NJ: Mathematica Policy Research, 1986.

Duan, N., et al. A comparison of alternative models for the demand for medical care. *Journal of Business and Economic Statistics* 1(2):115, April 1983.

Grannemann, T., et al. *Differential Impacts Among Subgroups of Channeling Enrollees*. Princeton, NJ: Mathematica Policy Research, 1986.

Greene, W. H. Estimation of limited dependent variable models by ordinary least squares and the method of moments. *Journal of Econometrics* 21(2):195, February 1983.

Heckman, J. J. Sample selection bias as a specification error. *Econometrica* 47(1):153, January 1979.

Hollister, R., P. Kemper, and R. Maynard. *The National Supported Work Demonstration*. Madison, WI: The University of Wisconsin Press, 1984.

Johnston, J. *Econometric Methods*. New York: McGraw-Hill, 1972, p. 207.

Maddala, G. S. *Limited-dependent and Qualitative Variables in Econometrics*. New York: Cambridge University Press, 1983.

Phillips, B., et al. *The Evaluation of the National Long Term Care Demonstration: The Survey Data Collection Design and Procedures*. Princeton, NJ: Mathematica Policy Research, 1986.

SECTION FIVE

A Case Study of the Research Process

CHAPTER FOURTEEN

Health Services Research as Process: A Case Study

A couple of years ago, the editors of *Health Services Research* were pleasantly surprised to receive for review an article prepared by Harold S. Luft, one of the more accomplished contributors to the field. This narrative, which follows, is an account of the history of a single research project literally from beginning to end, illustrating the many vicissitudes encountered during the process of research problem formulation, study design and execution, the analysis of findings, and their dissemination through formal publication.

This article illustrates the many serendipitous aspects of research, some positive and some negative, which can occur in even the most carefully designed projects. The project described is one that addresses two important aspects of the functioning of health maintenance organizations: selection effects and competitive effects. Luft describes the effort by the research team to develop a large, national data set whereby the impact of HMO performance in various markets could be determined. Through the course of the project, the investigators made a number of strategic decisions, one of which was to abandon the effort to develop the national database and to concentrate instead on the conduct of case studies of HMO behavior in particular localities.

This article does not focus on the findings of the research it describes, but on the process of conducting the research. One of the more interesting facets of this study is the way in which a team of researchers who set out to do an econometric modeling project using a large quantitative database ended up conducting a study that relied heavily on a set of qualitative data to answer the basic study questions. The article illustrates the way in which interdisciplinary research teams, when they work well together, actually sort out their various differences of perspective in seeking the best of all available methods relevant to a given research problem.

Papers such as this are rare in our field, for most of us would not take the time to recount the many decisions and dilemmas we face as we go about our craft. For this reason, the reviewers of this paper and the editors of *Health Services Research* considered it an important addition to the literature of our field. We regard it as an appropriate conclusion to this review of some of the more recent advances in the field of health care studies.

Health Services Research as a Scientific Process: The Metamorphosis of an Empirical Research Project from Grant Proposal to Final Report

Harold S. Luft

The process of health services research is rarely examined; attention is usually focused on results and policy implications. Large and small decisions made during the execution of a study, however, can have major impacts on its outcomes. This article describes a project that underwent major changes because of problems discovered in the basic data and threats to the valid interpretation of econometric results uncovered by qualitative case studies. Although the combination of difficulties encountered in this project may be unusual, it is likely that many similar problems and opportunities occur in other empirical studies.

Most health services research papers provide a rather straightforward discussion of the model to be tested, the data, methods used, findings, and implications of the results. While some research projects unfold according to schedule and reach useful conclusions as easily as the final papers suggest, others present many more difficulties and challenges.

This research was supported by Grant Number 18-P-97556/9-01 from the Health Care Financing Administration of the Department of Health and Human Services. The findings and interpretations offered are those of the author and do not necessarily reflect approval by HCFA.

Harold S. Luft, Ph.D. is Professor of Health Economics in the Institute for Health Policy Studies, School of Medicine, University of California, San Francisco. Address correspondence and requests for reprints to Professor Luft at the Institute for Health Policy Studies, School of Medicine, University of California, 1326 Third Avenue, San Francisco, CA 94143.

Sometimes the difficulties reflect poor decisions on the part of the investigator, so a certain reticence is to be expected. Yet a cursory reading of the literature might mislead a new investigator into believing that things should always go according to plan and that any deviations are attributable to researcher incompetence.

My research team and I recently completed the final report for a large research project that was designed to measure two effects of Health Maintenance Organizations (HMOs). The first, or selection effect, was the extent to which the lower observed hospitalization rates of HMO enrollees was due to the selective enrollment in HMOs of people who would use few hospital days even in the fee-for-service system. The second, or competitive effect, was the extent to which HMO development and growth led to cost-containing and hospital utilization-constraining responses by the fee-for-service system. The primary focus of the project was a large econometric model of hospital utilization across all 50 states encompassing the period 1947–1976. Three sets of dependent variables would be used: overall hospital utilization, as reported by the American Hospital Association; hospital utilization of Blue Cross enrollees; and hospital utilization of federal employees enrolled in Blue Cross. This econometric modeling was to be supported by a series of case studies to document how the anticipated selection and competitive effects took place. The original proposal allocated less than 15 percent of professional time to the case studies. Yet during the project, we decided to abandon the large econometric model; thereafter, our attention focused on the case studies and on an investigation of reasons why the available data were inappropriate for use in the econometric model. Because the data problems we encountered may have an impact on other research projects, we thought it appropriate to explain them thoroughly.

Although some of the problems encountered might have been specific to our project, they may help illustrate some important issues in the research process and, thus, be of more general interest. Therefore, this article focuses on the research process and pays little attention to the particular results of the project, which are available in the final report [1]. To provide the setting for this discussion of how a project was transformed, the first section of the article outlines the original project rationale and design. The second section discusses an important aspect of the design, the combination of quantitative econometric estimates with qualitative case studies. As in most empirical papers, we include a section on data collection, review, and analysis—but in this case, the focus is on the problems encountered during this usually mundane process. The fourth section explains how results from the case studies led to so much concern about how the econometric results would be interpreted that we dropped the latter analyses. A final section offers some lessons from the experience.

A Summary of the Original Project Design

One of the ideas implicit in an HMO's economic incentives is the reduction of expensive services rendered to realize financial savings for the plan and better coverage for the enrollee. Thus, people who select HMOs or who choose to remain in them over time may well require or prefer less expensive medical care. To the extent that this occurs, the observed differences in medical utilization of HMO and non-HMO members are the result of a true HMO effect (that is, what the HMO does to alter practice patterns) and a self-selection effect. The larger the selection effect, the smaller the fraction of the observed difference that is due to HMO incentives and the more illusory "savings" as measured by the differences in utilization between HMO and non-HMO enrollees. This may reduce the appeal of HMOs for cost-containment policy. For instance, the Seattle Model Cities Prepaid Health Plan Study indicated that the cost for enrollees in the Blue Cross/Blue Shield–type plan was 50 percent more than for those in Group Health Cooperative of Puget Sound. Adjusting for the higher pre-enrollment utilization patterns of the BC/BS enrollees, however, halves this differential to 25 percent [2]. Studies by Eggers and Prihoda [3] demonstrate a selection effect among new Medicare enrollees in prepaid group practices that is only partly explained by age, sex, and disability status.

Just as one should not focus on HMOs without considering the potential biases resulting from self-selection, one must also not assume that the conventional system is passive with respect to HMO development [4]. The history of prepaid group practice plans is replete with instances of bitter opposition by organized medicine in what must be seen as a competitive response. Those legal battles were won by the prepaid groups in the late 1940s, but a much more subtle form of competitive response is likely to have taken its place. To the extent that HMOs can offer more nearly complete coverage at comparable costs (either because of a true HMO effect or a self-selection effect), they will tend to expand at the expense of conventional health insurers such as Blue Cross and, indirectly, fee-for-service physicians. These insurers and providers might then try to respond to the HMO by controlling their own costs and thus retain their attractiveness to consumers. If our research led to the identification of a strong competitive effect arising from even relatively small market penetration, then the savings directly attributable to HMO enrollees might be multiplied severalfold by the indirect effects on people in the conventional system. With true externalities of this type, the case would be very strong for widespread HMO development, even with relatively small market shares.

All such policy considerations are superimposed on a medical care delivery system that is substantially more geographically diverse than those of most other countries. For instance, in 1973 there were 1,426 days of care per 1,000 population in the North Central region in contrast to 930 in the West [5]. Even more striking is the nearly twofold variation in days of care for Medicare beneficiaries—2,325 per 1,000 in Utah versus 4,571 in South Dakota [6]. These differences cannot be explained by age-sex differences, nor is weather an important determinant. While the life-styles of the Mormon population in Utah may account for their low Medicare utilization rates, it is noteworthy that four of the next five lowest states are Washington, Oregon, California, and Hawaii, all with substantial HMO enrollments. But, again, before one attributes too much to the competitive response explanation, one should also examine the roles of migration, hospital bed supply, long-term care facilities, physician supply, and other factors. Many of these are subject to policy manipulation, and yet little is known about their roles in explaining geographic differences in utilization. It should be noted, moreover, that these geographic differences are at least as large as those seen between HMOs and conventional plans and that current reimbursement policies make little effort to narrow them. Given this underlying view of the medical care system and the role of HMOs within the context of the larger system, the project was designed to answer two major questions. The first was the relative importance of self-selection in explaining the observed differences in hospital utilization between enrollees in HMOs and in conventional plans. The second question was whether the development and growth of HMOs engenders a competitive response by conventional insurers and providers that results in a decline in hospital utilization. In particular, the project would attempt to measure both the magnitude of such a competitive response and to provide examples of how such a response was implemented. Finally, as a by-product of the research design, the project would offer an explanation of the large differences in hospital utilization rates across the country and the changing patterns of use over time.

Rationale for Combining Case Study and Econometric Approaches

The selection and competition effects can be studied at various levels. Micro, or individual, studies involve data from a sample of people over time as they choose among and utilize the services of various health plans. Studies of this type include people in the Seattle Model Cities project [7], employees of various firms in Rochester, NY [8–10], Medicare beneficiaries [3,11], or the Rand Health Insurance Studies [12,13]. Another form of micro study involves detailed interviews and data collection among insurers and providers in an area to identify and document a competitive response to HMO development. This qualitative study approach has been used in Minneapolis-St. Paul [14]; Northern California and Hawaii [15]; and the Sacramento, San Diego, and Santa Clara areas of California [16]. Macro or aggregate studies use data on the hospital utilization of large population groups, holding various factors constant through statistical methods and, most importantly, drawing together historical data series to monitor over time the effects of the natural experiment of HMO development.

It is important to recognize that the alternative approaches are not completely interchangeable and that each has specific advantages and limitations. Micro studies of individuals can be very convincing in studying behavioral relationships, such as the influence of copayments on demand. Qualitative case studies are perhaps the best means of understanding *how* a phenomenon occurs and what subtle side effects result from an innovation. Findings from such studies can be very convincing in showing that a selection or competition effect does in fact occur. Very little can be said if no effect is measurable within the setting under study. This weakness is related to the case study approach. Not all HMOs are the same; in fact, there is even substantial variation in the operation and performance of the several Kaiser regions. Thus, a micro study in a single community provides little insight into whether similar communities would show larger or smaller responses. (For example, while the results of the randomized assignment of people to Group Health Cooperative of Puget Sound are quite convincing, they do not speak to their generalizability to other HMOs [13].) As will be seen below, however, there are times when negative results from several qualitative case studies can present a powerful argument.

Aggregate, or macro studies, while offering a less clear picture of *how* something happens, are well suited to determining *whether* something happens and the effect it has. In part, this is because studies can incorporate data from the entire relevant universe, e.g., all 50 states. Micro and macro studies obviously complement one another. Recognizing this relationship, our project was designed to pursue a macro-level analysis and to use those results in determining appropriate topics for a number of micro-level case study investigations. This was intended to allow us first to determine the magnitude of the selection and competition effects, and then to use those results to guide our investigation into *how* those effects take place.

At the aggregate level of study, the selection and competition effects are best analyzed with different populations. The selection effect takes place (if it occurs) within a given employee group that has repeated dual-choice options between HMOs and conventional coverage. The competition effect can be expected to involve all people with conventional coverage in a geographic area with a substantial HMO market share. In general, if the competitive effect leads to changes in practice patterns and insurance coverage, it will also influence people who do not have a dual-choice option. The research design examined behavior over time and across states (a time series–cross-section model) to provide sufficient variation in the data to separate the competition and selection effects.

If one examines a geographic area as a whole, there is no selection effect because all persons are included, irrespective of health plan, and the areawide utilization rate will depend primarily on the proportion of the population in the HMO (the competitive effect) and, to a small extent, the true HMO effect on its own enrollees. The utilization rate for the whole population is the weighted average of the experience for people with conventional (or no) coverage and the experience for HMO enrollees. Given the relatively small market shares of HMOs (at most, 15 percent in the period under study), and the likely size of the true HMO effect (probably 10–20 percent), the average will almost totally reflect the competitive effect. Overall hospital utilization in each state as reported by the American Hospital Association was to be used to measure the competitive effect.

The estimation of the selection effect can be best understood if one thinks of a firm that offers its employees the choice of a conventional insurance plan or HMOs where the latter are available. If there is no selection effect (and ignoring, for the moment, any competitive effect), then hospitalization rates among enrollees in the conventional plan should be independent of the proportion of employees who choose the HMOs. (Obviously, measured utilization rates will reflect geographic differences in the age and sex compositions of the employees and a host of supply factors, but the statistical estimation process was designed to hold constant those factors.) However, if employees who would normally be low users of hospital care disproportionately enroll in HMOs, then the hospitalization rates of enrollees in conventional plans will be *positively* related to the proportion of the firm's employees in the area who belong to HMOs.

If one is to measure the selection effect using cross-sectional data, one must also take into account the competition effect. While the selection effect is observed *within* a dual-choice population and depends upon the HMO's share of that employee group, the competition effect depends on the HMO penetration in the whole geographic area. This means that the observed utilization rate within an employee group for enrollees choosing conventional coverage will increase with the proportion of that group which chooses the HMO (the selection effect) and decrease with the proportion of total population in HMOs (the competition effect). The 1960–1975 experience of federal employees who chose Blue Cross/Blue Shield coverage was to be used to estimate this combined selection and competition effect. Blue Cross/Blue Shield coverage is available to all federal employees, but HMO options are available only in selected areas. More importantly, the proportion of federal employees who belong to HMOs in some areas exceeds the general HMO market share, thus reducing the problem of multicollinearity.

Finally, if one examines a population with conventional coverage, such as Blue Cross, without considering whether or not it has dual choice, the utilization rate will be in an intermediate position. There will be a negative competition effect stemming from the share that HMOs have of the total market and a positive effect related to the proportion of people subject to dual choice and, therefore, subject to self-selection. Estimates of the competition effect from this last group will be biased toward zero, or will be smaller than is truly the case. The use of three models allows the comparison of estimates, and the AHA and Blue Cross data go back far enough in time to predate almost all HMOs, so that the HMO influence can be tracked as HMOs come into being.

In the process of analyzing the separate data sets and estimating the general model, geographic differences in hospital utilization and the impact of HMO growth in local market areas will emerge. Case studies of these effects were planned to supplement the aggregate-level investigation and serve to strengthen the interpretation of the primary findings. In particular, using American Hospital Association and Blue

Cross data, trends in hospital utilization would be compared before and during the period when an HMO enters the medical market.

Hawaii, because of its geographic isolation, was thought to serve as a particularly valuable study. The Kaiser plan began there in the late 1950s, well after establishment of the California and Oregon locations yet sufficiently long ago to allow the observation of long-term effects. Furthermore, the relative dominance of Oahu in terms of population means that state data can be used with little error, and the state's geographic isolation virtually eliminates "border crossing." Additional case studies were planned to investigate further some of the variables identified by the regression analyses as well as those states that appeared to be outliers. Although the case studies were seen as important components of the original proposal, they accounted for only 15 percent of research staff time.

Data Collection, Review, and Analysis

In the initial design of the project, we recognized that the preparation of data from 50 states over a 30-year period would be a substantial undertaking and, therefore, that the first year was to be allocated to those tasks. The underlying documents had been identified prior to submission of the proposal, so the first stage of collection had been completed. However, we recognized that published data series have both documented and undocumented changes in methods and that errors may occur in the original source and in the various recoding processes.

Our approach was, first, to examine the source documents for consistency in definitions and for any footnotes or technical memorandums indicating changes in methods. Usually, all of the data for a single variable or group of variables would be available in a series of volumes from the same source, such as the Bureau of the Census or the American Hospital Association. Even in those instances, data occasionally had to be "patched in" from other volumes—for instance, data for Hawaii and Alaska in the years preceding statehood. Major changes in the health care system, such as Medicare, often had subtle impacts on data series. For instance, since 1966, health insurance coverage data have been differentiated between the under-65 age population and those 65 and over. In earlier years such differentiation was not routinely made, so we expended substantial effort in estimating a consistent time series.

One of the advantages of the broad time span is that occasionally there will be several independent estimates for the same variable—or at least what at first glance appears to be the same variable. The best available source of data for the number of physicians by state by year is the American Medical Association. The decennial census also provides state counts of physicians for 1940, 1950, 1960, and 1970. Closer examination of the definitions used by the two sources indicated potentially significant differences—the AMA focused on total or patient care non-federal MDs, while the census focused on physicians in terms of occupation—thus including those employed by the federal government as well as osteopaths and implicitly excluding persons holding an MD or DO license but not practicing medicine. An investigation of the alternate estimates provided by the two sources suggested reasonable comparability in the aggregate but substantial differences for a few states [17].

A second advantage of pooled time series-cross-section data is the ability to evaluate individual data points through consistency checks. After entering yearly data from the American Hospital Association, Blue Cross, and the Federal Employees' Health Benefits Program, the data were reorganized to produce a time series for each state or grouping. These data were then printed as tables and as graphs to identify any marked changes in patterns. A substantial number of errors were identified and corrected. A small proportion of these were data entry errors—due either to the keypunchers or to our coding. Some of the errors were typographical or arithmetic mistakes in the source documents. In other cases, changes in the classification of one or two hospitals in a state could result in major shifts in overall utilization variables. To check this, we tracked individual hospital listings in the annual *AHA Guide* issues and made a determination based on all the available data. Although such error checking requires substantial effort, it has been our experience that a small number of outliers, which are often erroneous, can have a major impact on regression results. Furthermore, once the research gets to the stage of regressions, the raw data are most difficult to check (see Mayer, 1980, for a discussion of data in economic research [18]).

Checking the data from Blue Cross and the American Hospital Association led to the observation of an apparent anomaly. The Blue Cross data exhibited a significant downward trend in hospital days and admissions per thousand enrollees over the last decade, but no such trend was apparent in the AHA data. Because Blue Cross plans account for one-third of all discharges among the under-65 age population, this divergence suggested either markedly different trends in use by the non-Blue Cross populations or an underlying data problem. Either situation could threaten the basic design of the project, which relied upon a comparison of the AHA and Blue Cross regressions to estimate the selection effect. It did not take long to surmise that the difficulties could be traced to the growth of duplicate health insurance coverage and sharp increases in utilization among Medicare disabled and Medicaid beneficiaries. (Duplicate insurance coverage leads to inflated enrollment estimates and, thus, to deflated use figures.) Developing the evidence to test these hypotheses was a bit more difficult, but it now appears that the growth in duplicate coverage accounts for about one-half of the diverging trends in hospital admissions [19].

Another phase of the data preparation resulted in the recognition of a different but related problem in the overall figures on health insurance enrollments. The Health Insurance Association of America (HIAA) prepares annual estimates of health insurance enrollment in each state, and these data have been published since the late 1940s. They are the only such state data available and have been widely used in previous studies. Upon examining the time series data for each state, it became apparent that 1973 represented a break in the series. The annual sourcebooks present the state data for the preceding year and a national time series. When the methods were changed, the national data were adjusted to make a consistent series, but no adjustments were made to state data for previous years. (See Health Insurance Institute [20]).

Footnotes in the documents indicated a change from employer-based to residence-based estimates. The person responsible for the data informed us that duplicate coverage was at the root of the problems. The HIAA has a formula to convert gross enrollment data obtained from the carriers to estimates of net enrollment. Although this formula is based upon national data, it is also applied to the state figures. The HIAA statisticians noticed that the resulting enrollment exceeded the under-65 age populations in some states and recommended a reallocation process. This problem may have been overlooked by most users of the data because the figures are published as total enrollments, rather than as percent covered, so one must obtain and divide through by the population estimates. This last step is usually done in the computer and the resulting ratio entered into the regression without detailed examination. The HIAA generously shared their worksheets with us so that we could recompute the 1973 and subsequent figures.

Fortunately, and quite by chance, about this time we became aware of the 1976 Survey of Income and Education (SIE), a household-based survey of a wide range of topics, including health insurance coverage. Unlike other surveys of health insurance, the SIE sample was designed to provide reliable estimates at a state level. This allowed a comparison of the HIAA and SIE estimates for 1976. The two were rather different, with an R^2 of only .3. Moreover, it appeared that much of the problem stemmed from the HIAA's adjustment technique for duplicate coverage. This led us to examine the factors that could explain duplicate coverage at a state level. We also developed synthetic estimates of net coverage by state and year for 1950–1976, using regressions based on the SIE and regional benchmarks from other surveys for 1953–1974 [21].

The synthetic estimates of insurance coverage would be adequate for use as independent variables in the utilization regressions. However, in order to adjust the Blue Cross enrollment figures with the synthetic estimates, we would have to assume identical duplicate-coverage patterns, both cross-sectionally and over time, for Blue Cross and all insurance carriers. Some Blue Cross plans were known to have exceptionally high or low duplicate-coverage rates, so this assumption was untenable. Moreover, the selection effect was to be derived by comparing the AHA with the Blue Cross and FEHBP estimates, which suffer from the same problem. Synthetic estimates may be used as an independent variable, but to use them as an adjustment to a dependent variable seemed unacceptable, especially when attention would be focused on *differences* in coefficients across data sets. Therefore, we reluctantly abandoned the analysis of the Blue Cross and FEHBP data and, hence, our attempt to separate the selection and competitive effects. The AHA data, however, seemed reliable, so we continued with preparations to estimate the competitive effect.

Interface of Macro and Micro Studies

In the original proposal, micro case studies were intended to complement the macro time series–cross-section regression estimate and provide a sense of how competitive and selection effects took place. Some micro studies were planned to explain outliers from the regressions, but others would be "freestanding" investigations of places where substantial competitive effects were thought to occur. There was little empirically based discussion of selection effects in the literature, so the case studies were to focus primarily on competitive effects. A separate grant from the California Policy Seminar was supporting an analysis of the medical care market in California [16]. Preliminary findings indicated active competitive processes, but for the two areas investigated in detail, Sacramento and San Diego, there was no convincing evidence of cost or hospital use containment stemming from the development and growth of the Kaiser Plan in the mid-1960s. These negative findings heightened our interest in micro studies of other parts of the country.

Hawaii was an area that immediately came to mind because of the relatively large Kaiser enrollment and low hospital use rates by both Kaiser and conventionally insured enrollees. Kaiser entered Hawaii in 1959, well after any postwar adjustments, yet long enough ago to allow the appearance of lagged responses. Hawaii's isolation and the population concentration in Oahu meant that state data could be used, thus allowing a richer set of source materials than is available at the metropolitan or county level. Data availability was an important consideration in the micro studies as travel funds were not available. Rochester, NY became a site for study with the publication of a report by the local health systems agency which attributed a sharp decline in hospital use by Blue Cross members to the competitive influence of local HMOs. The HSA Task Force went on to recommend that in recognition of the community's benefits from competition, Blue Cross forgive a $3.3 million loan to the major HMO [22]. Rochester was also interesting as a micro study because some earlier work on this project identified a clear selection effect among certain enrollees in the HMOs [2]. The choice of Minneapolis-St. Paul as a third site was based largely on the widespread attention given that area and the identification of the Twin Cities as a location almost unique in having a large number of HMOs competing with each other. A competitive process definitely was under way—the question we attempted to answer was whether evidence was there to suggest a cost-containing competitive outcome.

The research process in the case studies differed markedly from that of the larger project, which had a clearly defined model and data sources to test hypotheses. In the micro studies, the approach was similar to detective work—sometimes starting with an alleged relationship (Rochester), sometimes starting with the much more general question of whether a cost-containing effect was evident (Minneapolis-St. Paul). The available data ranged from published AHA data at the state, metropolitan area, or hospital level, to Health Systems Agency (HSA) statistics, to figures from local carriers. Unpublished data for Medicare and Medicaid beneficiaries were obtained from HCFA, state, and local officials. We even obtained data from the Defense Department concerning utilization at Tripler Army Hospital in Honolulu.

The range of data sources gives only a partial sense of our investigative approach. For instance, the Rochester HSA staff pointed to the refusal by local nursing homes to accept Medicare and Medicaid patients, thereby forcing them to back up in acute care hospitals, thus leaving no room for the under-65 Blue Cross enrollees [23]. If true, we should be able to observe increases in Medicare and Medicaid inpatient days, reductions in Medicare and Medicaid nursing home admissions, pressures on hospital occupancy, and offsetting declines in Blue Cross patient days, with the correct (that is, logically consistent) timing for these changes. Our results provide at least partial support for the "backup" hypothesis [24]. They also provide ample evidence of gaps and inconsistencies in the available data for all three areas. One quite successful approach that we used was to send on-site correspondents a first draft of our findings and interpretations using the best data available. They helped correct certain figures and often were able to provide important but previously unknown data sets.

The most disconcerting data problem arose in the analysis of Hawaii. Between 1971 and 1974, inpatient days in community hospitals, as reported by the AHA, fell by 24 percent. A substantial part of this decline was attributable to the closure of long-term beds in short-term hospitals. If a relatively small number of long-term care beds could alter statewide utilization rates, then might not similar changes explain some of the temporal trends in hospital use? Furthermore, might regional differences in the use of long-term beds within short-term hospitals explain some of the regional differences in utilization patterns? Since an analysis of regional and temporal patterns underlay the proposal estimation of the competitive effect from the AHA data, what impact might the unknown level and changes in long-term bed use have on the overall analysis?

At the same time that we were beginning to question the validity of the AHA data, the preliminary findings of the three micro studies raised further doubts about undertaking the time series–cross section study. In each area we found either little evidence of true reductions in hospital use or reductions in utilization more plausibly attributed to factors other than HMO competition [24]. The two California markets, San Diego and Sacramento, gave similar results. We were now in a quandary. The macro data analysis was supposed to estimate the *size* of the competitive effect, and the micro case studies were to explain *how* the effect took place. We now had five case studies indicating either no effect, or worse—a reduction in use that was roughly correlated with HMOs yet probably was due to other factors. If the macro regression estimates showed a statistically significant negative coefficient for

HMOs, how could we in good faith attribute the reductions in use to an HMO competitive effect when case studies of five promising locales showed no such effect? The nature of the negative results in Rochester, Hawaii, and Minneapolis-St. Paul reinforced our hesitancy to do the macro study. Careful analysis of each area showed how aggregate utilization data could be misleading, especially when examined over time by researchers looking for a competitive HMO effect.

The decision to abandon the time series–cross section model of state data was made somewhat easier by very preliminary results from a cross-section study of metropolitan areas. This piece of research had been designed to complement the larger study. Because it was a single cross section for 1976, it could neither provide much solid evidence about causation, nor could it separate the selection and competition effects. The preliminary results indicated no measurable competitive effect, further supporting the case studies. Work on that study had been halted in 1979 while awaiting estimation of the full model. We now chose to reexamine the SMSA regressions in lieu of the full-scale time series–cross section model. Although it would not provide the same detail and suffered in many ways from the same data shortcomings, the probable conclusions were at least worth a minimal effort.

The decision to abandon the time series–cross section analyses of the AHA data was difficult. Substantial time, energy, and money had been invested in preparing the basic data. The ambitious and complex model would be replaced by a series of case studies and a simple cross-sectional model similar to others in the literature. Unlike the Blue Cross and federal employee data, the AHA data were not massively flawed, and the model could still be estimated. The problem was that the case studies had generated doubt in our minds sufficient to make us unable to trust a simple interpretation of our own regression results. More importantly, if the regression findings were consistent with a competitive effect, there was a real likelihood—even if we tried to downplay their validity—that advocates for certain policy options would quote the results out of context. Rather than having to face the choice of later suppressing misleading findings or of spending time in the future correcting the misinterpretation of our results by others, we decided to spend the remainder of the project improving the case studies.

Lessons from the Experience

Most courses on research deal with formal methods and statistical techniques as applied to ideal sets of data. Yet, almost every empirically based researcher must deal with large and small decisions concerning problems, inconsistencies, and holes in the available data. Traditional methods courses are analogous to courses in architectural design that focus on the concept and grand scheme for a building. The creation of the structure, however, requires implementation of the design by a contractor who follows the architect's design, yet makes minor adjustments to accommodate irregularities in the materials, the need for supporting devices during construction, and the capabilities of the workers. Not surprisingly, the contractor's skills are acquired largely through apprenticeship and learning-by-doing, because the necessary judgment and "tricks of the trade" cannot be readily taught in the classroom or through books.

This description of the research process in one project is not meant to be an example of the best possible approach. Instead, it is intended as an example of one project that we hope may be directly useful to others or indirectly useful by encouraging other researchers to describe their own processes. At the risk of overgeneralization (and, perhaps, a little defensively), we suggest that some lessons for the future might be drawn from this case study. These lessons deal with secondary data sources, techniques in empirical research, and the general setting in which research is undertaken.

SECONDARY DATA SOURCES

Health services research is often done using secondary, or previously collected, aggregate data. For certain questions, such as the impact of HMOs on communities, one must use such aggregate information, and, unless massive funds are available to collect new data, secondary information must be used. Current trends in research funding suggest that inexpensive secondary data will be used even more frequently as researchers attempt to squeeze the maximum amount of analysis from ever smaller budgets.

By definition, secondary data are material that was collected by someone else for some other purpose, often a nonresearch purpose. In some cases, the unwary researcher may not realize that definitional and other problems may compromise the validity of the data. For instance, the American Medical Association's figures on the distribution of physicians generally omit osteopathic physicians, who often are fully licensed by states to substitute for MDs. The American Hospital Association classifies *hospitals* as long or short term, but until recently did not report separate utilization rates associated with long-term *beds* in short-term *hospitals*. The Health Insurance Association of America recognized the problems of duplicate health insurance coverage but lacked the data on which to make accurate estimates of net coverage at the state level. Insurance carriers generally have their marketing departments estimate enrollments, but since premium quotes can be based upon annual changes in total expenditures, there are no reasons to account accurately for duplicate coverage.

There are no simple techniques for identifying such underlying problems in the data. Among the approaches we used was the comparison of several independent estimates of the same underlying concept. Comparisons of AMA and census estimates of physicians highlighted the definitional problems. Different hospital use trends from Blue Cross and AHA data led to identification of the duplicate-coverage problem. The Survey of Income and Education provided a benchmark for the HIAA data. Another approach is to examine the data for internal consistency. Marked year-to-year changes in the hospital data by state pointed to the problem of individual hospital classification and the importance of long-term beds in short-term hospitals.

Some techniques are almost trivial—after the fact. Merely dividing the HIAA net enrollment estimates by the relevant population would have revealed several states with exactly 98 percent coverage. Not only is such a high level of coverage unlikely, but when five states have exactly the same level, something bears further investigation. Thus, scaling data to the appropriate rates can often be very informative. Simply printing out the raw data *and looking at the tables* often points out keypunch, coding, and source document errors. Unfortunately, such simple errors can have major and unnoticed impacts on regression results.

Careful reading of footnotes and methods sections associated with secondary data is imperative. Such sections usually describe what was done, but they seldom include warnings to the researcher about limitations and hazards in using the data. (This rarely reflects intentional deception because the data were not intended for nor prepared by researchers.) One way to approach the issue of data quality is to ask at each step where the information came from, how it was collected, and then, whether the data collection scenario is likely to result in the desired data for the research project. For instance, it is unusual for a complete census to be done to collect data. Rather, most data are themselves drawn from administrative or other records. In the few instances in which a census is done, one will need to know how the data are collected from the relevant universe and what that universe is. Even the decennial census, which is often perceived as the "gold standard" against which other data sources are to be measured, has an unknown degree of error due to undercounting of certain population groups.

TECHNIQUES IN EMPIRICAL RESEARCH

In a world of perfect data and simple models derived from unambiguous theory, it is a relatively simple task to choose the appropriate statistical tests for hypothesis testing. In the more complex world of empirical health services research, simple hypothesis testing has a substantial chance of producing incorrect results because of unrecognized problems with the data and model.

Perhaps the most important point is that the health care system is so complex and poorly understood that results *supporting* hypotheses are of relatively little value unless one can simultaneously *reject* all plausible alternative explanations. Our case studies of the competitive effects of HMOs all began with some evidence supporting the notion of a cost-containing competitive effect, yet alternative explanations of the available data seem more reasonable. In order to identify such alternative explanations, it is useful to think of medical care in systems terms and to look for analogs to double entry bookkeeping. Cost-containment for a population implies income reduction for providers, reductions unlikely to have gone unnoticed. Reduced hospital use by Blue Cross enrollees should be reflected in reduced hospital census and occupancy—unless other people have an increase in use. Altered incentives of IPAs should have their greatest impact on IPA enrollees, then on similar, conventionally insured patients of the same physicians, and, last, on publicly funded patients. If the results differ, then perhaps there are different causal relationships.

Given the paucity of simple yet crucial empirical tests, the conservative researcher should have several independent findings giving consistent results before reaching firm conclusions. Repeated studies using similar data and methods are less convincing than comparable results using markedly different methods. Our findings of no measurable cost-containing competitive effect in several case studies reinforce one another. These tentative conclusions from micro case studies are further strengthened by similar results from the aggregate metropolitan area analysis.

Regardless of the care one takes in collecting and preparing the data, errors are inevitable, so one should try to reduce the possibility that errors lead to substantially incorrect results. If sample sizes permit, split the data and estimate models twice; the results should be very similar. When possible, use estimating techniques that are insensitive to outlying observations, or at least examine the residuals from the regressions to make sure outliers are not due to errors. Surprisingly strong results bear careful scrutiny before you break out the champagne.

Finally, researchers should use the expertise and institutional knowledge of nonresearchers in the health care system. This is particularly true in case study microanalyses. Physicians, planners, and administrators often have an intuitive understanding of what is—or is not—occurring; yet it is difficult to incorporate this knowledge in a data collection scheme. Open-ended questions are sometimes fruitful, yet a barrier often appears between the researcher and practitioner that arises from the different ways a situation is conceptualized. One approach we have found useful is asking for comments on initial interpretations of data. The preliminary document serves as something concrete that elicits thoughtful commentary and suggestions. Some of the ideas lead down blind alleys, but these can be seen as alternative hypotheses that are rejected. Other ideas have been most valuable in redirecting our analysis and in providing qualitative support for quantitative findings.

IMPROVING THE RESEARCH ENVIRONMENT

The preceding discussion has focused on the metamorphosis of a research project and how one might be alert to the need for similar changes in other projects. However, one may ask whether such changes should be encouraged. It is our feeling that the original proposal was designed as carefully as possible and that the data problems we encountered could not have been reasonably anticipated. (The proposal was reviewed by several experienced researchers, none of whom pointed out the duplicate coverage problems.) We could have continued with the project, arguing either that the Blue Cross enrollment and utilization figures were the best available or that adjustment by the duplicate coverage rate would be sufficient. We could even have ignored the problem and done the project exactly as outlined in the proposal. Statistically significant results would have been obtained and interpretations offered—some reasonable and some obscure—and another piece of complex empirical research added to the literature.

We were most fortunate in having a project officer at HCFA, Benson Dutton, who treated the project like the grant that it was, rather than as a contract. He also listened to our analysis of the data problems and accepted our recommendations for reorientation. He trusted our judgment and was willing to let the overall project be evaluated on the basis of its products, not the degree to which it matched the proposal.

In an era of increasing calls for accountability in the expenditure of public funds, is it appropriate for granting agencies to take such a flexible approach with their grantees? We would argue that to eliminate such flexibility would almost certainly guarantee a sharp decline in the quality of the research. It is impossible to anticipate all of the potential problems that may occur in a project, irrespective of the amount of work that has gone into the planning. Although the primary focus of our discussion has been on the quantitative aspects of the project using secondary data, similar problems can occur with primary quantitative and qualitative data. For instance, some surveys have response rates that warrant only a discussion of reasons for the low response, rather than a detailed interpretation of the returned questionnaires. Similarly, qualitative case studies may find extremely limited access to certain sources or the perception among the respondents that the research questions totally miss the mark. To forge ahead with the original protocol casts aside a commitment to uncovering the truth.

If projects were terminated as soon as deviations became necessary, researchers would be under immense pressure to ignore warning signals in the data. Furthermore, the potential restrictions and attendant uncertainty would likely drive the most competent researchers to other fields. Occasionally, problems that occur are so serious that the project should not be continued at the same scale. But appropriate changes can be negotiated, and few researchers would want to commit several years to a project with known major flaws. It may be easier for everyone to abandon a major but flawed project if funds are made available for an orderly wind-down and presentation of the appropriate preliminary results, as well as for a discussion of the lessons of the project for other researchers.

How should the appropriate balance be struck between flexibility and accountability? The first step is to distinguish carefully those projects that should be treated like contracts from those that should be treated like grants. Contracts are most appropriate for projects with fairly straightforward approaches, such as data collection and preparation. Projects requiring more analysis and interpretation require more flexibility and thus the structure of a grant.

The second step is to develop a trusting relationship between the granting agency and the investigator. The agency should use peer review study sections and expert project officers to ensure that the investigators are competent; then the investigators should be trusted to do the best research possible. The investigator should be convinced that the agency will view a less-than-glowing progress report as an occasion for problem solving and possible redirection rather than as an opportunity to terminate the project. Formal and informal progress reports should be encouraged as opportunities to discuss preliminary results, interpretations, and midproject changes, rather than as moments of anxiety, posturing, and uncertainty.

If both the agency and investigator start with a presumption that the project will be carried to completion unless major problems occur, both parties are likely to be more open in discussing the relatively small changes that can improve substantially the quality of the research. It will not be easy to develop such a trusting environment, yet the importance of knowing more about the health care system in order to design appropriate national policy means that we must not only have more research but research more free of error.

ACKNOWLEDGMENT

I would like to thank Stephen McPhee, Susan Maerki, Joan Trauner, and an anonymous referee for helpful comments.

REFERENCES

1. Luft, H. S., S. C. Maerki, and J. B. Trauner. *Selection and Competitive Effects of Health Maintenance Organizations*. Final Report for Grant 18P-97556/9-01 from the Health Care Financing Administration. San Francisco: Institute for Health Policy Studies, University of California, San Francisco, September 1983. National Technical Information Service Numbers HRP 0906558 and PB 86-106762.
2. Luft, H. S. The Self-Selection Issue. In *Health Maintenance Organizations: Dimensions of Performance*. New York: Wiley-Interscience, 1981, pp. 40–57.
3. Eggers, P. W., and R. Prihoda. Pre-enrollment reimbursement patterns of Medicare beneficiaries enrolled in "at-risk" HMOs. *Health Care Financing Review* 4(1):55–73, September 1982.
4. Luft, H. S. Organizational and Environmental Factors in HMO Performance. In *Health Maintenance Organizations: Dimensions of Performance*. New York: Wiley-Interscience, 1981, pp. 342–80.
5. U.S. National Center for Health Statistics. Utilization of Short-Stay Hospitals: Annual Summary for the United States, 1976. *Vital and Health Statistics*, Series 13, Number 37. Department of Health, Education and Welfare Publication No. (PHS) 78-1788. Washington, DC: Government Printing Office, 1978.
6. Gornick, M. Medicare patients: Geographic differences in hospital discharge rates and multiple stays. *Social Security Bulletin* 40(6):1–20, June 1977.

7. Richardson, W. C., et al. *The Seattle Prepaid Health Care Project: Comparison of Health Services Delivery*. Springfield, VA: National Technical Information Service, PB 26-7488SET, 1976.
8. Roghmann, K. J., A. A. Sorensen, and S. M. Wells. Hospitalizations in three competing HMOs during their first two years: A cohort study of the Rochester experience. *Group Health Journal* 1(1):26–33, Winter 1980.
9. Berki, S. E., et al. Enrollment choice in a multi-HMO setting: The roles of health risk, financial vulnerability, and access to care. *Medical Care* 15(2):95–114, February 1977.
10. Berki, S. E., et al. Enrollment choices in different types of HMOs: A multivariate analysis. *Medical Care* 16(8):682–97, August 1978.
11. Eggers, P. Risk differential between beneficiaries enrolled and not enrolled in an HMO. *Health Care Financing Review* 1(3):91–99, Winter 1980.
12. Newhouse, J. P., W. G. Manning, C. Morris, et al. Some interim results from a controlled trial of cost sharing in health insurance. *New England Journal of Medicine* 305:1501–07, December 17, 1981.
13. Manning, W. G., A. Leibowitz, G. A. Goldberg, et al. A controlled trial of the effect of a prepaid group practice on use of services. *New England Journal of Medicine* 310(23):1505–10, June 7, 1984.
14. Christianson, J. B., and W. McClure. Competition in the delivery of medical care. *New England Journal of Medicine* 301(15):812–18, October 11, 1979.
15. Goldberg, L. G., and W. Greenberg. *The HMO and Its Effect on Competition*. Washington, DC: Federal Trade Commission, Bureau of Economics, 1977.
16. Butler, L. H., et al. *Medical Life on the Western Frontier, II. Further Evidence on the Competitive Impact of HMOs*. Berkeley: University of California, Institute of Governmental Studies, Monograph No. 6, 1980.
17. Maerki, S. C., and H. S. Luft. Is There a Doctor in the House? Estimating the Number of Physicians. Presented at the 107th Annual Meeting of the American Public Health Association, New York, November 7, 1979.
18. Mayer, T. Economics as a hard science: Realistic goal or wishful thinking? *Economic Inquiry* 18(2):165–78, April 1980.
19. Luft, H. S. Diverging trends in hospital utilization: Fact or artifact? *Medical Care* 19(10):979–94, October 1981.
20. Health Insurance Institute. *Source Book of Health Insurance Data*. Washington, DC: Health Insurance Institute, Annual.
21. Luft, H. S., and S. C. Maerki. Duplicate health insurance coverage: Determinants of variation across states. *Health Care Financing Review* 3(4):45–66, June 1982.
22. Finger Lakes Health Systems Agency, Task Force on Prepaid Care. *Health Maintenance Organizations in Rochester, New York: History, Performance, and Future Prospects*. Rochester, NY: Finger Lakes Health Systems Agency, January 1980.
23. Finger Lakes Health Systems Agency. *Task Force Report on the Hospital Back-Up of Long Term Care Patients*. Rochester, NY: Finger Lakes Health Systems Agency, November 1979.
24. Luft, H. S., S. C. Maerki, and J. B. Trauner. Competitive effects of health maintenance organizations: Another look at the evidence from

Hawaii, Rochester, N.Y., and Minneapolis-St. Paul. *Journal of Health Policy, Politics and Law* 10(4):625–58, Winter 1986.

Some Suggestions for Further Reading

There are no texts or compendia that cover all of the methods a health services researcher might make use of in studying the delivery of health care. This is due to the broad multidisciplinary nature of the field and the applicability of a wide range of techniques, from very simple, straightforward tabular and graphical displays of data to very complex, multi-level analyses combining several methods.

There are, however, some excellent texts and collections of papers that are applicable to certain specific methods and disciplinary approaches or that represent good summaries of a significant portion of the methods used in this volume.

One excellent text that provides an in-depth introduction to research and evaluation methods as they apply to health services organizations is Kaluzny and Veney's *Health Service Organizations*. A collection of papers that serves as a nearly complete compendium of statistical methodologies is the Sage University Papers, Series in Quantitative Applications in the Social Sciences. That series now includes more than 50 short volumes covering analysis, design, and sampling methodologies. A shorthand guide to choosing a particular statistical test is *A Guide for Selecting Statistical Techniques for Analyzing Social Science Data*, by Andrews et al., published by the Institute for Social Research of the University of Michigan.

A classical overview of some of the fundamental problems related to study design is Cook and Campbell's *Quasi-Experimentation: Design and Analysis Issues for Field Settings*. The standard texts for sampling have been and remain Kish, *Survey Sampling*, and Fleiss, *Statistical Methods for Rates and Proportions*, the latter presenting an excellent review of techniques for analysis.

Basic statistical analysis in the health sciences is introduced in the very readable text by Remington and Schork, *Statistics with Applications to the Biological and Health Sciences*. More advanced, multivariate methods are presented by Pedhazur in *Multiple Regression in Behavioral Research*; Neter, Wasserman, and Kutner in *Applied Linear Statistical Models*; and, from an epidemiologist's viewpoint, Kleinbaum, Kupper, and Morgenstern in *Epidemiologic Research*. A useful introduction to operations research techniques is provided by Eppen and Gould in their *Quantitative Concepts for Management*.

Geographic techniques for health services are covered by Meade, Florin, and Gesler in *Medical Geography*. Useful treatments of graphical presentations are found in Tufte's *The Visual Display of Quantitative Information* and in Tukey's *Exploratory Data Analysis*, which concentrates on problems of distributional tendencies.

BIBLIOGRAPHY

Andrews, F. M.; Klem, L.; Davidson, T. M.; O'Malley, P. M.; Rodgers, W. L., A Guide for Selecting Statistical Techniques for Analyzing Social Science Data. Second Edition. Ann Arbor, MI: Institute for Social Research, 1981.

Cook, T. D.; Campbell, D. T., Quasi-Experimentation: Design and Analysis Issues for Field Settings. Boston: Houghton Mifflin Company, 1979.

Eppen, G. D.; Gould, F. J., Quantitative Concepts for Management. Englewood Cliffs, NJ: Prentice-Hall, 1979.

Fleiss, J. L., Statistical Methods for Rates and Proportions (Wiley Series in Probability and Mathematical Statistics). Second Edition. New York: John Wiley & Sons, 1981.

Kaluzny, A. D.; Veney, J. E., Health Service Organizations: A Guide to Research and Assessment. Berkeley, CA: McCutcheon, 1980.

Kish, L., Survey Sampling. New York: John Wiley & Sons, 1965.

Kleinbaum, D. G.; Kupper, L. L.; Morgenstern, H., Epidemiologic Research: Principles and Quantitative Methods. New York: Van Nostrand Reinhold Company, 1982.

Meade, M. S.; Florin, J. W.; Gesler, W. M., Medical Geography. New York: The Guilford Press, 1988.

Neter, J.; Wasserman, W.; Kutner, M. H., Applied Linear Statistical Models: Regression, Analysis of Variance, and Experimental Designs. Homewood, IL: Richard D. Irwin, 1985.

Pedhazur, E. J., Multiple Regression in Behavioral Research: Explanation and Prediction. Second Edition. New York: Holt, Rinehart and Winston, 1982.

Remington, R. D.; Schork, M. A., Statistics with Applications to the Biological and Health Sciences. Second Edition. Englewood Cliffs, NJ: Prentice-Hall, 1985.

Sage University Papers, Series in Quantitative Applications in the Social Sciences. Beverly Hills, CA: Sage Publications.

Tufte, E. R., The Visual Display of Quantitative Information. Cheshire, CT: Graphics Press, 1983.

Tukey, J. W., Exploratory Data Analysis. Reading, MA: Addison-Wesley Publishing Company, 1977.

ABOUT THE EDITORS

GORDON H. DEFRIESE is Professor of Social and Administrative Medicine, and Professor of Medicine (in the Division of General Medicine) at the University of North Carolina at Chapel Hill, School of Medicine. In addition, he holds an appointment as Professor of Epidemiology in the UNC School of Public Health and as Professor of Dental Ecology in the UNC School of Dentistry. He took both his master's and doctoral degrees in the Department of Behavioral Science in the University of Kentucky College of Medicine. Since 1973, he has been Director of the Health Services Research Center at UNC. He is also Co-Director of the Robert Wood Johnson Clinical Scholars Program co-sponsored by the UNC School of Medicine and the Health Services Research Center. He is a past president of the Association for Health Services Research and the Foundation for Health Services Research. Dr. DeFriese is Editor of *Health Services Research*, the official journal of the Association for Health Services Research.

THOMAS C. RICKETTS, III, is Director of the Program in Health Policy Analysis, Health Services Research Center, the University of North Carolina at Chapel Hill. He received his Ph.D. from the Department of Health Policy and Administration of the UNC-CH School of Public

Health. He took a major part in the National Evaluation of Subsidized Rural Primary Care Programs and is the principal author of several articles concerning rural primary health care. Currently, he is project coordinator for a study of practice variations among North Carolina physicians being conducted in cooperation with the North Carolina Medical Society and project coordinator for the National Evaluation of Community Clinical Oncology Programs. He is secretary of the North Carolina Health Council, Inc., and a member of the American Public Health Association, the Association for Health Services Research, and the North American Primary Care Research Group. He serves as Associate Editor of *Health Services Research*.

JANE S. STEIN is Associate Director for Data Management and Director of the Program on International Health at the Health Services Research Center, the University of North Carolina at Chapel Hill. She is also a research associate of the Center. She received her masters of science degree in Operations Research and Systems Analysis from UNC-CH. Ms. Stein has served as co-principal investigator of a longitudinal study of the effects of fathers' unemployment on the health of children and of a study comparing the cost effectiveness of asthma treatment by different medical specialties. Ms. Stein is a charter member of the University of North Carolina's Advisory Committee for Academic Computing and has served as data management consultant on many of the Center's research projects. She is a member of the Association for Health Services Research, the National Association for Public Health Policy, and the American Public Health Association.